Manual of Clinical Child and Adolescent Psychiatry

Revised Edition

Manual of Clinical Child and Adolescent Psychiatry

Revised Edition

Edited by
Kenneth S. Robson, M.D.
Professor and Director
The Institute of Living
University of Connecticut
Division of Child and Adolescent Psychiatry
Hartford, Connecticut

American Psychiatric Press, Inc.

Washington, DC
London, England

Note: The authors have worked to ensure that all information in this book concerning drug dosages, schedules, and routes of administration is accurate as of the time of publication and consistent with standards set by the U.S. Food and Drug Administration and the general medical community. As medical research and practice advance, however, therapeutic standards may change. For this reason and because human and mechanical errors sometimes occur, we recommend that readers follow the advice of a physician who is directly involved in their care or the care of a member of their family.

Books published by the American Psychiatric Press, Inc., represent the views and opinions of the individual authors and do not necessarily represent the policies and opinions of the Press or the American Psychiatric Association.

Manufactured in the United States of America on acid-free paper
97 96 95 94 4 3 2 1
Revised Edition

American Psychiatric Press, Inc.
1400 K Street, N.W., Washington, DC 20005

Library of Congress Cataloging-in-Publication Data
Manual of clinical child and adolescent psychiatry / edited by Kenneth S. Robson. — Rev. ed.
p. cm.
Rev. ed. of: Manual of clinical child psychiatry. c1986.
Includes bibliographical references and index.
ISBN 0-88048-528-0 (alk. paper)
1. Child psychiatry. 2. Adolescent psychiatry. I. Robson, Kenneth S. II. Manual of clinical child psychiatry.
[DNLM: 1. Child Psychiatry. 2. Mental Disorders—in infancy & childhood. 3. Mental Disorders—in adolescence. 4. Adolescent Psychiatry. WS 350 M2935 1994]
RJ499.M2635 1994
618.92′89—dc20
DNLM/DLC
for Library of Congress 93-28362
CIP

British Library Cataloguing in Publication Data
A CIP record is available from the British Library.

Contents

Section II: Approaches to Treatment

Section III: Consultation and Special Clinical Problems

List of Tables and Figures

Tables

Figures

Contributors

Marie Armentano, M.D.
Instructor in Psychiatry, Harvard Medical School; and Coordinator, Adolescent Substance Abuse Services in Child Psychiatry, Massachusetts General Hospital, Boston, Massachusetts

George W. Bailey, M.D.
Medical Director, The Kellar Center, Fairfax, Virginia; and Clinical Associate Professor of Psychiatry, Georgetown University Medical Center, Washington, DC

Robert I. Berkowitz, M.D.
Assistant Professor of Psychiatry and Pediatrics, Philadelphia Child Guidance Clinic, University of Pennsylvania School of Medicine, Philadelphia, Pennsylvania

James R. Brasic, M.D., M.P.H.
Research Assistant Professor of Psychiatry, Developmental Neurobiology Unit, Division of Child and Adolescent Psychiatry, Department of Psychiatry, New York University Medical Center and Bellevue Hospital Center, New York, New York

Joae G. Brooks, M.D.
Child Psychiatrist, Staff, Beth Israel Hospital, Boston; Assistant Clinical Professor of Psychiatry, Harvard Medical School, Boston; and private practice of child psychiatry, Brookline, Massachusetts

Terrell Clark, Ph.D.
Psychologist, Harvard Medical School, The Children's Hospital, Tufts University, Boston, Massachusetts

Barbara J. Coffey, M.D.
Director, Psychopharmacology and Tourette's Clinics, McLean Hospital; and Instructor in Psychiatry, Harvard Medical School, Boston, Massachusetts

Lee Combrinck-Graham, M.D.
Associate Professor of Clinical Psychiatry, University of Illinois at Chicago, Evanston, Illinois

Margaret P. Gean, M.D.
Deputy Chief, Division of Child and Adolescent Psychiatry, New England Medical Center; and Associate Professor, Tufts University School of Medicine, Boston, Massachusetts

James C. Harris, M.D.
Director of Developmental Neuropsychiatry and Associate Professor of Pediatrics, Psychiatry, and Mental Hygiene, Johns Hopkins University School of Medicine, Baltimore, Maryland

Joseph J. Jankowski, M.D.
Associate Clinical Professor of Psychiatry and Pediatrics, Tufts University School of Medicine; and Director of Child Psychiatry Consultation/Liaison and Emergency Services, New England Medical Center Hospitals, Boston, Massachusetts

Michael S. Jellinek, M.D.
Chief, Child Psychiatry Service, Massachusetts General Hospital; and Associate Professor of Psychiatry [Pediatrics], Harvard Medical School, Boston, Massachusetts

Robert A. Lobis, M.D.
Senior Director, Child and Adolescent Psychiatry, The Institute of Living; and Assistant Clinical Professor, University of Connecticut School of Medicine, Hartford, Connecticut

Ourania Madias, M.D.
Psychiatrist, Harvard Community Health Plan/McLean Hospital-Child Services, Boston, Massachusetts

Sid Mondell, Ph.D.
Psychologist, Massachusetts General Hospital, Harvard Medical School, Boston, Massachusetts

Steven L. Nickman, M.D.
Assistant in Psychiatry and Director, Adoption and Custody Unit, Child Psychiatry Services, Massachusetts General Hospital; and Clinical Professor of Psychiatry, Harvard Medical School, Boston, Massachusetts

Stephen G. Porter, M.D.
Assistant Clinical Professor of Psychiatry, Tufts University School of Medicine; and Director, South Boston Court Clinic, Boston, Massachusetts

Judith E. Robinson, M.D.
Assistant Professor of Child Psychiatry and Director, Outpatient Child Psychiatry Service, New England Medical Center Hospitals, Boston, Massachusetts

Kenneth S. Robson, M.D.
Professor and Director, The Institute of Living, University of Connecticut, Division of Child and Adolescent Psychiatry, Hartford, Connecticut

Kreig D. Roof, Ph.D.
Clinical Fellow in Neuropsychology, Division of Child and Adolescent Psychiatry, Vanderbilt University, Nashville, Tennessee

P. S. B. Sarma, M.B., B.S.
Associate Professor and Director of Child Psychiatry, Department of Psychiatry, University of Health Sciences, The Chicago Medical School, North Chicago, Illinois

Maria Sauzier, M.D.
Lecturer in Psychiatry, Harvard Medical School, Boston, Massachusetts

Alberto C. Serrano, M.D.
Professor of Psychiatry and Pediatrics and Associate Chairman, Department of Psychiatry, University of Pennsylvania School of Medicine; and Medical Director, Philadelphia Child Guidance Clinic, Philadelphia, Pennsylvania

Michael G. Tramontana, Ph.D.
Associate Professor of Psychiatry and Director of Child Neuropsychological Services, Division of Child and Adolescent Psychiatry, Vanderbilt University, Nashville, Tennessee

V. Susan Villani, M.D.
Medical Director, Gaebler Children's Center; and Clinical Instructor, Harvard Medical School, Boston, Massachusetts

J. Gerald Young, M.D.
Professor of Psychiatry, New York University School of Medicine, New York, New York

Preface

The first edition of this manual appears to have been a useful addition to the literature in child and adolescent psychiatry. As originally designed, its major purpose was to introduce practical, core knowledge to clinicians entering the specialty. This goal remains unchanged.

Since its original publication in 1986, knowledge about child and adolescent psychiatry has expanded, and its practice has become more complex. Whether in training or in practice, there is less time to reflect, more information to master, and less clarity and certainty about integrative principles and unifying models of either development or psychopathology.

Other medical specialties depend on a base of epidemiologic studies to inform their practices; in child and adolescent psychiatry, such studies have only recently gained prominence. The brilliant efforts of Michael Rutter (1988, 1989) and his colleagues to shed light on childhood conditions and their natural histories are at the center of the epidemiologic perspective. Such studies show enormous promise in establishing the scientific basis of child and adolescent psychiatry.

However, no factual knowledge can be effectively used if the skill and art of talking to children with empathy, sensitivity, respect, and a sense of humor are not the "keys" to diagnostic "locks." Psychodynamic models that underscore the importance of play, fantasy, impulses, defenses, and symbolic processes continue to be invaluable aids to competent diagnostic efforts.

I am even more convinced that there is growing difficulty for child and adolescent psychiatrists to master the fundamentals of basic, high-quality, clinical care of children, adolescents, and their families. It is hoped that this second edition will continue to facilitate that task. More extensive coverage of the current state of the field is provided elsewhere (Garfinkel et al. 1990; Lewis 1991; Noshpitz and King 1991; Rutter and Hersov 1985).

References

Garfinkel BD, Carlson GA, Weller EB (eds): Psychiatric Disorders in Children and Adolescents. Philadelphia, PA, WB Saunders, 1990

Lewis M (ed): Child and Adolescent Psychiatry. Baltimore, MD, Williams & Wilkins, 1991

Noshpitz JD, King RA: Pathways of Growth: Essentials of Child Psychiatry, Vols 1 & 2. New York, Wiley, 1991

Rutter M: Epidemiological approaches to developmental psychopathology. Arch Gen Psychiatry 45:486–495, 1988

Rutter M: Pathways from childhood to adult life. J Child Psychol Psychiatry 30:23–51, 1989

Rutter M, Hersov L (eds): Child and Adolescent Psychiatry: Modern Approaches. Oxford, England, Blackwell Scientific Publications, 1985

Section I

Diagnostic Assessment

1

Introduction to Diagnostic Assessment

Kenneth S. Robson, M.D.

The Nature of Childhood Psychopathology

In approaching the diagnostic process in child and adolescent psychiatry, the relationships among developmental phenomena, psychopathology, and systems of classification (nosology) are frequently confused (Shapiro 1983). Furthermore, the models underlying these three clinical arenas are blurred by the patchwork use of terms, concepts, and schools of thought that obscures clarity of thinking.

To begin, normative development and mental health are synonymous in childhood. Development may be defined as a progressive process resulting from the interplay between biological maturation and environmental influences. Growth, consolidation of functions, mastery, and integration—all aspects of development—are the central core of healthy functioning in childhood. Conversely, all forms of psychopathology in childhood and adolescence involve varying degrees of developmental deviance. Whether catastrophic and relatively fixed (as in autism and childhood schizophrenia) or minimal and transient (as in the adjustment disorders of the preschool child), these developmental deviations result from some combination of biological, psychological, and sociocultural factors. The goal of the diagnostic process is to identify these pathogenic factors clearly, particularly those subject to some form of modification. The aim of all therapeutic interventions is to eliminate or alter these "pathogens" to facilitate development.

Models of development in the child psychiatric literature are offered by seminal theorists such as Sigmund Freud, Anna Freud, Melanie Klein, Erik Erikson, Donald Winnicott, Heinz Werner, Jean Piaget, Heinz Kohut, Margaret Mahler, and Robert White (Bemporad 1980). Each of these authors and others have made significant contributions to particular areas of development, or particular points of view across the continuum of the life cycle. A distillate of Erikson's (1963) epigenetic cycle and stages of development and Anna Freud's (1963) concepts of developmental lines provides a useful template of development against which to view the disturbances of childhood and adolescence.

Erikson (1963) conceived of development as a series of specific tasks generally conforming to more or less discrete ages in childhood and adolescence. Failures in one stage of development leave "unfinished business" for subsequent stages. For example, an infant who fails to establish "basic trust" during the first year of life will be plagued by distrust in later relationships. Erikson's model is cross-sectional and assumes, in general, that all aspects of development are delayed or advanced in unison. Anna Freud (1963), on the other hand, elaborated a series of longitudinal developmental lines or systems that, while closely related to one another, may and often do proceed at different rates in relation to chronological age, developmental interferences, and pathogenic conditions. These lines include cognition and interpersonal relations. Indeed, it is clinically true that children referred for psychiatric evaluation exhibit differential progress in certain lines of development. The 5-year-old with precocious speech who is encopretic illustrates the usefulness of this model.

If one loosely combines the cross-sectional and longitudinal concepts of Erikson and Anna Freud, the result is a kind of "exoskeleton" of development that seems to be a useful vehicle for clinical thinking and the integration of other developmental issues, lines, and systems. This perspective is illustrated in Figure 1–1. Within this diagram the

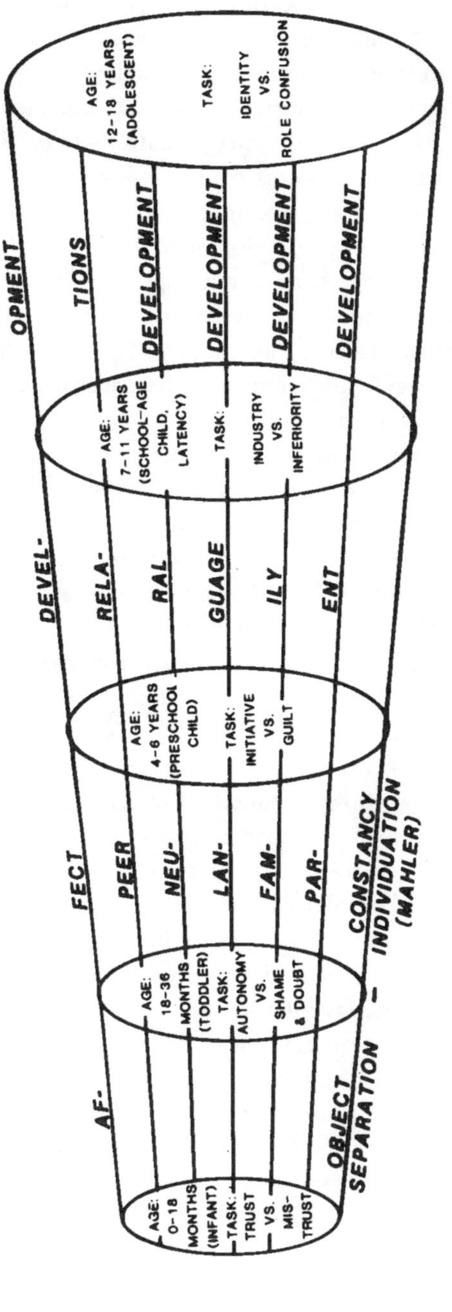

Figure 1–1. “Exoskeleton” model of development combining the cross-sectional and longitudinal concepts of Erikson and A. Freud.

cross-sectional phases/tasks of Erikson are supported by the developmental lines of Anna Freud. Both models relate to one another but view the process of development from differing perspectives. Such an ideogram also permits the student of child and adolescent psychiatry to insert and incorporate particular authors (e.g., Klein, Winnicott, and Mahler) and subsystems of development (e.g., central nervous system maturation, affect tolerance) into one construct.

The relationship of development to pathology is complex and sometimes confusing. At times developmental deviance itself, particularly in the less serious disorders seen in preschoolers (e.g., reactions to stress and transient sleep, toileting, and behavioral disturbances) represent "pathology" without intrinsic disease process. Other conditions such as Tourette's syndrome, autism, and schizophrenia more closely approximate the traditional medical model of illness; massive and persistent developmental arrests are always present. In these latter disorders the pathologic process seems to have its own line of development that weaves its way, like a vine, into the interstices of normal developmental potential, eroding and stifling as it grows. In still other syndromes, such as attention-deficit/hyperactivity disorder, the teasing out of developmental issues as apart from pathologic process may be evident only with the passage of time. Some children with attention-deficit/hyperactivity disorder at age 5 or 6 years may be asymptomatic in all respects by adolescence; others progress into borderline states or frank psychosis in puberty. But again, all childhood disorders are either defined or accompanied by some developmental skewing.

Normal developmental progress requires optimal and sensitively modulated levels of internal and external stimulation delivered by an empathic, nonintrusive, and respectful caretaking environment. In general, every child referred for psychiatric evaluation or treatment suffers from excessively intense internal and external stimulation and some degree of empathic failure in the caretaking environment. Excessive stimulation may arise from too much or too little excitement or arousal, or, as is more usual in clinical practice, both. The functional result within the child is the same: *flooding* of the child's ego so as to interfere with or prohibit developmental processes. The brain-damaged or constitutionally hypersensitive child, for example, is easily stressed or disorganized by normal levels of environmental noise, physical handling, or the internal stimulation of puberty. On the other hand, parental overstimulation, whether seductiveness and physical excess or neglect and abrupt withdrawal, so floods the inner world of the child that various patterns of developmental deviance are inevitable. These include poor separation-individuation, cognitive disruption, impulse-control problems, and more grave disturbances.

From his vast clinical experience, Donald Winnicott (1967) described two fundamental modes of relatedness that respectively interfere with or enhance development. The "orgiastic" mode is characterized by poor respect for interpersonal boundaries, peaks and valleys of stimulation and contact, and recurrent flooding of the developing child's ego. The "ego-relatedness" mode is an opposite mode that empathically modulates stimulation levels, observes interpersonal separateness, and creates the quiet space so essential for the crystals of development to take their shape. Within the schema being described here, the orgiastic mode is to some extent present in all forms of childhood psychopathology, and ego-relatedness is to some extent the therapeutic goal. Adult manifestations of overstimulation and empathic failure are manifest in such problems as "intensity"; poor impulse control; lability of self-esteem, affects, and relationships; and narcissistic concerns.

This manner of describing and understanding psychopathology does not eliminate the need for precise understanding of pathologic phenomena of every variety (e.g., neurologic, biochemical, perceptual, cognitive, and interpersonal). Nor does it bypass rigorous differential diagnoses and the use of the *Diagnostic and Statistical Manual of Mental Disorders*, Fourth Edition (DSM-IV) (American Psychiatric Association 1994). Rather, it weaves such data together as they affect the envelope of internal and external "atmospheric" conditions surrounding the child. Empathic caretaking and modulated levels of stimulation are the critical clinical principles, the "thermostats," by which the child psychiatrist gains understanding of the broad picture of psychopathology, designs therapeutic interventions, and assesses their success. This perspective of development and childhood psychopathology views internal or external conflict as relatively unimportant in causing pathologic states. In most instances a child's conflicts such as those over the expression of aggression or "oedipal concerns" will resolve themselves in the context of empathic parenting and appropriately modulated levels of stimulation. The clinical usefulness of this point of view will be discussed in subsequent sections of this manual (Chapters 2, 6, 7, and 8). Some aspects of this perspective on childhood psychopathology are summarized in Figure 1–2.

Within Figure 1–2, examples of external overstimulation and empathic failure coexist, as is the case in clinical practice. Indeed, overstimulation is always associated with empathic failure. In the therapeutic side of clinical practice, one addresses one or both problems in relation to such considerations as timing, stability, and depth of the therapeutic alliance with parents. In general, environmental overstimulation and empathic failures contribute to the larger variance in their effects on developing psychopathology.

The Medical Model in Child Psychiatric Diagnosis

Like the history of child and adolescent psychiatry itself, the diagnostic process involved in the clinical appraisal of childhood disorders involves data from several disciplines, including pediatrics, psychoanalysis, education, social work, clinical child psychology, and child development (Group for the Advancement of Psychiatry 1966). Not surprisingly, a multiplicity of philosophies, systems, and nosologies have emerged to cover and confuse the diagnostic landscape. The dominant role of clinical medicine and its models in American child and adolescent psychiatry is a recent trend. As a result, the beginning clinician, usually trained in general psychiatry as well as other medical specialties, is often anxious and confused about both where and how to begin. Furthermore, the knowledge and skills of experienced nonphysician colleagues (e.g., social workers, child-care staff, clinical psychologists) may threaten the sense of "seniority" and clinical competence established in the general residency before starting child psychiatric training. In addition, to play with children as an essential part of one's medical work can seem initially incongruous or even alarming. Such concerns in the entry-level child and adolescent psychiatry resident are to some extent inevitable, generally short-lived, and a

Figure 1–2. The pathophysiology of childhood disorders.

OVERSTIMULATION

Internal (child)

“Hyperacusis” to sound, talk, etc.
Central nervous system hypersensitivity (second degree) to brain damage
Impulsivity
Erotization of physical contact
Intolerance of affects
Rejection sensitivity
Panic anxiety
Poorly regulated and labile self-esteem
Rigid ego ideal
Overly harsh conscience
Impatience and inability to delay gratification of wishes
Narcissistic entitlement

External (parents)

Seductive and erotizing physical contact and closeness
Abrupt withdrawal in anger
Emotional unavailability (as in depression or schizoid states)
Frightening behavior (physical or emotional)
Open bathroom doors
Persistent and inappropriate teasing
Child sleeping in parent’s bed
Extreme and age-inappropriate expectations
“Intrusiveness” and lack of respect for child’s boundaries
Physical and sexual abuse
Open bedroom doors
Communal toileting and bathing

EMPATHIC FAILURES

Misunderstanding of child’s behavior
Difficulty in accurately identifying child’s inner states
“Spoiling”
Misperception of child’s capacities in reaction to age
Misreading child’s needs
Difficulty in treating child as separate person (i.e., treating child as “selfobject”)
Need for child as sustaining object
Rigid replaying of one’s own parents unempathic caretaking
“Identification with the aggressor”

DEVELOPMENTAL DEVIANCE IN SPECIFIC PATHOLOGIC STATES

part of the identity reorganization that accompanies the acquisition of new skills. It is useful to keep in mind that the psychiatrist completing both general and child residency training is the true physician "generalist" in the field. One of the particular pleasures of the specialty is the capacity to exercise psychiatric skills across the entire life cycle in relation to individual children, adolescents, adults, parents, marital couples, and families.

A clear conception of the systems of classification underlying child psychiatric diagnostic work guides learning and reduces ambiguity. The data relevant to any clinical syndrome or entity are best gathered from the biopsychosocial "pool." The interaction of biological, psychological, and social variables in the etiologies of pathologic conditions in childhood, although not always obvious, is consistently true. Furthermore, although not all child psychiatric diagnoses are readily classified as disease entities, the traditional medical model is sufficiently broad to integrate all varieties of childhood psychopathology. The use of this model is also consistent with the diagnostic classification of DSM-IV. The organization of clinical data within the standard medical case history described in this chapter encourages clear and rigorous diagnostic thinking, sound treatment planning, well-executed write-ups, authoritative case presentations, and effective communication with medical colleagues. In diagnosing childhood psychopathology, the use of a biopsychosocial perspective focused through the lens of the medical model and DSM-IV is strongly recommended.

The Case History

The database gathered in child psychiatric diagnosis is substantially larger than in general psychiatry. Because the child patient can provide only limited information, the child psychiatrist must turn to others (i.e., parents, teachers, agency staff, medical colleagues). Furthermore, because assessments of current life functioning are so essential for both diagnostic process and treatment planning, in-depth data from the child's family and institutional affiliations (e.g., schools, foster homes, therapeutic settings, courts) are required. Assembling these data in a concise and logical format, however, is difficult. Furthermore, in time one learns that certain data are irrelevant in most instances. Careful, tactful working on the clinician's part is necessary to elicit data from expectably defensive parents. A diagnostic template such as that described in the next section of this chapter is extraordinarily valuable to the beginning clinician; it provides a kind of clinical road map to the diagnostic process. The case history format that follows has proven useful to child and adolescent psychiatry residents, general residents, medical students, and other professional trainees. The order in which data are organized and presented in this schema is designed to maximize clear diagnostic thinking; this order should be maintained. For example, the elaboration of the family history before developmental history places the latter immediately in the context of the child's world. Because divisions of child and adolescent psychiatry frequently utilize many forms for recording diagnostic data, this case history format can be modified when necessary. As a tool this format is especially helpful in determining which data to gather; organizing those data; developing differential diagnostic thinking; facilitating treatment planning; and communicating results clearly to parents, colleagues, courts, schools, and so on, and within teaching settings.

Child Psychiatric Case History Diagnostic Format

With experience, the clinician soon learns shortcuts to the most valuable data, particularly in the early stages of a diagnostic workup when decisions regarding treatment and hospitalization must be made.

Chief complaint/presenting problem. A few sentences concisely summarizing the primary reason and source of the referral. Include the child's name, parents'/family's name, sex, age, race, religion, and birth order. The precise reasons for the referral—in the words of the referral source—should be used whenever possible. If this is not the first referral to the service, that fact should be noted.

Present illness/precipitating stress. A brief description of the interpersonal, intrapsychic, and environmental circumstances leading up to the development of the chief complaint/presenting problem and referral. This section of the workup is obviously more relevant to situations with an *acute* onset and should include illness, loss of a family member, moves, and developmental changes (e.g., weaning, menarche). The *absence* of precipitating stresses is significant and should be noted.

Family history, family composition, and home environment. A concise but thorough description beginning with the current family composition and including three generations. A family tree offers a rapid visual presentation of complicated data (Figure 1–3).

The database should include names, birth dates, parental marital history, dates of separations, hospitalizations, divorces, deaths, abortions, and stillbirths; both month and year of these events should be specified. Family history of medical conditions, major mental illness, "nervous breakdowns," tics, alcoholism, drug addiction, seizures, and mental retardation should be noted. These data can be appended to the family tree and are helpful in establishing any possible genetic base for a psychiatric illness. In addition, brief summaries of each parent's life events should be added, and events pertaining to their own development emphasized.

A description of the house or apartment—including neighborhood, number of rooms and floors, and location of child's and parents' rooms, siblings' rooms, and bathrooms—should be gathered. Toileting and bathing style and customs (e.g., bathroom doors open, nudity, bathing together) can be noted.

Developmental History

Pregnancy. Parity and gravid status of mother at time of conception, medical complications, weight gain or loss, attitudes of parent(s) toward pregnancy, well-being of mother, any complicating life events, preference for girl or boy.

Labor and delivery. Medical complications (e.g., fetal distress, jaundice), birth weight, Apgar scores if available (request birth records if any question about complications or prematurity), mother's feelings

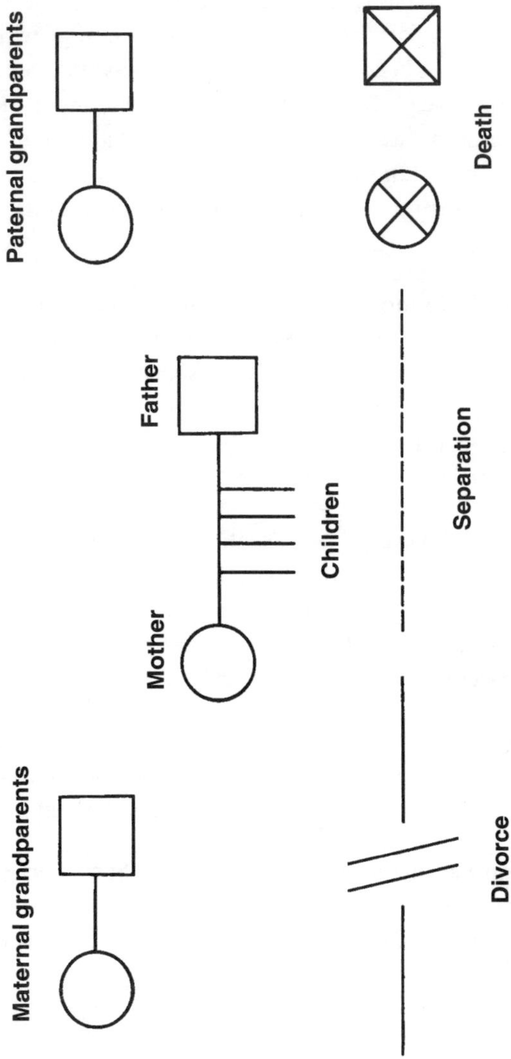

Figure 1–3. Descriptive symbols used in composing a family tree.

surrounding her impression of baby (e.g., family resemblance, personality characteristics), choice of baby's name, maternal depression, anergy.

Infancy (0–18 months). Medical problems first 18 months, feeding patterns, irritability, sleeping patterns, rocking and head banging, onset and intensity of stranger anxiety (being strange with people) and separation protest behavior, unusual fearfulness and unusual sensitivity to loud noises (e.g., blender, vacuum cleaner, sirens, unfamiliar settings), indiscriminate response to others, "cuddliness" with mother and others, onset and nature of speech *(crucial)*, gross motor milestones (e.g., sitting, walking), prolonged separations, and parental illness.

Toddler (18–36 months). Onset and success of toilet training; presence and nature of externally directed aggression including temper tantrums, fears, and night terrors; socialization; separation behavior; sleeping patterns and whether child sleeps in parental bed (and frequency); speech development; development of autonomy and self-control; contest "struggles."

Preschool (3–5 years). Socialization, adjustment to nursery school and kindergarten, peer relations, fears, impulse control, curiosity, assertiveness, soiling/smearing, enuresis, management of aggression, masturbation, coordination, clumsiness, nightmares, whether child sleeps in parental bed (and frequency).

Latency (6–11 years). Peer relations (e.g., best friends), interests, hobbies, sports, cognitive gains, impulse control, coordination, clumsiness, separations (e.g., camp) and reactions to them.

Puberty and adolescence (12–16 years). Secondary sexual characteristics, masturbation, menarche, alcohol, tobacco, drugs, regressions in learning and/or behavior, depression, withdrawal, peer relations.

School History

Current school. Name and address of school, grade, names of teachers (homeroom, guidance counselor, principal), grades (request report cards), and any changes within the past year in grades and/or behavior in school. If involved in present or past special education program, obtain summaries.

School history. Adjustment to first school experience, separation problems, school refusal ("phobia"), behavior problems, failing or acceleration.

Medical History

Date, place, and physician carrying out most recent physical examination and results; all significant illnesses, operations, and injuries since birth with dates, hospital(s), and outcome; history of allergies and current use of medications.

Interviews With Child and Mental Status Examination

A concise but thorough description of observations during interviews. Include general appearance and behavior, relatedness, dominant mood/affect, coordination and movement, speech and language, perception/cognition, play, conscience/impulse control, self-concept (see Chapter 2). For practical purposes in write-ups or presentations, a summary of those aspects of the mental status examination and interview content is essential for differential diagnosis and disposition.

Interviews With Family

Description of family. Members present, number and dates of interviews.

Summary of interviews. Seating arrangement(s) (draw), quality of interactions, key reactors, major themes, quality of communication, ability to listen to one another, respect for separateness, prevailing mood and affect, degree of concern for one another, "enmeshment/disengagement," family's view of child's problem (will family support or resist therapy for child), manner in which family has managed child's problem to date.

Auxiliary Data

Psychological testing, neurologic evaluations, laboratory data.

Formulation

A brief but salient synthesis of all previous biopsychosocial data, the intent of which is to convey the chronological internal and external event-related development of the child's problem. This summary, a critical portion of the workup, should include biogenetic factors; primary conflict(s); psychosexual level of development (see A. Freud 1963; Erikson 1963); primary defenses utilized ("ego strength"); degree that problem is ego-syntonic or ego-alien, internalized, acute or chronic.

The formulation should include relevant family data such as stage of family development (Zilbach 1979); style of family functioning (Minuchin 1974; Skynner 1976); family defenses, preoccupations, losses, and shifts; and quality of object relations. Identification and listing of primary problem facilitates treatment planning.

Diagnosis

The diagnostic considerations should flow naturally from the formulation and conform to that database. Differential diagnoses should be listed, and a working final diagnosis noted in relation to DSM-IV.

Plan

This is a brief description of the therapeutic plan, including psychotherapy, medication, school modification, and environmental manipulations.

Furnishing the Office Playroom

The psychiatric assessment of a child can be conducted in virtually any setting. Whether schoolroom, hospital bedside, the child's own home, or the office playroom, the critical variables are the comfort of the examiner and the quality of contact with the child. Valuable diagnostic data can be gathered rapidly and accurately by the physician who can and should relax, enjoy, and explore the clinical process spontaneously. Hence, in most respects, the attitudes and behaviors of the diagnostician are the most important "furnishings" in successful clinical work. Nonetheless, the office playroom is a major workspace and deserves attention.

In some clinical settings, office and playroom are separate from one another. Although some clinicians prefer such an arrangement, it is by no means necessary. The combined space has the advantage of flexibly encouraging play and/or verbal interchange for children of all ages. Such an arrangement is useful in family meetings where both "adult" and "child" space is required. In addition to adult-size desk and chairs, a smaller table and chairs to match for younger children are helpful. Personal and homey touches—such as an electric water heater for instant coffee, cocoa, and soup and a jar or box with crackers or nuts—create a pleasant atmosphere, are useful diagnostic tools in their own right, and facilitate alliance formation with both children and parents. Hospitality and informality need not be incompatible with professional competence. A cup of coffee for an anxious parent can establish a sense of safety and comfort that is work enhancing. Photographs of the diagnostician's spouse and children probably do *not* belong in the office playroom.

A bulletin board is almost essential for children's drawings. A calendar and maps of the local city, state, and country are useful diagnostic and therapeutic aids. Space to keep the projects and products of children in therapy may be located in the examiner's desk or on a shelf. Shoe boxes can serve the same purpose and, when identified by the child's name, can lend privacy and continuity to clinical work.

Obviously, some collection of toys and games is important. The beginning clinician is well guided by the principle that "less is more." Most children brought to the child psychiatrist suffer from some form of overstimulation (particularly in the American culture). Too many bright, novel, and interesting objects often lead to chaos, overactivity, and a nervous and harried examiner. *The most valuable diagnostic tool is one's self.* Material objects, especially in excess, complicate and confuse the diagnostic process. Furthermore, the uses and limitations of various play objects should be kept in mind. They are not present to entertain or distract (either examiner or child); their primary purposes are, in order of importance,

- To serve as a medium for contact/relatedness with the child
- To inform the diagnostician about cognitive, affective, and perceptual capacities or deficits
- To facilitate developmental progress in therapies

At the same time, selecting items that are of interest to or that are skill areas of the examiner is perfectly reasonable as long as they are not used to protect his or her own sense of competence against the natural anxieties of beginning clinical work with children.

Some practical items from which to make selections, by age, are as follows:

- *Infant/toddler (1–3 years).* One or two dolls, large rubber or Nerf ball, pull or push toy such as large wooden train with cars that connect.
- *Preschool (4–5 years).* Drawing and construction materials (crayons, felt-tip markers, paper, scissors, stapler, paste, and adhesive tape), dollhouse, hand and finger puppets, family figurines, anatomically correct dolls, toy guns, toy soldiers, Lincoln Logs or Tinker Toys, Matchbox cars, simple card games (e.g., Go Fish, War, Old Maid) on large decks with pictures, simple board games (e.g., Candyland, Chutes and Ladders), books, Play-Doh, old newspapers, water paints.
- *School-age (6–12 years).* Books, deck of cards, Nerf basketball set, soft rubber dart gun, Velcro darts and target, games (e.g., chess, checkers, Othello, Score Four, dominoes, Labyrinth, tabletop sports games), model building equipment (penknife with retractable blade, Duco cement, cutting board), cassettes for tape-recording stories and play.

Some of these items are useful starters. All may be used by any age group (including adolescents), depending on the level of development or the phase of treatment or play therapy. Whenever possible, it is best to keep one's play equipment behind cabinet doors to avoid overstimulation. The examiner needs to encourage spontaneity and to maintain control.

References

American Psychiatric Association: Diagnostic and Statistical Manual of Mental Disorders, 4th Edition. Washington, DC, American Psychiatric Association, 1994

Bemporad J: Child Development in Normality and Psychopathology. New York, Brunner/Mazel, 1980

Erikson EH: Childhood and Society. New York, WW Norton, 1963

Freud A: The concept of developmental lines. Psychoanal Study Child 18:245–265, 1963

Group for the Advancement of Psychiatry: Psychopathological Disorders in Childhood: Theoretical Considerations and a Proposed Classification. New York, Group for the Advancement of Psychiatry, 1966

Minuchin S: Families and Family Therapy. Cambridge, MA, Harvard University Press, 1974

Shapiro T: The borderline syndrome in children: a critique, in The Borderline Child. Edited by Robson K. New York, McGraw-Hill, 1983, pp 11–29

Skynner ACR: Systems of Family and Marital Psychotherapy. New York, Brunner/Mazel, 1976

Winnicott DW: The location of cultural experience. Int J Psychoanal 48:368–372, 1967

Zilbach J: Family development and familial factors in etiology, in Basic Handbook of Child Psychiatry, Vol 2: Disturbances of Development. Edited by Noshpitz J. New York, Basic Books, 1979, pp 62–87

2

Diagnostic Assessment: Technical Considerations

Kenneth S. Robson, M.D.

In child and adolescent psychiatry, less is often more in all aspects of clinical work. The natural force and momentum of growth and development are powerful allies to the clinician and increase the likelihood of modest change leading to significant therapeutic results. Skillful management of diagnostic assessments can prove to be substantial interventions in the life of a child. Thus, even more than in general psychiatry, the alert diagnostician needs to couple a therapeutic stance with clear but flexible goals in the evaluation of children. These goals tend to separate into first-stage and second-stage issues.

Goals of the Diagnostic Process

First-Stage Diagnostic Issues

- To establish whether emergency intervention is required (see Chapters 15 and 16).

- To develop positive contact with the referral source.
- To explore financial issues sufficiently to consider their relevance in the evaluation (see "Parent Interviews" later).
- To decide who should be involved in the initial clinical session.
- To gather as much clinical data as necessary from the family, child, and other agencies to reach a preliminary diagnosis sufficient to make decisions regarding a working plan of treatment; extended diagnostic evaluations; or referral elsewhere. Decisions to treat or refer are often possible long before comprehensive diagnostic data are available or necessary.

Second-Stage Diagnostic Issues

- To refine and elaborate preliminary diagnostic impressions via clinical contacts, psychological testing, laboratory tests, and school consultation.
- To define the developmental needs and deficits of the child clearly (i.e., separation from parents, establishment of autonomy, enhancement of peer relations, and the means to address them).
- To integrate all existing data into a comprehensive treatment plan. Given the nature of child and adolescent psychiatry, such treatment planning is complex and resembles good choreography—timing is critical! For example, a child's need for intensive psychotherapy, a therapeutic school, or psychoactive medication may be quickly evident to the clinician but not recommended until parental support for such steps is established.

The Clinical Approach in Child and Adolescent Psychiatry

The resident in general psychiatry, and in other medical specialties, learns a professional bearing with patients and families that may encourage formality and relative distance. In child and adolescent psychiatry, such a bearing may complicate work with children and parents. A comfortable but appropriate informality is likely to be more effective.

Pleasantness, small talk and chattiness, and *active* efforts to help new and always anxious patients feel at ease are compatible with excellent care. For example, offering parents coffee or soup on a cold day can accelerate alliance formation and the diagnostic process. Further, one's own personality, life experiences, memories, interests, and beliefs are valuable assets to be thoughtfully, professionally, and comfortably used rather than obscured. Being "one's self" is not unprofessional. The child psychiatrist's capacity to play and enjoy it *belongs* in the clinical process. A few points:

- Parents are not patients. They are parents and should be treated as respected collaborators.
- Children like to know, and usually assume, that the doctor knows something about their world in the small ways that matter. Take every chance to reacquaint oneself with the activities, life space, and mundane details of children of all ages (e.g., current sports heroes, television programs, breakfast cereals, movies, slang, drug names, shoe brands).
- Children are not little adults. Those who can relate like adults (i.e., sitting and talking) often don't need to.
- Reacquaint oneself with one's own childhood memories. Although at times painful, this is extraordinarily useful in developing empathy and clinical skills. Children often believe that adults cannot understand them and were never children themselves.
- Enjoy the work and expect anxiety, confusion, and occasional embarrassment as natural and temporary aspects of the job.

Referral of Children

Unlike adults, children and even most adolescents rarely refer themselves for psychiatric care. They are in some sense captives of the family, foster care, or institution serving them in loco parentis. Further, the resistances to referral, particularly in biological families, are probably more powerful than is the case with individual adult patients. The child is enmeshed in a complex network of relationships in which a change may be perceived as threatening to an entire family system.

In the normal course of events, growth and development impose a loss on parents that is always difficult. In pathological situations, where children often serve as inappropriate but sustaining figures for a parent, the potential, and usually unconscious, threat of separation may color the referral process with danger. In addition, the inevitable, intense feelings of guilt and failure on the part of parents create further encumbrances to successful referral. For these reasons, the clinician's first and most essential task in the diagnostic process is to establish a sympathetic, empathic, nonjudgmental, and supportive stance with the family member making the referral. An early assessment of the "power structure" affecting the child's life is always useful and sometimes necessary. For example, a father who must pay the bills may need contact with the diagnostician if the referral is to succeed.

Because of the resistances to referral in biological families, most initial contacts or referral suggestions are made by other people involved in the child's life. In order of usual frequency, these include teachers/schools; social service agencies; courts; and pediatricians, family practitioners, and other mental health professionals. Sensitivity to the needs and feelings of these referral sources is equally important. Prompt return of telephone calls and letters of acknowledgment, progress, and planning should be habitual.

There are often many "hidden agendas" in referrals of children. This is particularly true when multiple referral sources are involved (e.g., school and parents, or agency and parents). As noted earlier, the politics of referrals are often complex. In relation to the question of who should be seen first—child, parents, family, or referral source—it is generally useful to retain flexibility. The clinician usually can establish the most critical party with whom to initiate contact in the first meeting. Parents may need to "check out" the clinician first. Perhaps the child, as repository of all family psychopathology, can serve as the only acceptable entry point. Such needs must be understood and respected. In rare instances parents may insist, generally defensively, that the child be seen first because the child is "the patient." If that is not the case, with preadolescent children it is helpful in an initial visit to see the parents alone briefly to establish contact, then the family together, and then to spend some time alone with the child before his or her next visit. Adolescents more often are seen alone initially, although "enmeshed" families may require a group session or sessions in some instances. Premature insistence on a rigid diagnostic format may lose the referral. The beginning clinician will profit from exploring a variety of formats with the collaboration of an experienced clinician.

The Clinical Diagnostic Interviews

"Agency" Referrals

In clinic settings, and increasingly in private practice, children are referred by courts, lawyers, special educators, and agency staff in state welfare offices. Such referrals are complex, often involving adversarial and fiscal issues between agencies and biological or foster families with conflicting ideas about the child's best interest. Questions of custody, abuse, and "fitness" are common. Support for a special educational placement may be deemed too costly and unnecessary. The clinician who accepts such a referral without first clarifying the issues may waste extraordinary amounts of time while limiting the usefulness of the assessment. In situations of this kind, it is wise to establish *beforehand*

- Who are all of the interested parties, what are their respective roles in the child's life, and "who wants what from whom"?
- What are the limits and characteristics of your role in the evaluation (e.g., clinical evaluator, consultant, potential expert witness)? To whom will you have access? The diagnostician needs maximal leeway and data and may wish to see biological parents and foster parents, for example. In general, the safest and most important role for the child psychiatrist is as evaluator of and advocate for the child involved.
- Is the case now in litigation or is that route anticipated? If so, will you be expected to testify? Can and should you?
- What financial arrangements are involved if court time is likely to occur?

Careful prior assessment of these issues, whether by telephone or in person, is the prerogative of the child psychiatrist. Numerous cases of this kind may not be appropriate referrals but are difficult to interrupt once initiated.

Parent Interviews

The decision to have one's child evaluated is difficult to reach and is fraught with anxiety for most parents who feel exposed, vulnerable, and certain of their presumed failure. To be sympathetic and empathic but not prematurely reassuring is useful. Whenever possible it is wise to leave the details of an evaluation (e.g., precise number of sessions with parents and child) open. A general description of the format, however, is comforting. Mentioning that meeting with the entire family at some point in the diagnostic process would be helpful can facilitate that part of the evaluation. Ordinarily one or two meetings with a parent or parents, one or two meetings with the child, auxiliary data gathering when indicated (e.g., psychological testing, laboratory tests), and a wrap-up session with parents (and sometimes the child) suffice to reach first-stage decisions.

Financial questions often arise in an initial telephone contact. The influence of fiscal realities on clinician options and planning is increasingly powerful and is in many cases a limiting factor in accomplishing evaluations or treatment. For example, many third-party payers have annual maximums, particularly for outpatient work; to use up these monies in an extensive evaluation may deprive the child of treatment. Psychological testing may be delayed in many situations where its cost would compromise treatment options. A diagnostic hospitalization, generally considered in relation to questions of serious disturbance, may sometimes be justified on economic as well as clinical grounds because inpatient insurance coverage is usually more extensive. Finally, in many clinics and hospitals, limits on "bad debt" and "free care" control levels of fee adjustments and length of stay. The diagnostician needs to be well informed about local fiscal regulations and relate them to initial planning with parents from the outset.

Another question facing the evaluator arises when the referred child is involved in a separated or divorced family. Generally, but not always, the custodial parent makes the first contact and probably should be seen alone first. Although the participation of the noncustodial or estranged parent may be essential, it is ordinarily wiser to meet the referring parent first. In such situations, however, the diagnostician may be told that the other parent has "no interest" in the child or the evaluation. Such is often far from the case, and circumspection and patience are advised.

Assuming that parent(s) sessions have been scheduled, certain guidelines can be helpful. A semistructured interview style is useful. Permitting parents to share their own perceptions of the child and their own anxieties can provide much useful data. Often specific details of developmental history are mentioned spontaneously and can be briefly explored without disrupting the spontaneous flow of material.

At some natural break point in the parent interviews, the gathering of specific developmental family history data is essential. Let the chief complaint guide and prioritize the areas to pursue. For example, where depressive concerns are part of a referral, a detailed family history of alcoholism and affective disease and the child's sleeping patterns are more imperative than neuromotor milestones or toilet training. Because the diagnostic process is frequently the beginning of treatment in many instances, the documentation of certain data can be delayed and treated as second-stage phenomena.

It is of enormous practical significance to assess and document in a preliminary way, while gathering both family and developmental history, the levels of stimulation to which the child is exposed or responds (see Chapter 1). Questions such as whether the child sleeps in parental beds, bathes with parents, and likes physical contact are useful and nonthreatening. Are doors kept open or shut? Are transitions such as from home to school in the morning and bedtime at night calm and low intensity or abrupt and disruptive? Do mealtimes facilitate pleasant modulated contact among family members or do chaos and agitation prevail? These data can play a major role in increasing understanding and therapeutic leverage.

Given limited time, there are three functional areas of a child's life that provide enough data for first-stage decisions regarding the degree of impairment and the need for therapeutic interventions: 1) school competence (work), 2) the presence and quality of peer relationships (love), and 3) level of personal distress (e.g., depression, anxiety) (play). Interviews that focus on these areas in sufficient detail are cost-effective. Of course, there are situations where a child who functions well in these areas may need to be taken into treatment because of family dysfunction externalized onto a relatively healthy child.

Most parents will want to know about diagnosis and prognosis early in the evaluation, often before the child is seen. Both premature reassurance and dire predictions should be avoided.

If not brought up spontaneously, the question of what to tell the child about the evaluation is important to address. Parents can be told that evaluations do not damage children or create problems that were not there already. Children can be told directly that they are going to see a doctor who helps with worries and problems, identifying the specific issue with the child (e.g., school problems, depression, separation anxiety). Parents should be discouraged from lying to a child about the nature of the evaluation.

Increasing numbers of children are referred and brought to the diagnostician by persons in loco parentis such as foster parents, social workers affiliated with state agencies or institutions, child-care staff, and lawyers. Data from such sources, and from schools and teachers as well, are obviously as critical as that from parents in intact families. The diagnostician may modify the principles and practices described above in such instances, but the aims of the data gathering are, of course, the same.

Family Interviews

With the possible exception of those catastrophic conditions of childhood apparently dominated by biological determinants (e.g., autism, pervasive developmental disorders, Tourette's syndrome, major depression), the interpersonal environment of the child plays a dominant role in both hindering and facilitating developmental process. To see this environment in action during the diagnostic evaluation is, therefore, extraordinarily important. An observant clinician can note, in a single family session, crucial aspects of the child's world that can include

- His or her role in the family (e.g., scapegoat, "pseudo-parent" to a mother or father, lover)

- The quality of parental relatedness and the meaning of an absent parent or lost object
- The mode of relating in the family as "enmeshment" or "disengagement" (Minuchin 1974) and the primary family affect (Fleck 1980)
- Developmental arrests or pathology in other family members
- Some sources of symptomatology in the child and, from these data, specific goals for subsequent therapeutic intervention

Without being a family therapist, the diagnostician can relatively quickly learn to use "family work" in a flexible manner in both the evaluation and treatment of children. Further, the introduction of family sessions during the diagnostic phase can facilitate subsequent use of this approach in therapies that follow. A diagnostic family session is strongly recommended (Serrano 1979). Some principles to guide the clinician follow:

- Family sessions are stressful, and extra efforts to put family members at ease should be made. The clinician must be active.
- Invite all members to attend and always include infants.
- Use a room large enough to accommodate adults and young children; the latter need space to move about, "peel off," and return to the central group. Some play materials such as crayons and paper should be readily available.
- Schedule 1.25–1.5 hours for such sessions.
- Encourage communication but make it clear that no one has to talk about anything they would rather not. Similarly, forbid physical injury or destruction of property.
- The data from such meetings are vast. An observant clinician will not try to catch all interactions but rather the central issues of seating arrangements, dominant affect(s), and mode of relatedness. One will learn more by expecting less.

Child Interviews

For the beginning clinician, interviews with children are anxiety provoking. The world of childhood, especially if one is not a parent, seems to be a foreign country. Further, the clinician must unlearn in many respects the posture assumed with adult patients, who generally can talk and often observe themselves. Finally, the affects of children are intense and often quite uncomfortable to experience, including the reawakened traumas of one's own childhood years. Anxiety is to be expected.

Another source of confusion to the clinician is the presence of play as a communicative mode. When one is accustomed to following the complexities of adult thought and speech, play as a form of action (even more so when alternating with speech in the verbal child) is difficult to follow. A common error is to search for too much meaning in every sequence of play. Most play sequences derive from real-life experiences, not fantasies, and are better understood as communications about past or current realities. The best guide to the content of any child interview is the child's affect. Generally, if the clinician can gain a sense of the prevailing emotion (e.g., anxiety, terror, sadness, depression, anger, despair, agitation), play and other forms of communication fall readily into place and seem to make sense. To achieve this stance the main effort should be simply to join the child, be with him or her—that is at once the easiest and hardest of tasks. To strain at it, however, never works. To try for less in this regard is usually to gain more. The stories that children have to tell are basic ones—to listen is enough to know that they feel afraid, discouraged, mad, or unloved. One cannot diagnose a child without first establishing contact. Do not look for "mysteries." The central issues are generally self-evident.

It is important not to substitute toys, games, complicated psychological tests, or rigid interview techniques for spontaneous interchange with the child. A *few* pieces of age-appropriate play materials (see Chapter 1) will suffice to facilitate rapport. Selecting two or three age-appropriate play items before the interview provides an orientation for the child and reduces the likelihood of stimulus overload in both patient and diagnostician.

The more formal categories of data to be observed are as follows:

General appearance and behavior. Size, habitus, weight, coloring, gait, dress, grooming, facial expression, ease or difficulty coming with examiner and separating from parents, eyeglasses, physical defects, "oddness."

Relatedness. Style and quality of contact with the examiner, availability or genuineness of child, depth of contact, shallowness, precociousness, use of eye contact, seductiveness and excessive use or avoidance of physical contact, rate of relatedness (indiscriminate and immediate or avoidant and fearful). Change in depth of relatedness over time (within or across interviews) is especially important to note.

Dominant mood/affect. Depression (include suicidal ideation or plans), discouragement, apathy, anxiety, fear, panic, drivenness, anger, irritability; excitement, helplessness, optimism; blunting, shallowness, lability of affects.

Coordination and movement. Clumsiness (examine for "soft" neurological signs, see Chapter 3), agility, level of activity, stiffness of bearing and gait, hand-eye coordination, abnormal involuntary movements including tics, tremors, choreoathetosis, spasticity, and oral-buccal movement when evaluating for tardive dyskinesia. Minor physical anomalies may be noted (Waldrop and Halverson 1971).

Speech and language. Vocabulary, expressive clarity, use in interpersonal communication; idiosyncrasies including punning, neologisms, echolalia, pronominal reversal; modulation of tone and intensity; paralinguistic richness versus "tin woodman" or metallic quality of speech; stuttering, complexity and age appropriateness of verbal expressions; precocity of language.

Perception/cognition. Integrity of vision and hearing; orientation to time, place, and person; confusion; attention and capacity to concentrate; level of intelligence and obvious learning impairments (capacity to read and do math problems can be examined); quality of thinking: logicality, organization, concreteness, ability to use symbolization and abstract thought, evidence of primary process; presence and durability of reality testing; content of thought: repetitive themes, preoccupation, richness, impoverishment, ability to fantasize at age-appropriate level; constriction or inhibition of thought.

Play. Spontaneity, choice of materials/activities, ability to involve examiner, capacity to sustain interest and elaborate themes, anxiety, and "play interruptions" (the abrupt cessation of a play sequence in relation to anxiety-provoking material); repetitive sequences.

Conscience/impulse control. Rigidity or laxity of conscience, stability of impulse control.

Self-concept. Self-esteem, identifications, gender preference and perception. Asking a child to draw himself or herself is very helpful in this regard.

In time the beginning diagnostician will develop a style in conducting interviews with a child. In training it is especially useful to observe experienced clinicians interviewing one's patients; if not offered, it can be requested. In any event, the integration of these data may seem a staggering task. This task is simplified if one distills from the mental status examination its essential aims—namely, to become informed about 1) the overall integrity of the child's neuromotor and cognitive apparatus, 2) the child's capacity for relatedness, and 3) the status of his or her development vis-à-vis chronological age and the evenness or unevenness of major developmental "lines."

A general appreciation of each of these areas in conjunction with the stigmata of specific syndromes (e.g., the tics of Tourette's syndrome, vegetative signs of depression, thought disorder in schizophrenia) provides the diagnostician with ample information for the elaboration of differential diagnosis. However, data from the physical neurological examination, laboratory tests, and psychological assessments may also be necessary. Approaches to these data are described in Chapters 3, 4, and 5. The integration of these data and their communication to others are discussed in Chapter 6.

References

Fleck S: Family functioning and family pathology. Psychiatric Annals 10:17—35, 1980

Minuchin S: Families and Family Therapy. Cambridge, MA, Harvard University Press, 1974

Serrano AC: A child-centered family diagnostic interview, in Basic Handbook of Child Psychiatry, Vol 1: Development. Edited by Noshpitz J. New York, Basic Books, 1980, pp 624–630

Waldrop MF, Halverson CF: Minor physical anomalies and hyperactive behavior in young children, in Exceptional Infant, Vol 2. Edited by Hellmuth J. New York, Brunner/Mazel, 1971, pp 343–380

3

Physical and Neurological Examinations and Laboratory Studies

P. S. B. Sarma, M.B., B.S.

Child and adolescent psychiatric disorders are frequently associated with a number of medical findings in the physical appearance, physiological systems, and laboratory test data of the individual. These findings may simply accompany the psychiatric disorders without etiological significance. On the other hand, they may have more direct and significant relationships with psychiatric disorders in one or more of the following ways:

- Direct causal relationship (e.g., phenylketonuria and mental retardation)
- Indicator of deviation or insult at a specific point in development (e.g., first-trimester–related congenital anomalies)
- Indicator of predisposition to certain syndromes (e.g., low levels of dopamine β-hydroxylase and certain conduct disorders) (Bowden et al. 1988)
- Indicator of recent insult to the nervous system (e.g., high lead levels in the blood)
- Probable indicator of prognosis (e.g., luteinizing hormone [LH] and follicle-stimulating hormone [FSH] patterns in clinically im-

proved anorexia nervosa)

- Indicator of side effects from overzealous or even optimal treatment (e.g., electrocardiogram [ECG] changes associated with tricyclic antidepressant treatment)
- Features of the psychiatric disorders themselves (e.g., multiple superficial lacerations of the wrist in the histrionic and depressed adolescent girl or the low levels of growth hormone secretion seen in psychosocial dwarfism)

In the following pages the relevance of and indications for the use of established procedures are discussed. Some new procedures that are helpful in the comprehensive psychiatric examination of children and adolescents are also described.

The Physical Examination

Most children and adolescents seen for evaluation in the office do not need to disrobe in order to undergo a rapid, selective physical examination. General indications for a complete physical examination include

- *Major* psychiatric disturbances
- *Early onset* of the disturbance in the developmental spectrum
- Suspicion of *physical or sexual abuse* of the child
- Suspicion of *substance abuse*
- Suspicion of *anorexia nervosa or bulimia*
- Presenting problems that are clearly *physical* in nature (e.g., pain, loss of weight)

Since every physician is trained to perform a physical examination, the details of this procedure will not be dealt with here. In the preschool age and in the early grade school age, it is advisable to record height and weight data routinely as well as the percentile scores. Heart rate and blood pressure should be recorded to compare against changes from the future treatments. Assessment of the integrity of the visual and auditory systems is especially important at all ages. These tests are generally performed in schools. However, if there is any doubt about the reliability of school reports, or if the reports are not available, it is advisable to use the Snellen chart for vision. Audiological screening is indicated for all children with problems in language skills, learning impairments, pervasive developmental disorders, or autism.

It is important that the child and adolescent psychiatric physician be familiar with the dysmorphic features associated with the following conditions and with minor physical anomalies in general:

- Fetal alcohol syndrome, which can present with small head size, short palpebral fissures, drooping eyelids, epicanthic folds, maxillary hypoplasia, joint anomalies, cleft palate, capillary hemangioma, altered palmar creases, low birth weight, small-for-gestation size, a variety of cardiac anomalies, and significant delays in cognitive development.
- Fragile X syndrome, which can present with mental retardation, coarse facial features, large ears, prominent lower jaw, and large testicles.
- The various features associated with the long-recognized chromosomal anomalies such as Down's syndrome, Klinefelter's syndrome, Turner's syndrome, and those associated with tuberous sclerosis, neurofibromatosis, Prader-Willi syndrome, hypothyroidism, hyperthyroidism, and Lesch-Nyhan syndrome are important for the child psychiatrist to be aware of since the above conditions often have associated behavioral and/or cognitive deficits (see Chapter 22).

Minor Physical Anomalies

In the last 20 years, minor physical anomalies (MPAs) have elicited increased attention in psychiatry. There have been reports of high MPAs in low-incidence, high-severity syndromes like autism (Gualtieri et al. 1982; Walker 1977) and schizophrenia (Green et al. 1987; Gualtieri et al. 1982). There have also been reports of a relationship to more common syndromes like hyperactivity (Gualtieri et al. 1982; Waldrop et al. 1968) and subgroups of alcoholic patients (Gualtieri et al. 1982).

MPAs are indicative of first-trimester influences during intrauterine life or genetic influences or both. Although hundreds of malformations related to various parts of the body have been cataloged well by Smith (1976), the MPA descriptions given by Waldrop and colleagues (Waldrop and Halverson 1971; Waldrop et al. 1976) are particularly useful to the psychiatric clinician and are listed below. For excellent descriptions and illustrations, the reader is referred to their original reports.

- Fine electric hair (hair that simply will not comb down)
- Two or more hair whorls (either two or more distinct hair whorls near the crown of the head or a line that is an inch or more in length)
- Head circumference that is at least one standard deviation (SD) outside the normal range
- Epicanthic folds (where the upper and lower lids join the side of the nose, the point of union is partially or completely covered by a fold. This often leads to complete or partial invisibility of the lacrimal caruncle on direct view)
- Hypertelorism (distance between the eyes is greater than normal after accounting for racial differences)
- Low-set ears
- Adherent earlobes
- Malformed ears
- Asymmetrical ears
- Soft and pliable ears
- High-steepled palate (the roof of the palate forms an angle or is narrow and flat, instead of being dome shaped)
- Furrowed tongue (tongue has one or more deep grooves, usually not along the center line)
- Tongue with smooth-rough spots due to localized thickening of the epithelium (also known as "geographic tongue")
- Curved fifth finger (usually curved "inward"—toward the other fingers)
- Single transverse palmar crease
- Third toe longer than the second toe. (This is said to be a normal finding in children under age 3 years, but uncommon in elementary school children)

- Partial syndactyly of two middle toes
- Big gap between the first and second toes (the gap at the base should be more than half the width of the second toe)

Waldrop and Halverson (1971) reported that three items—two or more hair whorls, soft and pliable ears, tongue with smooth-rough spots—were not more common in schizophrenic patients. Gualtieri et al. (1982) did not score the items fine electric hair and two or more hair whorls in their study because these cannot be scored for black subjects. They dropped the following items because of poor reliability: low-set ears; asymmetrical ears; soft and pliable ears; syndactyly of two middle toes. By scoring and weighting the remaining items according to the system of Waldrop and Halverson, Gualtieri et al. obtained a mean MPA score of 2 ± 0.9 in a group of symptom-free children and 2.8 ± 0.9 in a group of hyperactive children. In that study, autistic children obtained a score of 3.7 ± 0.9.

Based on the above, an unweighted MPA score of 3 or higher among the following 10 items can be considered significantly high: head circumference out of normal range, epicanthic folds, hypertelorism, adherent earlobes, high-steepled palate, furrowed tongue, curved fifth finger, single transverse palmar crease, third toe longer than second toe, and big gap between first and second toes.

At this time, there are no clear data linking specific MPAs to central nervous system dysfunction. However, the association of a high number of MPAs with autism, Down's syndrome (Epstein 1989), and schizophrenia is strongly suggestive of a link.

Neurological Assessment

It is clear that dysfunctions of the brain are related to significantly higher incidence of psychiatric disorders in children (Rutter 1983). Therefore, it is advisable that a psychiatric evaluation of a child makes proper use of the "windows" that are available to assess brain function. These windows generally represent different and progressively more complex levels of assessment in terms of the time involved and costs. It is important that the clinician evaluating a child has basic neurological assessment skills and is knowledgeable regarding the more complex investigations as well as the indication for suggesting or ordering these investigations. Kaufman et al. (1992) summarized these data.

Neurological Examination

A quick screening version of the traditional neurological examination is described in Appendix 1.

Minor Neurological Signs

Even in the absence of positive findings in a traditional neurological examination, an examination for minor neurological signs can, at times, uncover areas of dysfunction or developmental delay. Although the clinical significance of these signs is controversial, there is increasing evidence for their utility in "signaling" a neurodevelopmental component in some child psychiatric disorders, as illustrated by the following example. In a number of cross-sectional studies, boys with academic problems have been found to manifest certain soft signs significantly more frequently than control subjects (Adams et al. 1974; Myklebust 1973; Peters et al. 1975; Sarma 1989; Shaywitz et al. 1984).

In a longitudinal study, there was evidence for a higher number of soft signs in low-birth-weight children who had perinatal complications. Those who had a higher number of soft signs at the time of follow-up at age 8 years manifested a greater prevalence of academic and behavioral problems (Hertzig 1981). In another longitudinal study, boys with dysgraphesthesia and dysdiadakokinesis at age 7 years manifested a similar picture on follow-up at age 16. At age 16, these boys seemed to manifest a higher prevalence of depressive symptomatology compared with control subjects (Shaffer et al. 1985).

There is considerable evidence from neuropsychological studies that even in the presence of "normal" gross neurological status, there can be evidence of higher brain dysfunctions in psychiatric syndromes (Golden et al. 1983; Tramontana et al. 1980).

Although a comprehensive neuropsychological examination or one of the neuroimaging procedures described later in this chapter can give information regarding subtle brain dysfunctions, they are fairly expensive and should be used sparingly and judiciously in today's economic climate. An examination for soft neurological signs might be helpful in identifying subtle brain dysfunctions. If further delineation is necessary, more expensive procedures can be considered. Most soft-sign studies to date have involved a large number of items in a battery that discourages the clinician from using them on a regular basis. Furthermore, many of these items have poor reliability. After reviewing the various studies, I constructed EXAMINS (Examination for Minor Neurological Signs), which is described in Appendix 2.

Electroencephalogram (EEG)

The EEG has an important place in the neuropsychiatric evaluation of children. In every child manifesting unexplained temper tantrums; episodic violence; rage attacks; episodic hyperactivity; sleepy spells; vague auditory, visual, olfactory, or gustatory hallucinations; or amnesic or fugue states, an EEG with a sleep record and activating procedures of hyperventilation and photic stimulation is absolutely essential to rule out temporal-lobe-related or other seizure phenomena. The recording of cerebral electrical activity is of value in the documentation of seizures and the assessment of interictal cerebral activity. EEG is helpful in the evaluation of abnormalities of mental status due to metabolic disorders (e.g., hepatic) or infectious diseases (e.g., subacute sclerosing panencephalitis, herpes encephalitis, Creutzfeldt–Jakob disease). EEG has also been used to evaluate behavioral disorders to determine whether a behavior in question may be a manifestation of a seizure disorder such as the automatisms associated with temporal lobe epilepsy. During the last several years a number of new approaches to EEG recording and advances in equipment have expanded the value of EEG in assessing disturbances in behavior. These include the following:

Prolonged EEG recording. To extend the recording time and increase the likelihood of recording abnormalities of cerebral electrical activity, prolonged EEG recording techniques have been developed.

A major value is to allow for a correlation between clinical and electroencephalographic events—that is, to distinguish between episodic behavioral outbursts of a dyscontrol nature from those of temporal lobe epilepsy, and repetitive stereotyped behaviors as seen in autism from seizure phenomena. With the addition of physiological monitors, these systems allow for recording of ECG, respirations, and eye movements, allowing for a variety of electrophysiological and clinical correlations and for accurate sleep trend analysis (see below). Three methods are available. Although in each case the patient wears an EEG transmitter, the recording techniques differ in their method of transmitting the signal. With cable telemetry, the transmitter is connected directly to the recording device. Radio telemetry permits more freedom of movement. Video monitoring via split screen may be added following the recording of the direct correlation between behavior and EEG activity. Patients undergoing these evaluations are restricted to the laboratory or hospital.

Ambulatory EEG monitoring. Ambulatory EEG monitoring using cassette recordings allows the patient complete freedom of activity in the setting in which the EEG is recorded. The patient wears a small recording device similar to a small portable tape player. This device permits the correlation between behavior and EEG activity in the setting in which it usually occurs and observations by those who have been concerned about the behavior (e.g., by teachers in the classroom). In addition to previously mentioned benefits, ambulatory EEG monitoring with cassette permits evaluation of such classroom behaviors as inattentiveness by distinguishing seizure-related inattentiveness from daydreaming or deliberate avoidance behaviors. With this technique, recording of sleep studies can take place at home in a more natural setting than in a sleep laboratory.

EEG sleep studies. EEG recorded during prolonged periods of natural sleep allows for an evaluation of a number of sleep disorders such as sleep apnea, disorders of transitional stages (e.g., somnambulism, night terrors), and other unusual nocturnal events. Direct correlation with behavior can be made. A sleep trend analysis permits quantitative evaluation of sleep stages. Rapid-eye-movement-latency evaluations may be helpful in predicting sensitivity to tricyclic antidepressants.

Brain Electrical Activity Mapping (BEAM)

BEAM provides computer synthesis of EEG frequencies in various regions of the brain and pictorial representation of these patterns. Furthermore, evoked potential patterns during various cognitive activities can be recorded. For example, the P-300 wave pattern during active listening and counting versus during passive listening to noises in the headphones can be recorded and compared with normative data for the same age and gender. This strategy is being used increasingly to identify the electrophysiological disturbances in various psychiatric disorders. In the near future, BEAM might become a diagnostic tool.

Neuroimaging Procedures

Since brain structure and function are the areas of concern in many psychiatric disorders, the rapidly advancing technology of the scanning (neuroimaging) procedures has a lot of potential in the systematic study of psychiatric disorders in children and adolescents. These procedures include computed tomography (CT), magnetic resonance imaging (MRI), also known as nuclear magnetic resonance (NMR), single photon emission computed tomography (SPECT), and positron-emission tomography (PET). For detailed descriptions of the technical aspects of these procedures and excellent reviews of the studies conducted in psychiatry, the reader is referred to the text edited by Andreasen (1989).

The following is essential reading for the child and adolescent psychiatrist. Lucid descriptions of these procedures and discussion of their applications in child and adolescent psychiatry have been provided by Kuperman et al. (1990). A critical evaluation of the cost-benefit ratio of such procedures in child and adolescent psychiatric practice is presented by Woolston and Riddle (1990).

CT. CT involves X rays directed at many angles toward the tissues of interest. The computer reconstructs the images picked up by radiation sensors after the X rays have passed through the tissues. When a contrast study is required, an intravenous iodine contrast medium is injected, and this can be particularly useful in identifying vascular malformations. CT is relatively lower in cost (compared with MRI), is widely available, and can be helpful in identifying gross structural abnormalities, calcifications, and vascular malformations. The disadvantages are the radiation exposure and limited clarity of intracranial structures, particularly if the posterior fossa contents (e.g., cerebellum) are of particular interest.

MRI. MRI involves no radiation or potentially allergenic contrast medium. It can provide visualization in three dimensions and without the interference of the bone image. MRI provides much sharper images of various parts of the brain, compared with CT.

The technology, briefly, is as follows. The magnetic resonance of the hydrogen atoms of tissues is used for producing their images. The protons are first aligned by a high-strength magnetic field. They wobble (precess) like a spinning top. Then a radio signal at the same frequency at which the protons are precessing is added. This tips the protons into a different axis, so that their magnetic moment changes direction. The signal stops; the protons, however, are resonating for a period of time (like a tuning fork), and this signal is measured as it gradually diminishes or relaxes to the original state. Pathological processes will affect the relaxation time because of the change in the number of hydrogen atoms (e.g., more fluid) or because of changes in the size of the tissue (e.g., the size of the caudate nucleus). The white matter of the brain returns to its original net magnetization more quickly than the gray matter and so it produces a stronger, brighter signal.

MRI is ideal for identifying demyelinating lesions, which are not likely to show in CT. Brain atrophy can be picked up much more clearly because of the better fluid-solid contrast and better gray-white matter contrast. However, it requires the subject to lie immobile in a cavelike tube for more than 30 minutes, and it cannot be used in the presence of metallic foreign bodies. Nor can it provide dynamic images of the working brain.

SPECT and PET. Dynamic imaging of the working brain can be accomplished either through regional cerebral blood flow measurement (accomplished by SPECT) or through measurement of regional glucose utilization (accomplished by PET).

PET is very sensitive, but is also very expensive (because it requires a cyclotron nearby). Therefore, PET will be limited to a few select research centers for the foreseeable future, in view of the severe constraints being placed on funding for medical care. SPECT, on the other hand, is relatively less expensive and can provide color images representing gradations of regional cerebral blood flow, providing functional measurements, which can add more meaningful information to images of structural pathology (Andreasen 1989) obtained by CT or MRI.

Laboratory Investigations

Laboratory procedures in child and adolescent psychiatry have the advantage of being highly standardized in relation to physiological, biochemical, and structural deviations. However, they add to the expense of medical care and have to be used selectively on the basis of relevant clinical findings. They cannot substitute for a thorough and accurate clinical examination. The last decade has witnessed a major growth in the available laboratory procedures in child and adolescent psychiatry; the indications for and significance of current procedures are discussed below.

Blood Count

A complete blood count (CBC) is advisable in children who have not had one in the past 6 months. A baseline CBC is essential before initiating all forms of pharmacotherapy.

The most recent broadening of the Centers for Disease Control criteria (AMA News 1991) for a diagnosis of acquired immunodeficiency syndrome (AIDS) includes "fewer than two hundred CD4 lymphocytes" (p. 12). Whether this applies to children is not clearly stated at this time.

Blood Chemistry

A baseline blood chemistry including liver enzymes is advisable whenever any potentially long-term pharmacological treatment is initiated.

Before initiating treatment with medications that are excreted in the urine (e.g., dextroamphetamine, methylphenidate) or those that can affect the kidney function (e.g., lithium), it is advisable to have a baseline assessment of kidney function, by ordering serum creatinine, blood urea nitrogen, and electrolytes.

When Lesch-Nyhan syndrome is suspected, further confirmation is provided by high uric acid levels.

Iron-deficiency anemia has been reported to be associated with pica and at times subsides when the iron deficiency is treated (Petersdorf et al. 1983). In mentally retarded individuals in institutions, a low zinc level has been, at times, associated with pica and responds to zinc supplementation (Lofts et al. 1990).

Although some interesting findings regarding norepinephrine metabolism have been described in childhood psychiatric disorders (Rogeness et al. 1988; Zametkin and Rapoport 1987), they have not reached the level of clinical utility at this time.

Lead level should be ordered in children who have cognitive dysfunction, particularly in the presence of current or past history of pica (Needleman and Gatsonis 1990).

When there is a history or suspicion of substance abuse or of the influence of intoxicants, a toxic screen should be ordered. In these subjects, possible liver damage should be looked for.

Folic acid deficiency should be considered in children who have been on anticonvulsants.

Blood level monitoring of tricyclic antidepressants and most anticonvulsants is quite well established in clinical practice.

When evaluating children with autism, pervasive developmental disorder, or mental retardation, it is important to recognize that an occasional child with phenylketonuria that was not picked up in the newborn screening can present with these features.

Urinary Investigations

Every child presenting with enuresis should have a urinalysis to rule out urinary tract infection and diabetes. An intravenous pyelogram and voiding cystourethrogram can be helpful in identifying factors involved in daytime enuresis. Appropriate urinary tract evaluation for sexually transmitted diseases is indicated in children who have been sexually abused and in children who have engaged in sexual activity.

Urine amino acid qualitative screen is indicated in children with significant cognitive dysfunctions.

Some uncommon metabolic disorders can present with psychiatric symptoms. Acute intermittent porphyria can present with abdominal pain, peripheral neuropathy, and mental changes. In the urine, there are usually high levels of porphobilinogen and aminolevulinic acid. Hartnup disease can present with photosensitive skin rash, intermittent ataxia, and psychotic behavior. Hartnup disease is associated with high levels of the following amino acids in the urine—threonine, tyrosine, and histidine. Wilson's disease can present with dystonia, ataxia, and various emotional-behavioral features. During the symptomatic state, there is a high excretion of copper in the urine. Even in an asymptomatic state, patients who are homozygous for the gene can usually be identified by high copper excretion in the urine (range of 2,000 g/24 hours) induced by penicillamine (Tu 1991).

Chromosome Studies

When children present with features suggestive of specific chromosome abnormalities, chromosome studies can provide confirmation of the diagnosis. It is, however, important to specify in the order that we are considering fragile X syndrome, if that is the suspected condition, because the laboratory has to use highly specific procedures (folate and thymidine deficient medium) for detecting the fragile X chromosome.

Neuroendocrinological Investigations

The dexamethasone suppression test, although not necessary for the diagnosis of affective disorder, can be useful in the decision, in complex syndromes, to use pharmacotherapy and in determining the degree of recovery and the chances for relapse (Evans et al. 1987). In children, 0.5 mg (or 1.0 mg in adolescents) of dexamethasone is given orally at 11:00 P.M., after a baseline blood drawing at 8:00 A.M. for cortisol level. The following day, blood is drawn at 4:00 P.M. for cortisol level and a level of 5.0 μg/dl is considered positive (failure to suppress cortisol secretion). A positive test is not a valid indicator of neuroendocrine abnormality for up to 2 weeks after drug or alcohol abuse or during treatment with anticonvulsants or psychotropic medications.

Evaluation of thyroid function for hyperactivity is indicated in recent weight loss, warm and moist hands, tachycardia, and high emotionality, particularly in a teenager who is not abusing drugs. Evaluation of the thyroid function for hypoactivity is indicated in the presence of lethargy, weight gain, or cognitive deterioration. This can be a side effect of lithium treatment.

Assessment of pituitary function is indicated in patients who manifest precocious puberty or delayed puberty, in individuals with markedly deviant growth patterns, in patients with anorexia nervosa or bulimia nervosa, and in patients with treatment-resistant affective disorders.

A number of neuroendocrine challenge procedures have been used in neuropsychiatric research (e.g., thyroid-stimulating hormone [TSH] response to thyrotropin-releasing hormone [TRH] challenge; growth hormone response to clonidine challenge). In view of the continually unfolding role of endocrine functions in psychiatric disorders (Jensen and Garfinkel 1990), we can reasonably expect that in a few years some of these challenge procedures will become useful in the clinical practice of child and adolescent psychiatry.

In addition to its role in the dexamethasone suppression test, cortisol levels can be indicators of "arousal." As we develop increasing familiarity with salivary cortisol level and its correlations to serum levels and to high arousal states, it can become a very useful and noninvasive measure with utility in subgrouping disruptive behavior disorders, with treatment implications (McBurnett et al. 1991).

ECG

A baseline ECG is advisable for children before starting treatment with lithium or tricyclics. During the course of treatment, when significant increase in dosage of tricyclics is ordered (e.g., beyond 2 mg/kg/day), it is advisable to monitor the cardiac status with ECG, approximately 1 week after the increase.

Appendix 1

Neurological Examination of Children

The aim of the psychiatric clinician generally is to do a fairly rapid neurological screening examination that will identify significant cognitive or other neurological dysfunctions. It is impractical to do a funduscopic examination as part of such a screening.

Cognitive Screening

In children under age 6 years, the "language" and "fine motor–adaptive" sectors of the Denver Developmental Screening Test (Frankenburg et al. 1973) can be helpful for cognitive screening. The examiner draws a line at the child's age and checks to see if the child passes those three items in each sector that fall to the left of the age line.

In children between ages 6 and 12 years, reliable data regarding the child's academic functioning can help to rule out cognitive dysfunction. In the absence of such reliable data and/or psychological test results, the examiner might find the following reading and spelling tests helpful as quick screening instruments.

Reading. The child is presented a sheet with the following letters, numbers, and words typed in characters 1 cm high: A C D L M N; 5 8 6 3 2 1; NO, CAT, DOG, MOTHER, CLOWN, SCHOOL, BEGAN, WANTED, AFTER. The examiner starts with a *base of 4.5 years* and gives 1 month additional credit to each correctly identified letter and number. Each correctly sounded word is given additional 4 months credit.

Spelling. The examiner asks the child to print the following words: cat, dog, man, book, read, bird, horse, cross, circle, square, and diamond. Testing can be stopped when the child makes two consecutive mistakes. From a *base of 6 years,* the following additional credits are given to each correctly spelled word—4 months each for the words cat, dog, and man; 6 months each for the other words.

Reading or spelling scores that are more than 1 year below the child's chronological age should elicit concern about a possible cognitive dysfunction and should lead to a more thorough evaluation.

In the examination of teenagers, the Mini-Mental State Exam (Folstein et al. 1975) can be helpful.

When there is a suspicion of cognitive dysfunction, the head circumference should be measured.

Cranial Nerves

First nerve. This is rarely impaired in children. If the examiner decides to test smell, substances familiar to the child (e.g., chewing gum) should be used.

Second nerve. Most school-age children will have undergone vision screening through the school. For younger children, matching pictures or letters can be a quick screening approach. The Snellen chart can be used for color vision. Observation of the child during the earlier reading and spelling tasks can indicate visual acuity problems if the child seems to strain his or her eyes to focus on the material or if the paper is held too close to the eyes.

Third, fourth, and sixth nerves. The presence of a persistent head tilt in a child is often indicative of extraocular movement deficits. The position of the eyes at rest, on distant gaze, and on lateral gaze during ocular pursuit of a pen or finger should be observed. Any asymmetry during these procedures is indicative of extraocular movement deficit. Significant drooping of the upper eyelids suggests depression, fatigue, or ptosis. Downward deviation of the eyes at rest and paralysis of upward gaze are common in hydrocephalus. Sixth nerve weakness (impaired lateral deviation) can be associated with increased intracranial pressure. Nystagmus should be checked for and described (horizontal or vertical; worse on looking in which direction).

Fifth nerve. Generally the motor functions of the fifth nerve can be screened by observing the chewing movements of the child. The jaw will deviate to one side if there is a dysfunction. It is generally not necessary to test the sensory component.

Seventh nerve. This can be screened by observing movements of the face, during smiling, raising eyebrows, puffing out the cheeks, and so on, in a playlike activity. Taste sensation generally can be assessed by history.

Eighth nerve. *Hearing*—The functional hearing of preschoolers can be screened by careful observation of their spontaneous speech. School-age children can generally cooperate in individual testing of each ear, using a wristwatch. Almost all states have mandatory hearing screening in the schools. When in doubt, a repeat screening or audiological evaluation can be requested.

Vestibular function—A history of ataxia or vertigo or the finding of nystagmus might raise the index of suspicion.

Ninth and tenth nerves. A brief examination of the pharynx with the mouth open can be helpful in checking the symmetrical shape of the soft palate. Nasal quality of the voice or history of difficulty in swallowing liquids will raise the index of suspicion regarding these nerves.

Eleventh nerve. Presence of a shoulder droop, inability to shrug both shoulders, or difficulty in turning head to the opposite side should raise the index of suspicion.

Twelfth nerve. Careful observation of the tongue for asymmetry during rest and during side-to-side movements can help identify dysfunction. Fasciculations should be looked for.

Extremities

A quick screening of the tone, power, and coordination of the arms and legs can be accomplished usually by the following:

- Observe the gait of the child and, if the child is age 5 years or older, have the child walk on toes and then on heels.
- Ask the parent about shoe sizes to find out if one foot is considerably smaller than the other.
- Children who are age 5 or older should be able to hop on one foot a few times. They might want to hold on to the wall or furniture under age 7.
- Have the child touch the tip of his nose with the tip of the index finger of a hand—first with the eyes open to imitate the examiner and then with the eyes closed. Look for significant missing of target or tremors.
- Have the child hold both your hands in a handshake position and squeeze your hands. Ask the child to maintain the squeeze pressure steady. In children under age 8 years, having them squeeze two of the examiner's fingers (index and middle together) will be easier for the child to do. Significant weakness or tremors can be easily identified.

Deep tendon reflexes can be elicited in a playful manner in most children. In young children, it is important to make sure that the head is in the midline and not turned to one side, because the asymmetric tonic neck reflex (ATNR) can be still operative.

Sensory testing is very difficult to do in a reliable manner in young children. Graphesthesia is described in Appendix 2.

Any positive findings in the screening examination should lead to a careful and comprehensive neurological examination by a clinician who is experienced in the procedure.

Appendix 2

Examination for Minor Neurological Signs II (EXAMINS II)

This procedure originally consisted of 18 items. Pilot studies were conducted with the aim of identifying those items that had good reliability and occurred more frequently in boys with academic problems, compared with boys with no academic or behavioral problems. Now it consists of 8 items with satisfactory reliability (kappa ≥ 0.75), requiring no more than 10 minutes to administer and score.

Although these items have been validated in small-scale clinical studies, correlations of these minor neurological signs to neuropsychological or neuroimaging findings have not been established so far.

A well-developed 8-year-old is able to pass all the items. The mnemonic "GRAP SEED" can help the clinician to remember the items. *Any time a child fails a particular item of this group, the item is repeated. Only if the item is failed on second trial, is it marked as fail or impaired.*

1. Graphesthesia. First, the examiner writes the following numbers on the table with the blunt end of a pen or with the examiner's index finger, so that the child is familiar with the way the numbers 2, 3, 4, 6, 7, and 8 are written by the examiner. The examiner makes sure that the child is able to recognize these numbers when they are written on the table. Then the child is asked to place his hands on the table with palms up, to keep his eyes closed, and to guess what numbers are being written on his palms. The examiner alternates between the two hands in different orders. The numbers are written in characters that are about 2 inches in height with the stylus of a pen without ink.

Pass: If the child makes no more than one mistake in the test involving 12 trials (6 numbers on each palm).

Graphesthesia is an item that has been found to be significant in a number of studies (Adams et al. 1974; Myklebust 1973; Peters et al. 1975).

2. Right–left identification. The examiner states the following to the child, "I am now going to check if you know your right and left. I will ask you to do something with your right or left hand. I will then repeat it. Please listen carefully and do it after I am finished repeating." The examiner then gives the following instructions:

- "Touch your right ear with your left hand."
- "Touch your left shoulder with your right hand."
- "Touch your right knee with your left hand."
- "Touch your right knee with your right hand."

Pass: If the child is able to do it right three of the four times. Do not give feedback to the child about if he was right or wrong until after the item is scored.

This item was modified from the earlier version to improve its reliability (Peters et al. 1975).

3. Arm dominance. The examiner asks the child to write his name on a piece of paper. Then the examiner asks the child to throw an imaginary baseball. If there is some uncertainty, the child is asked to demonstrate these activities with each arm so the examiner can determine which side is better at each task.

Pass: If there is a clear dominance of the same arm for both activities. The side of arm dominance is recorded.

Boys who are right-handed writers, but left-handed throwers, appear to be at risk for academic problems (Sarma 1989).

4. Passive head turning. The child is helped to stand comfortably with feet slightly apart and with the arms held out in front at the shoulder level. The child is told that the examiner will stand behind the child and turn the child's head from side to side. The child is instructed to leave his head loose so the examiner can turn his head, but the child is not to let his arms or body turn. The head is turned to each side from the midline and from side to side. If the child appears to be moving the head voluntarily, he is instructed not to assist the examiner in moving the head, but to leave the head loose. The freedom to move the head in a 150-degree range is assessed. The examiner observes the hands to see if either hand crosses the midline when the head is turned.

Pass: If both the following criteria are met: a) there is no significant resistance to passive turning of the head and, b) neither hand crosses the midline while the head is being turned.

This item is infrequently positive (Peters et al. 1975) (child fails the item), but when it is positive, it is generally associated with significant neurodevelopmental problems.

5. Speech. The child is engaged in sufficient informal conversation to permit assessment of clarity of speech. Then the child is asked to repeat the following words, one at a time, after the examiner: "Wisconsin," "Virginia," "Kentucky," "Oklahoma," "Pennsylvania," "Washington," "Massachusetts."

Pass: If the child repeats all but one of the statements clearly, the way they were stated. Here, it is important to make sure that the examiner pronounces them in the generally accepted manner.

This item was modified from Peters et al. (1975).

6. Eye symmetry. Symmetry of the eyes during eye tracking and during alternate focusing on a distant object and on a pencil held about 3–6 inches in front of the forehead (pencil is held upside down to provide a clear field of vision) is looked for.

Pass: If there is no asymmetry during lateral gaze or during convergence. In some children, one eye will start drifting out after initial convergence. If this is persistent, it is scored as fail.

This item was modified from Peters et al. (1975).

7. Eye tracking. The child is asked to follow the top of a pen or pencil (held about 12 inches from the face) with the eyes, without turning the head. The pencil is moved in such a way that lateral gaze on each side to a 60-degree angle is tested. Irregular ocular pursuit, jerky movements while crossing the midline, and any persistent overshooting or undershooting is looked for.

Pass: If the ocular pursuit is smooth without persistent overshooting or undershooting.

This item was derived from Levine et al. (1983).

8. Diadakokinesis. The process of tapping the table with the palm and the dorsum of the hand alternately is demonstrated to the child, and the child is encouraged to practice this for about 10 seconds with each hand. Then the child is asked to do it as rapidly as possible with one hand. The examiner counts the number of times the child taps the table with the palm in 10 seconds. The examiner also observes for frequent loss of rhythm. The procedure is then repeated with the other hand.

Pass: If an 8-year-old taps the table with each hand at least 10 times in 10 seconds; 9-year-old . . . 11 times in 10 seconds; 10-year-old . . . 12 times in 10 seconds . . . up to 16 times in 10 seconds for a 14-year-old. There should not be repeated loss of rhythm.

Sometimes, a child who is very eager to please might attempt this task too rapidly and miss the rhythm. The examiner can advise the child to go a little slower. This leads to the child attaining criterion without loss of rhythm. This item has been found to be significant in many studies (Adams et al. 1974; Levine et al. 1983; Peters et al. 1975; Shaywitz et al. 1984).

The above-described abbreviated EXAMINS includes sensory, motor, cranial nerve, and lateralization items and has been quite useful to the author in the neuropsychiatric examination of children. Nevertheless, further studies are needed to establish its validity.

References

Adams RM, Kocsis JJ, Estes RE: Soft neurological signs in learning disabled children and controls. Am J Dis Child 128:614–618, 1974

AMA News: Vol 34, August 19, 1991, p 12

Andreasen NC (ed): Brain Imaging: Applications in Psychiatry. Washington, DC, American Psychiatric Press, 1989

Bowden CL, Deutsch CK, Swanson JM: Plasma dopamine—β-hydroxylase and platelet monoamine oxidase in attention deficit disorder and conduct disorder. J Am Acad Child Adolesc Psychiatry 27:171–174, 1988

Epstein CJ: Down syndrome (trisomy 21), in The Metabolic Basis of Inherited Disease, 6th Edition. Edited by Schriver CR, Beaudet AL, Sly WS, et al. New York, McGraw-Hill, 1989, p 292

Evans DL, Nemeroff CB, Haggerty JJ, et al: Use of the dexamethasone suppression test with DSM-III criteria in psychiatrically hospitalized adolescents. Psychoneuroendocrinology 12:203–209, 1987

Folstein MF, Folstein SE, McHugh PR: Mini-Mental State: a practical method for grading cognitive state of patients for the clinician. J Psychiatr Res 12:189–198, 1975

Frankenburg FK, Dodds JB, Fandal A: Denver Developmental Screening Test. Denver, CO, LADOCA Project and Publishing Foundation, 1973

Golden CJ, Moses JA, Coffman JA, et al: Clinical Neuropsychology. New York, Grune & Stratton, 1983

Green MF, Satz P, Soper HV, et al: Relationship between physical anomalies and age at onset of schizophrenia. Am J Psychiatry 144:666–667, 1987

Gualtieri CT, Adams A, Shen CD, et al: Minor physical anomalies in alcoholic and schizophrenic adults and hyperactive and autistic children. Am J Psychiatry 139:640–643, 1982

Hertzig ME: Neurological "soft" signs in low-birth-weight children. Dev Med Child Neurol 23:778–791, 1981

Jensen JB, Garfinkel BD: Growth hormone dysregulation in children with major depressive disorder. J Am Acad Child Adolesc Psychiatry 29:295–301, 1990

Kaufman DM, Solomon GE, Pfeffer CR (eds): Child and Adolescent Neurology for Psychiatrists. Baltimore, MD, Williams & Wilkins, 1992

Kuperman S, Gaffney GR, Hamden Allen G, et al: Neuroimaging in child and adolescent psychiatry. J Am Acad Child Adolesc Psychiatry 29:159–172, 1990

Levine MD, Meltzer LJ, Busch B, et al: The pediatric early elementary examination: studies of a neurodevelopmental examination for 7–9 year old children. Pediatrics 71:894–903, 1983

Lofts RH, Schoreder SR, Maier RH: Effects of serum zinc supplementation on pica behaviour of persons with mental retardation. Am J Ment Retard 95:103–109, 1990

McBurnett K, Lahey BB, Frick PJ, et al: Anxiety, inhibition and conduct disorder in children, II: relation to salivary cortisol. J Am Acad Child Adolesc Psychiatry 30:192–196, 1991

Myklebust HR: Identification and diagnosis of children with learning disabilities: an interdisciplinary study of criteria, in Minimal Cerebral Dysfunction in Children. Edited by Walzer S, Wolff PH. New York, Grune & Stratton, 1973

Needleman HL, Gatsonis CA: Low-level lead exposure and the IQ of children: a meta analysis of modern studies. JAMA 263:673–678, 1990

Peters JE, Romine JS, Dykman RA: A special neurological examination of children with learning disabilities. Dev Med Child Neurol 17:63–78, 1975

Petersdorf RG, Adams RD, Braunwald E, et al (eds): Harrison's Principles of Internal Medicine, 10th Edition. New York, McGraw-Hill, 1983

Rogeness GA, Maas JW, Javors MA, et al: Diagnoses, catecholamine metabolism and plasma dopamine-β-hydroxylase. J Am Acad Child Adolesc Psychiatry 27:121–125, 1988

Rutter M (ed): Developmental Neuropsychiatry. New York, Guilford, 1983

Sarma PSB: Mixed-handedness and achievement test scores of grade school children. Percept Mot Skills 68:839–846, 1989

Shaffer D, Schonfeld I, O'Connor PA, et al: Neurological soft signs—their relationship to psychiatric disorder and intelligence in children and childhood adolescence. Arch Gen Psychiatry 42:342–351, 1985

Shaywitz SE, Shaywitz BA, McGraw K, et al: Current status of the neuromaturational examination as an index of learning disability. J Pediatr 104:819–825, 1984

Smith DW: Recognizable Patterns of Human Malformation, 2nd Edition. Philadelphia, PA, WB Saunders, 1976

Tramontana MG, Sherrets SD, Golden CJ: Brain dysfunction in youngsters with psychiatric disorders: application of the Selz-Reitan rules for neuropsychological diagnosis. Clinical Neuropsychology 2:118–124, 1980

Tu JB: Overlooking Wilson's disease (letter). J Am Acad Child Adolesc Psychiatry 30:154, 1991

Waldrop MF, Halverson CF: Minor physical anomalies and hyperactive behaviour in young children, in Exceptional Infant, Vol 2: Studies in Abnormalities. Edited by Hellmuth J. New York, Brunner/Mazel, 1971, pp 343–380

Waldrop MF, Pedersen FA, Bell RQ: Minor physical anomalies and behaviour in preschool children. Child Dev 39:391–400, 1968

Waldrop MF, Bell RQ, Goering JD: Minor physical anomalies and inhibited behaviour in elementary school girls. J Child Psychol Psychiatry 17:113–122, 1976

Walker HA: Incidence of minor physical anomaly in autism. Journal of Autism and Childhood Schizophrenia 7:165–176, 1977

Woolston JL, Riddle MA: The role of advanced technology in inpatient child psychiatry: leading edge or useful aid? J Am Acad Child Adolesc Psychiatry 29:905–908, 1990

Zametkin AJ, Rapoport JL: Noradrenergic hypothesis of attention deficit disorder with hyperactivity: a critical review, in Psychopharmacology: The Third Generation of Progress. Edited by Meltzer HY. New York, Raven, 1987, pp 837–842

4

Psychological Testing

Sid Mondell, Ph.D.
Terrell Clark, Ph.D.

Psychological testing is an important component of the child's diagnostic evaluation and a complement to other sources of data. Testing is also used in school or vocational assessments, in pretreatment baseline evaluations, and for a variety of research purposes. There are several forms of psychological testing, including

- Cognitive (IQ) tests
- Educational (achievement) tests
- Tests of visual-motor skills
- Children's drawing tests
- Projective personality tests

Psychological tests distinguish themselves from other forms of interview data through their attention to standardized administration, the use of reference or norm groups, and the presence of carefully researched studies of their reliability and validity.

The skills and knowledge necessary for the administration and interpretation of these tests require extensive training and clinical experience. "Psychologists" and "professional psychologists" refer to a doctoral-level (Ph.D., Ed.D., or Psy.D.) professional who has received a degree from a regionally accredited graduate school in the fields of clinical, counseling, educational, or school psychology. The careful clinician is urged to collaborate with professionals with the highest levels of training, education, and experience.

Psychological testing has its historical roots in World War I when research studies on the nature of intelligence led to the development of test instruments. The U. S. Army "Alpha" test was such a prototype and was used to sort out quickly the suitability of men being conscripted into the military services. Since that time, the concept of standardized tests to sort, type, or describe people relative to some reference group has flourished. Psychological research led to the evolution of the tests used today and continues to develop tests, paving the way for new formats and revisions of existing tests that will be used tomorrow. As people, times, and reference groups change, so must these instruments (Groth-Marnat 1984).

Indications for Use of Psychological Testing

In general, the indications for or advantages of using psychological testing as part of the diagnostic evaluation of children and adolescents include the following:

- In particularly complex and complicated diagnostic evaluations, psychological testing provides data of a qualitatively different nature from interviews and history. The additional data, with reference to norm groups, standardization, and objective or quantitative scoring, may shed new light and contribute valuable pieces to the diagnostic puzzle. In some cases testing may reaffirm impressions gleaned from other sources of information; in other instances it may raise new questions, concerns, a child's hidden strengths, or suspected but unconfirmed vulnerabilities that were not obtained in prior evaluation.
- Some diagnostic information (e.g., IQ, cognitive functioning, educational achievement, the presence of learning disability) is definitively assessed *only* by psychological testing. Although mental status

evaluation or interview may suggest estimates, actual quantitative scores may be obtained only through competently administered testing.

- Psychological testing may be required or mandated by law. PL 94-142 (1975), or its state equivalent, which mandates individual educational planning for students with special needs, requires psychological testing specifically to assess cognitive, educational, and psychological functioning.
- In forensic evaluations, courts and lawyers often favor testing and quantitative scores. Testing is often perceived by courts as more "objective" due to a standardization of administration, scoring, and interpretations.
- Testing is often helpful in persuading parents to accept treatment recommendations or diagnostic impressions of their child. The perception of objectivity and standardization can help in such situations.
- Test data are often useful in establishing a quantitative or "objective" baseline for a child before some changes (educational, social, or therapeutic) are introduced.

Psychological testing is generally perceived by children and adolescents as a pleasant, helpful, or even growth-enhancing experience. Most children enjoy the testing experience and "feel good" or even relieved at its completion. At times, symptom improvement results following the testing, a so-called testing cure. Improvement may result from placing appropriate attention and concern on a previously neglected problem. In other cases, psychological testing and follow-up feedback to the parents and the child leave an individual or family system ripe for therapeutic interventions by again drawing appropriate attention and concern to problems requiring further work, recognition, or elucidation.

Limitations of Testing

Included among the limitations of psychological testing are the following:

- Not all tests may be given to all children. Tests vary as to specific age ranges and appropriate references or standardization in regard to age or other relevant characteristics.
- Tests generally have lower reliability and thus are less valid for preschool children (below age 6). One must qualify test results with these children and take into account various factors that may have lowered or altered a given "performance" relative to the child's true competence or "inherent nature."
- Testing in general is highly language dependent. Thus, its usefulness is more limited with children who have major verbal handicaps, who are preverbal, or who speak a primary language different from the psychological tester.
- Testing can be frightening and perceived as overly intrusive or humiliating by a minority of children and, especially, their parents. Timing administration and recommendations become important in such instances.
- Testing can be "forced" or administered without the active cooperation and participation of the child.
- If a child becomes mute, obstinate, or otherwise uncooperative, valid test results cannot be obtained. Children who are in altered states of consciousness, who are heavily sedated or medicated, or who are in physical restraints cannot be tested.
- Children should not be "overtested." Retesting within 1 year's time is rarely optimal and may prove invalid because of practice effects. Annual testing is a similar misuse of psychological testing. Prior consultation before referral with a professional psychologist is recommended where the advisability of testing, given a previous record of testing for the child, is questioned.
- Psychological testing, although often covered by mental health insurance policies, is an expensive procedure. For every hour of administration with the child present, a psychologist may spend another 1–3 hours scoring, interpreting, and writing up results. This time investment results in relatively high costs that must be individually weighed against the need and the patient's family's ability to afford the service.

Cognitive Assessment

The appraisal of children's intellectual functioning plays an important role in clinical child psychology. What is actually measured through intelligence testing and what comprises "intelligence" are sources of both academic and political controversy. There is a strong positive correlation between measured IQ and achievement in school. The development and exercise of cognitive abilities and learning go hand-in-hand for most children. In conducting intelligence testing, a well-trained, qualified clinical psychologist will observe the child's manner, style, behaviors, responses, and appearance. How the child executes items on the test instruments and how the child relates to the examiner are diagnostically important and bear on the evaluation as much as how well the child scores on the tests administered.

There are a number of individually administered tests of intellectual functioning used in clinical practice. The most popular and widely used of these are the Wechsler scales, which have three versions. The Wechsler Preschool and Primary Scale of Intelligence—Revised (WPPSI-R) (Wechsler 1967) is appropriate for use with young children ages 4–6. The Wechsler Intelligence Scale for Children—III (WISC-III) (Wechsler 1974) is designed for youngsters ages 6–16. For those ages 16 and over, the Wechsler Adult Intelligence Scale—Revised (WAIS-R) (Wechsler 1981) is used.

The Wechsler scales are among the best of intelligence tests available for clinical use. Their reliability and validity have proven to be stable over time in comparison with other respected tests of intellectual functioning and academic achievement. The Wechsler scales are composed of a number of subtests, some of which emphasize knowledge of vocabulary, auditory comprehension, and verbal reasoning. Others rely more heavily on visually presented information and manipulation of pictures, puzzles, and objects in largely nonverbal reasoning, perceptual, organizational, and problem-solving tasks. Scores yielded on the Wechsler scales include a Verbal Intelligence Quotient, Performance Intelligence Quotient, and Full Scale Intelligence Quotient, as well as incrementally comparable scaled scores for each of the individual subtests. The following summaries provide a description of the subtests of the WISC-III:

Verbal Scale Subtests

- *Information:* Assesses familiarity with basic facts in topics such as history, geography, and science.
- *Similarities:* Assesses logic, verbal reasoning, and ability to explain associations and relationships.
- *Arithmetic:* Requires solution of so-called word problems through mental computation without paper and pencil.
- *Vocabulary:* Requires explanation or formulation of definitions of the meaning of words.
- *Comprehension:* Assesses responses to questions regarding exercise of common sense, social judgment, and practical knowledge.
- *Digit span:* Provides an alternate or optional subtest in which repetition of random series of numbers is required.

Performance Scale Subtests

- *Picture completion:* Involves ability to differentiate essential from nonessential details and visual memory as well as recognition of pictures of common objects and animals.
- *Picture arrangement:* Involves sequencing of pictures into logical order and involves ability to note cause-effect relationships and to interpret social situations.
- *Block design:* Assesses perceptual-organizational skills, reasoning, and problem-solving abilities required to reproduce geometric patterns using colored cubes.
- *Object assembly:* Involves perception of part-whole relationships; manipulation of puzzle pieces; and problem-solving, organizational, and visual-spatial skills.
- *Coding:* Assesses speed and accuracy of performance in this paper-and-pencil task involving associational learning and manipulation of arbitrary visual symbols.
- *Mazes:* Provides an alternative or optional subtest involving visual-motor planning and integration skills.

The WPPSI-R and WAIS-R are composed of similar types of tasks and subtests. The titles of the subtests on these scales differ slightly.

Naturally, the levels of item difficulty are designed to challenge individuals in their respective age groups. On all versions of the Wechsler scales, the average scaled score is 10. Scaled scores above 7 and below 13 comprise the average range. Very low values would be in the range of 1–3 and very high values would be those above 16.

Two relatively new tests of cognitive development and intellectual functioning are gaining in popularity among psychologists for use with very young children. These are the McCarthy Scales of Children's Abilities (McCarthy 1972) and the Kaufman Assessment Battery for Children (Kaufman and Kaufman 1983). The Merrill-Palmer Scale of Mental Tests (Stutsman 1948) and the newer Extended Merrill-Palmer Scale (Ball et al. 1978) are also widely used in the assessment of preschool-age children.

To augment diagnostic information gained from administration of the more comprehensive tests of intelligence, such as the Wechsler scales or the Stanford-Binet Intelligence Scale (Thorndike et al. 1986), psychologists might choose also to examine vocabulary development, sophistication of human figure drawings, or responses on brief screening measures. Tests utilized for these purposes might include the Peabody Picture Vocabulary Test—Revised (Dunn and Dunn 1981), Goodenough-Harris Drawing Test (Harris 1963), Developmental Test of Visual-Motor Integration (VMI) (Beery 1989), Slosson Intelligence Test (Slosson 1983), and Ammons Quick Test (Ammons and Ammons 1962).

Children who display extraordinary physical or mental disabilities (e.g., blindness or visual impairment, deafness or hearing impairment, cerebral palsy, severe mental retardation, infantile autism, extreme language and communication disorders) often demand extraordinary skills on the part of the psychologist conducting the evaluation. Some of the more specialized tests that might be utilized include the Leiter International Performance Scale (Leiter 1979), Columbia Mental Maturity Scale (Burgemeister et al. 1972), Progressive Matrices (Raven 1965), Pictorial Test of Intelligence (French 1964), Haptic Intelligence Test for Adult Blind (Shurrager and Shurrager 1964), and Hiskey-Nebraska Test of Learning Aptitude (Hiskey 1966). Not all psychologists are experienced in administering and interpreting results from these tests, nor in evaluation of youngsters with such handicaps.

What types of diagnostic information can be obtained from tests of cognitive development and intellectual functioning? One type of score is an intelligence quotient (IQ). Normative data from most tests have been statistically manipulated such that the "average" IQ is 100. Scores within one standard deviation of the mean are considered to fall within the average range. Scores that differ from the mean by more than one standard deviation (in either direction) are considered to be significant and thereby indicative of relative strengths or weaknesses.

There are various classifications of intelligence offered by authors of these intelligence tests. Generally, the levels of classification parallel those outlined in Table 4–1.

Another type of score that may be obtained is a mental age (MA) or age equivalency score. Understanding the concept of MA is intricate. The relationship between MA and chronological age is not a static one. That a 3-year-old earns an MA of 4 years may be indicative of superior-level intellectual potential, whereas an 11-year-old passing tests at the 12-year age equivalency level may simply be demonstrating average-level functioning. Also, a mentally retarded 15-year-old who earns an MA of 8 years is not likely to resemble a typical third grader in learning style, intellectual curiosity, or repertoire of functional and adaptive skills. There is usefulness to the notion of age equivalency scores, but their meaning requires interpretation and explanation by an experienced clinician.

Table 4–1. Classifications of intelligence as measured by IQ tests

Measured IQ	Classification	Incidence
≥ 130	Very superior	Top 2% of population
120–129	Superior	
110–119	Bright or high average	
90–109	Average	Middle 50% of population
80–89	Dull or low average	
70–79	Borderline	
<70	Mentally defective	Bottom 2% of population
50–69	Mild retardation	
25–49	Moderate retardation	
< 20–24	Severe retardation	

Analyses of results from various tests administered and of responses to items within various segments of given tests yield valuable information regarding cognitive ability, learning style, and relative talents and deficits. The ability to interpret test protocols and profiles is the key area of expertise for skilled psychologists. One needs to understand more than a global estimate of cognitive ability (the IQ) when psychological testing is requested for a child. The influence of factors such as ethnic and family background, educational experiences, emotional adjustment, physical disabilities, organic impairments, specific learning disorders, and environment must be considered. The contribution of such factors is often reflected in the content of children's responses and revealed in analysis of the results of testing.

Although comprehensive assessment of cognitive skills is necessary in many clinical situations, an office screening of these functions can be a useful diagnostic tool. Such a screening device should never substitute for a full-scale study but can be taught to the beginning child psychiatrist by an experienced clinical psychologist.

Academic Skills

All children should have entered school by age 6. Although many begin formal educational experiences at age 3 or 4, most participate in some kind of kindergarten experience, either public or private. A simple way to determine what grade a child "should" be in is to subtract 5 from the child's chronological age. Thereby, 6-year-olds are generally first graders, 8-year-olds are third graders, and so on.

School is the consuming arena in which children between ages 5 or 6 and 16–18 must grow, prove themselves, flourish, and succeed. Failures experienced in school are likely to be dramatically expressed in other spheres of the child's life. Likewise, trauma, disappointment, illness, upset, anger, anxiousness, and defeat in any aspect of a child's existence usually spill over into the school setting and affect academic, social, and interpersonal performance there. Understanding the school experience of children is therefore crucial to effective diagnosis and treatment of this age group.

At no age is school seen as merely a playground. Both from the children's and the teachers' points of view, the responsibility of schooling is far more serious than that. There are rules to be obeyed and there are lessons to be learned. Beginning with shapes, colors, letters, numbers, community helpers, animal products, and parts of the body, the content of curricula quickly escalates to the complexities of grammar, set theory, main ideas, supporting details, world geography, dates in history, chemical structures, and transportation and communication systems. The demands on 7-year-olds in the classroom would astound most adults. Even so, the majority of children capably meet these demands and perform at least adequately in the school setting.

Although one encounters variations among local school districts, the following represents a fairly typical curricular progression through the elementary grades:

Kindergarten

- Recognizing, naming, and forming letters
- Spelling and printing first and last name
- Counting at least to 20
- Recognizing, naming, and forming shapes
- Identifying (by name and function) instruments such as clock, calendar, thermometer, and ruler

First Grade

- Reading
- Beginning phonics (short vowels, long vowels, single consonants)
- Basal texts
    - Preprimer (50–75 words)
    - Primer (100–175 words)
    - First-grade–level reader (250–350 words)
- Comprehension skills
    - Story titles
    - Locating specific facts or information

- Spelling and writing
    - Common spelling rules or conventions
    - Mastery of approximately 100 words
    - Recognizing and printing letters

- Math
    - Counting at least to 50
    - Simple addition and subtraction
    - Simple fractions ($\frac{1}{2}$, $\frac{1}{3}$, $\frac{1}{4}$)
    - Telling time by the hour
    - Naming values of coins

Second Grade

- Reading 2^1- and 2^2-level readers (950–1,700 words)
- Phonics, including consonant blends and digraphs (e.g., ch, st, ck), vowel digraphs (e.g., ai, ea, oa), and *r*-controlled vowels (e.g., ar, ir).
- Comprehension skills
    - Main idea
    - Sequence of events
    - Author's intent

- Spelling and writing
    - Mastery of approximately 300 words
    - Correct formation and spacing of all uppercase and lowercase letters

- Math
    - Counting by 2s and 10s
    - Reading 2-digit numerals
    - Column 2-digit numerals
    - Column addition and subtraction
    - Place valuc

- Telling time by hour, half-hour, and quarter-hour
- Fractions ($\frac{2}{3}$, $\frac{5}{8}$)
- Measuring by the inch and half-inch and/or by centimeters

Third Grade

- Reading 3^1- and 3^2-level readers (1,900–3,300 words)
- Mastery of phonics
- Structural analysis (prefixes, suffixes, roots)
- Decoding skills
- Comprehension skills
    - Describing skills
    - Anticipating conclusions
    - Comparing authors' styles
- Spelling and handwriting
    - Cursive writing introduced
    - Short compositions and formal letters of correspondence
    - Use of dictionary and alphabetization
    - Spelling rules: formation of plurals, common phonograms, affixes (change of verb tense, adding *ly*)
- Math
    - Counting by 3s and 5s
    - Identifying 3-digit and 4-digit numerals (100s and 1,000s)
    - Adding and subtracting with regrouping (carrying and borrowing)
    - Simple multiplication
    - Finding lowest common denominator among fractions
    - Adding sums of money and making change

Fourth Grade

- Reading
    - Fourth-grade–level reader (2,800–3,500 words)

- Emphasis shifts from oral to silent reading
- Having "learned to read," priority becomes "reading to learn"
- Comprehension and content become most important

- Spelling and writing
  - Exclusive use of cursive handwriting
  - Approximately 2,000 spelling words mastered
  - Considerable written production expected (compositions, reports, term projects)

- Math
  - Roman numerals
  - Times tables committed to memory
  - Division introduced

Fifth Grade

- Reading
  - Fifth-grade–level reader (4,500–6,000 words)
  - Study skills emphasized (outlining, summarizing, note taking)
  - Rate or speed of silent reading increases

- Spelling and writing
  - Proofreading and self-correction of spelling and punctuation
  - Continued emphasis on reports, compositions, projects, essays
  - Volume of written output increases considerably

- Math
  - Division with remainders
  - Computations with fractions
  - Geometric principles (diameter, area, polygons)
  - Use of instruments (metric ruler, compass, barometer)
  - Units of measure (equivalents and conversion)

Sixth Grade

- Reading
  - Sixth-grade–level reader (6,000–8,500 words)
  - Use of primary reference materials encouraged
  - Literature and classics assigned
- Spelling and writing
  - More than 3,000 words mastered
  - Original short stories, poems, compositions expected
  - More lengthy detailed reports and term projects
- Math
  - Division with 2-digit or 3-digit divisors
  - Simple algebraic expressions
  - Measurement, time, money skills mastered
  - Decimals and percentages

Assessment of Academic Skills

If a child is experiencing difficulties with school learning, the assessment of academic competencies and school function *begins* with obtaining information about the child's level of academic achievement. Is the child achieving on a level commensurate with expectations for age and grade level? Sources for verifying such information would include parental report, consultations with the child's teacher or school principal, school records and report cards concerning the child, and possibly referral for formal assessment through individually administered achievement tests. Such testing may be available on referral through the local school system. On occasion, it may be preferable to request achievement testing through an agency or clinic independent of the school system. Should there be a discrepancy between the child's measured level of academic achievement and age- or grade-level expectations in one or more of the basic subject areas, further investigation and assessment to help determine the reason for the discrepancy are definitely warranted.

Review of the child's school history may reveal a checkered record of school attendance. Lengthy or frequent absences from school usually adversely affect school performance. Moves resulting in transfer from one school to another may contribute to setbacks and poor academic progress. Inadequate preparation for entering the school experience may account for some youngsters' extraordinary difficulties with acquiring language, learning to read, understanding numbers and developing quantitative skills, producing legible writing, or attending sufficiently well to learn in a standard classroom setting. Slow cognitive development or limited intellectual potential may underline a child's poor academic achievement.

Previously undetected physical conditions—such as some degree of hearing impairment, visual defects, metabolic disorders—may account for a child's difficulties with learning. Factors such as investment, social adjustment, emotional maturity, family harmony, friendship networks, and attitude toward the value of school should also be explored as these may directly affect the child's performance in school.

If the presenting complaint includes problems with performance in school, the following questions should be considered:

- What is the child's school history (age at which school enrollment began, attendance record, any changes in school placement, promotions or retentions, disciplinary actions, parent-teacher conferences)?
- What is the child's academic achievement profile? Is the child demonstrating achievement commensurate with expectations for age and grade placement?
- Is there any reason to suspect specific learning disabilities?
- Do you suspect globally lower cognitive functioning or intellectual brilliance?
- Do you suspect developmental delay or deviance?
- Are there physical conditions or medical concerns that may be contributing to or interfering with reported school performance?
- Are there social or emotional factors that may influence reported school performance?

Sources of information for addressing such questions would include

- Parental interview
- Review of school records
- Telephone contact or interview with school personnel (teacher, principal, guidance counselor, school nurse)
- Results from academic achievement testing
- Results from individually administered psychological and diagnostic educational testing
- Child interview

What is it that an educational specialist assesses when conducting an evaluation of a child's academic skills? Diagnostic tests of reading include measures of word recognition, decoding, and comprehension of written material. Auditory and visual-perceptual skills and memory skills would also be assessed. Proficiency with both oral and silent readings—including reading rate, fluency, and phrasing—would be measured. Assessment of math or number skills might cover sequencing, seriation, memory, conservation, visual-spatial organization, numeration, reasoning skills, and computation skills. The application of math skills to concepts of time, measurement, and money and to the solution of verbally presented problems also enters the comprehensive assessment of the child's ability to deal with numbers. Factors such as established handedness, type of pencil grasp, sitting posture, orientation of paper, letter formation, figure drawing, spacing, legibility, speed, and fluency enter the assessment of handwriting skills. Ability to recognize graphemes (letters and symbols), sequencing and memory skills, understanding of syllabication, and synthesis skills all enter the diagnostic evaluation of spelling—beyond demonstration of how many words a child can spell aloud or on paper. Throughout the evaluation of academic competencies, an astute evaluator will be observing for indications of learning style. Matching recommended instructional approaches, materials, and techniques to a particular child's demonstrated propensities or style of learning is the major contribution that an educational specialist can make.

Some of the frequently used and popular measures of academic achievement clinicians may encounter are highlighted in Table 4–2.

Maintaining successful performance in school is important not only to future life goals but also to the confirmation of self-worth and to the establishment of confidence in the growing child. Complaints about achievement and adjustment in school are common among those youngsters referred for mental health evaluations and services. Concerns about a child's school performance should be taken seriously and investigated through interviews, phone contacts, school records, and referral for formal evaluations where indicated. A significant discrepancy between a child's measured level of academic achievement and what is generally expected of students at the same age and grade level signals the need to refer for more elaborate and sophisticated diagnostic evaluation of the child's learning abilities and style.

Assessment of Visual-Perceptual-Motor Skills

Assessment of perceptual-motor skills comprises an area of specialized testing often conducted by trained psychologists. Development of adequate visual-perceptual, visual-memory, eye-hand, and integrative skills contributes to the child's competency in learning and performing certain academic tasks (principally reading and writing). Deficits in these skills may reflect organically based learning disabilities or impairments. The ability to integrate visual and motor functions requires simultaneous processing of several stimuli and the smooth coordination of receptive, organizational, planning, and expressive capacities. Assessment of such skills, therefore, presumes to provide some reflection of the integrity of the central nervous system.

Assuming that visual acuity has been checked through an eye examination, visual-perceptual skills constitute the first level of assessment. Accurate reception of visual image and interpretation of visually presented information should be tested under conditions that do not require a motor response. The child's responses to some of the items on the Wechsler scales may provide an indication of visual-perceptual skills. A popular assessment tool is the Motor-Free Visual Perception Test (Colarusso and Hammill 1972). Portions of the Detroit Tests of Learning Aptitude (Baker and Leland 1967) may also be used to assess

Table 4–2. Academic achievement tests and diagnostic tests of educational attainments

Test	Reference	Age/grade	Description
Wide Range Achievement Test—R	Jastak and Wilkinson 1984	5–adult, K–post-12th	Brief screening measure of letter and word recognition, spelling and writing, and number and computational skills
Peabody Individual Achievement Test—R	Markwardt 1989	K–12th	Individually administered test of achievement in word recognition, reading comprehension, spelling, math, and general information
Woodcock-Johnson Psycho-educational Battery	Woodcock 1977	3–adult	Lengthy instrument containing multiple subtests designed to measure achievement in academic and basic learning skills
Gray Oral Reading Tests	Gray 1967	1st–12th	Yields descriptive and diagnostic information about competency of oral reading skills
Woodcock Reading Mastery Tests	Woodcock 1973	K–12th	Contains five subjects: word identification, word comprehension, word attack, passage comprehension, and letter identification

Spache Diagnostic Reading Scales	Spache 1981	1st–8th	Individually administered test of oral reading, paragraph comprehension, word recognition, and decoding skills
Durrell Analysis of Reading Difficulty	Durrell and Cutterson 1987	1st–6th	Lengthy assessment of skills necessary for competency with reading; contains 13 subtests
KeyMath Diagnostic Arithmetic Test	Connolly et al. 1971	preK–6th	Contains 14 subtests organized into 3 major areas of assessment: content (numeration, fractions, geometry, symbols), operations (addition, subtraction, multiplication, division, mental computation, numerical reasoning), and application (word problems, missing elements, money, measurement, time)
Morrison-McCall Spelling Tests	Morrison and McCall 1923	1st–12th	Dictated spelling test that yields grade-level score and records types of errors made
Test of Written Spelling	Larsen and Hammill 1976	1st–12th	Assesses both predictably (regular) spelled words and unpredictable spelling (nonregular) of words

visual-perceptual skills, visual-memory, and visual-motor integration skills.

By far the most widely used tests of visual-motor capabilities are the Visual Motor Gestalt Test (Bender-Gestalt) (Bender 1938) and the VMI. The Bender-Gestalt has been in use clinically since the 1930s. It consists of nine classic geometric designs to be copied on paper. The accuracy of the child's efforts in drawing the figures, the organization of the figures on the paper, the size, the symmetry, and the formation are all considered in scoring and interpreting performance on this test. What the child reproduces can be used as an indicator of maturational level and may provide insight into possible organic dysfunctions.

The VMI has been in use since the 1960s. Again, copying geometric designs on paper is required. However, the test consists of 24 figures arranged in ascending order of complexity reflecting a sequential development according to age-level criteria. On the VMI, the test format is more highly structured than on the Bender-Gestalt. Criteria for scoring children's performance are well delineated in the VMI test manual, which also contains suggestions for remedial procedures should results of testing indicate deficiencies.

Neither the Bender-Gestalt nor the VMI are timed. Contrasting a child's performance on timed versus untimed tasks can often yield interesting diagnostic information. One subtest of the Detroit Tests of Learning Aptitude involves demonstration of eye-hand speed and precision. Performance on the coding or digit symbol subtests of the Wechsler scale may also be interpreted in light of speed and accuracy under timed conditions. Portions of some educational tests involve copying words, sentences, or symbols within given time constraints. Such tasks may prove useful as a practical measure of a child's ability to perform complex tasks requiring visual-motor integration skills under circumstances resembling conditions in a classroom.

Children's Drawings

Children's drawings have occupied an important place in the psychological testing battery. These easily administered tests are readily accepted by children. Drawing is a well-established route of communication with children. Materials (a pencil or crayons and some plain white paper) are of minimal cost and maximum availability in most settings.

Purposes of and Indications for Children's Drawings

- To begin a test battery as a means of establishing rapport with the child and putting the child at ease.
- To obtain a quick, rough, screening-level estimate of personality-related concerns, fine motor control and visual-motor integration, skills, intelligence, and ability to attend to a task or details.
- To assess very young children or children with expressive language difficulties: drawings are relatively nonverbal and are not compromised or limited by the child's verbal expressive abilities.

Limitations of Children's Drawings

- The major limitation of drawings is when their use exceeds their screening-level, rough estimate, hypothesis-generating capacities.
- The use of drawings is also limited by perceptual or fine motor handicapping conditions (e.g., children with severe neuromaturational delay or motor spasticity).

Varieties of Children's Drawings

The common varieties of drawings used and their interpretations are discussed below.

Human figure drawings (draw a person or draw a child) are generally administered individually, providing the child with a pencil, eraser, and plain white paper. Crayons are sometimes provided as a variation, but pens are rarely used. Instructions are generally kept simple, such as: "Please make me a drawing of a complete, whole child (or person)." Following the drawing of the child as a person, one variation is to request a drawing of the opposite-sex child or person to the one first drawn. Another variation is to make an inquiry regarding the person/child drawn, asking about his or her age, name, sex, person from real life the drawing may resemble, and so on.

In the *house/tree/person test,* a child is asked to draw pictures of a house, a tree, and a person (in any order) on separate pieces of plain paper. The use of crayons for color is a popular variant. Interpretations of the drawings are derived through their study as displaced or "projected" self-referents. Interpretation takes into consideration the following:

- The "mood" suggested by the drawing
- The implied competence and "stature"
- The age and sex portrayed relative to the age and sex of the child
- Body parts that appear to be overemphasized or neglected relative to the portrayal in the rest of the drawing
- Erasures or other evidence of confusion, distortion, or misrepresentation, a possible indication of anxiety regarding some part of the body and its perceived ability to function
- General line quality—whether tentative, light, vague, dark, or pressured, or moderate and assured—a possible indication of self-esteem and self-assurance
- Motor control, perceptual accuracy, distortion, and other signs of "organicity" or neuromaturational delay

For a *kinetic family drawing,* the child is instructed: "For this drawing I would like you to draw a picture that includes everyone in your family doing something." If the child questions whether extended family should be included, it can be left to the child's discretion. If the child questions whether he or she should be included, the child's own inclination should be noted, but the child should be instructed to do so. If the child is not included in the drawing, that should be noted, but then the child should be instructed to include himself or herself. If the child asks whether the family should be doing something together or individually, the decision may be left to the child's discretion. The names, ages, sexes, and activities (if unclear) of all persons represented in the drawing should be recorded.

Interpretation of the family drawing is based, in part, on the consideration of the following elements:

- Who is included or omitted
- The activities: whether engaged in together or individually, competitive or cooperative, their nature, and quality
- Who is mutually engaged with whom, who is separated, who is "involved," who is "distant"
- What alliances exist, either of a supportive or tension-producing nature
- Relative "closeness" in family relations as represented by physical distance between family members, interactions, who's facing whom, who is physically cut off from whom
- Activities and person placement as an indication of perception of family roles vis-à-vis the child

Projective or Personality-Based Assessments

Projective or personality-based psychological testing originated close in time to cognitive testing. Projective testing, although studied extensively and empirically validated, rests on one basic theoretical principle: that given a sufficiently ambiguous stimulus, a subject's response will be the result of his or her own projected personality. Expressed another way, the picture reveals the nature of the artist; the story reveals the nature of the author; the percept reveals the nature of the perceiver. Thus children, in their responses to ambiguous but standardized test stimuli, can reveal to the trained observer needs, concerns, coping styles, ability to integrate and tolerate affect, capacity to test reality, and perceptions of oneself and others.

Purpose and Indications for Projective Testing

- Projective testing may be useful as another piece of independent data (apart from history, mental status, play interview) in the differential diagnosis of psychiatric problems. This is particularly true in complex situations in which it is otherwise difficult to assign weights to various factors or diagnostic data being observed or being reported.

- Major psychopathology, including thought disorder, affective disorder, or other psychiatric disorders, is usually revealed through projective instruments.
- Projective tests can help in the assessment of suicidal risk and other impulse disorders: how pressing and conscious the concerns and ideation are and how they relate to other aspects of personality functioning.
- Projective tests may provide a perspective on overall personality functioning: coping and defensive styles, adequacy of defenses, strength of various affects, integration of affect, and frightening thoughts or affects being defended.
- Projective tests may help clarify a child's self-perception and perception of significant others, whether the perception is conscious or not.
- "Opening up" an otherwise verbally or behaviorally constricted child may result from projective tests. These tests may function as a "window" on personality and psychological functioning when other avenues appear closed.
- The relative role of affective or emotional factors in other behavioral concerns, symptoms, academic problems or peer/socialization difficulties can be assessed.
- Projective testing may be "politically" helpful in justifying (e.g., courts or educational boards) special needs or residential therapeutic placement.

Limitations of Projective Testing

- Children must voluntarily participate and cooperate to a maximum extent for the testing to yield useful data. In the case of flat refusals to participate, no data can be obtained.
- A child with extreme emotional constriction or severely impaired relatedness would yield data of dubious quality or validity.
- Projective testing is not fully independent of verbal expressive abilities, which places limits on its usefulness under the following conditions:
    - Extremely young children with no or very limited language skills or abilities.

  - Moderately to severely retarded children with limited language skills or abilities.
  - Children with major expressive language problems; any results with such classes of children, if possible at all, would require careful, qualified interpretation.

- Projective testing may be experienced as anxiety arousing to some children. In actuality, this would be true of only a small minority and would more likely affect older adolescents than younger children.
- Results are likely to be inadequate if tests are given, scored, or interpreted by other than a qualified professional psychologist.
- Cost may be a limiting factor. Projective tests require time to administer, score, interpret, and write up. Insurance, ability to pay, and its necessity must be carefully considered and weighed.

Types of Projective Testing and Possible Interpretations

There are many classes of projective tests; the major ones are discussed below. These tests tend to vary in 1) the age of the child for which it is appropriately given, 2) the degree of structure or ambiguity of the test stimuli, 3) the types or areas of information that are specifically elicited, and 4) the specific kinds of interpretations that can potentially be made.

Drawings. Children's drawings were discussed earlier in this chapter. As projective tests, they tend to have particularly rich potential to tap self-related concerns such as self-esteem and body image. Family perceptions, relations, and role perceptions are also revealed. As projective tests, children's drawings are a rich source of hypothesis, but absolute interpretations are difficult and rest on corroborating data obtained elsewhere in the test battery.

Incomplete sentence tests. There are many forms of child and adolescent incomplete sentence tests. Among the most popular is the Rotter Incomplete Sentences Blank (Rotter and Rafferty 1950). In all versions of this test, the child is asked to complete a list of sentence stems that have no endings. Examples might be "Howard was sorry after he______" "Ray thought that his mother should______," or "April felt that her future______." Responses are checked for themes, sequencing of material, and unusual or unique sentence endings.

Incomplete sentence tests are helpful in learning the following kinds of information:

- Indications of stresses, pressures, needs
- More conscious emotional concerns
- Worries, fears, anxieties
- Additional self- and family-related perceptions
- General indication of reality testing and orientation
- Some indication of affective pulls, coping styles, and typically used defenses

Rorschach (inkblot test). The Rorschach (Rorschach 1921) has been used with children of all ages, adolescents, and adults. The test plates or inkblots are the same in all cases; however, the administration (to some extent) and interpretation (to a larger extent) vary depending on the person's age. This test is generally not administered to children under age 4 or 5. The Rorschach uses the least structured and most ambiguous projective test stimuli available. It consists of 10 cards presented serially. These cards vary in black and white versus color content as well as in form ambiguity. The child is instructed to look at the cards and describe what they resemble. Responses and behavior are carefully recorded. One or sometimes two detailed inquiries regarding the initial percepts are necessary to complete scoring and interpretation.

The Rorschach yields the following kinds of information:

- Reality testing, accuracy, orientation, and adequacy under various emotional conditions
- Defenses, their uses and adequacy
- Ability to handle and integrate affect
- Presence of strong affect states and how they may be experienced
- Indications of suicidality

- Object relations: orientation and receptivity to interpersonal relations
- Creativity, emotional resourcefulness, and ability to integrate affect and cognition

Children's Apperception Test and Thematic Apperception Test. Apperception tests are a standard part of most projective batteries. The Children's Apperception Test (CAT) (Bellak and Bellak 1961) is used most often with children from ages 3 to 7; the Thematic Apperception Test (TAT) (Murray 1943) is used from ages 8 and up. The CAT is composed of 10 cards depicting various younger animal-figures engaged in a variety of activities with adult counterparts. Pictured themes include nurturance, family competition, sibling rivalry, socialization, toilet training, and handling of aggression.

The TAT is composed of a wide variety of cards to be used by men, women, boys, or girls. The psychologist is free to choose (usually 10) cards that have thematic material of greater relevance to the case. Cards are drawings that depict children and adults in various poses, activities, interactions, and postures. Themes run a gamut of affective states and interpersonal dilemmas. However, the drawings are sufficiently ambiguous to have a wide variety of perceptions possible on any given card.

For both apperception tests, the child is generally instructed to tell a story from his or her own imagination, using the card as a stimulus. If not included spontaneously in the story offered, the tester may inquire about perceptions regarding what is happening in the story, who the various characters might be, what each of the characters is thinking or feeling, and what would happen next or be the ending of the story.

A wide range of interpretations regarding reality perceptions, coping styles, affective stresses, and perception of oneself and significant others is potentially available in the scoring or analysis of apperception test responses. Apperception tests provide corroborating evidence from a range of other tests such as drawings, sentence completions, and the Rorschach. Since they are somewhat more structured than the Rorschach, they are not as sensitive to reality distortion potential or less conscious issues and material. However, responses to these tests may suggest potential for emotional functioning under more favorable, more clearly structured situations and environments.

Other projective tests. A number of other, less frequently used, projective tests are available for children and adolescents. Among them are the Education Apperception Test (Thompson and Sones 1973), which assesses adjustment to specific educational environment situations, and the Blacky Pictures (Blum 1950), an older picture test for children that attempts to assess psychosexual development. New projective tests appear in research and are occasionally published when research is favorable. An example of such a test is the Roberts Apperception Test for Children (McArthur and Roberts 1982) for children, which attempts to assess adjustment to more contemporary interpersonal events in children's lives.

The Tasks of Emotional Development Test (Cohen and Wilke 1979) may be the most popular "other" projective test. It consists of 12 cards depicting photographs of children and adults in various situations or problem confrontations. Separate sets of cards exist for latency-age boys and girls, as well as adolescent boys and girls. Similar to the apperception tests, children are asked to make up a story about what is happening. Children's responses to the test allow for the detection of areas of specific concern in psychological developmental tasks, reality distortions, affective pressures, coping styles, and self-other perceptions. However, the cards favor the perception of feelings for and expectations regarding the specific tasks of

- Peer socialization
- Parental nurturance
- Peer aggression
- School achievement
- Conscience and impulse control
- Separating from parents
- Sex role identification
- Sibling rivalry
- Accepting limits from parents
- Handling parental intimacy

- Conflict resolution with parents
- Developing a self-identity

Empirical/objective personality measures. Empirical or objective personality measures are generally used less often with children than with adults. These tests are generally in the form of a long list of true-false or yes-no answers. Scoring is objective in that one's pattern of responses is compared with that of groups of "known" type. Normative data are derived through strict empirical data collection. Scoring of such tests is often done by computer and yields a computerized "personality profile."

The Minnesota Multiphasic Personality Inventory (Hathaway and McKinley 1989) is the best known and most widely used of such tests. It is composed of more than 500 true-false questions. Norms have been developed for adolescents to whom the test may be administered. There are no "child" norms; this test is not used with preadolescents. When appropriate and valid, scoring will yield a personality profile as well as an indication of how high or low an individual scores (above, below, or within normal limits) on a number of scales. These include hypochondriasis, depression, hysteria, psychopathic deviate, masculinity/femininity, paranoia, psychasthenia, schizophrenia, mania, and social introversion.

Another similar objective measure growing in popularity in research and clinical use is the Personality Inventory for Children (Wirt et al. 1977). In this test, it is the *parent* who responds to a list of 600 true-false questions regarding perceptions of the child. Profiles and state scores falling within or outside of "normal" limits have been developed, including, for example, depression, self-concept, anxiety, reality distortion, peer relations, conscience development, activity level, somatic complaints, school adjustment, and family discord.

A final, related instrument, the Vineland Adaptive Behavior Scales (Sparrow et al. 1984)—a recent revision of the older Vineland Social Maturity Scale (Doll 1965)—exists in three versions to assess adaptive behaviors, strengths, and weaknesses in children from birth to age 19: 1) a survey form for screening, placement, and diagnostic purposes; 2) an expanded form for developing specific educational or treatment plans; and 3) a classroom edition. In all forms, a semistructured 30- to

60-minute interview is administered to parents or primary caregivers. Scores, normed with percentile ranks, are available in the following adaptive domains: communication, daily living skills, socializations, motor skills, and an adaptive behavior composite. This screening test is not in widespread clinical practice because it requires both application and sustained clinical exposure.

Conclusion

Interpretation of data gained in projective or personality-based assessments is a complex art and science at present. Therefore, conclusions are best drawn with consultation of an appropriately trained professional.

References

Ammons RB, Ammons CH: Quick Test. Missoula, MT, Psychological Test Specialists, 1962

Baker HJ, Leland B: Detroit Tests of Learning Aptitude. Indianapolis, IN, Bobbs-Merrill, 1967

Ball RS, Merrifield P, Stott LH: The Extended Merrill-Palmer Scale Instruction Manual. Chicago, IL, Stoelting, 1978

Beery KE: The Developmental Test of Visual-Motor Integration: Administration, Scoring and Teaching Manual, 3rd Edition, Revised. Cleveland, OH, Modern Curriculum Press, 1989

Bellak L, Bellak SS: Children's Apperception Test (C.A.T.) Manual, 4th Edition. Larchmont, NY, CPS, 1961

Bender L: A Visual Motor Gestalt Test and Its Clinical Use. Albany, NY, American Orthopsychiatric Association, 1938

Blum GS: The Blacky Pictures. Santa Barbara, CA, Psychodynamic Instruments, 1950

Burgemeister BB, Blum LH, Lorge I: Columbia Mental Maturity Scale. Cleveland, OH, Psychological Corporation, 1972

Cohen H, Wilke D: Tasks of Emotional Development Test. Bensenville, IL, Scholastic Testing Service, 1979

Colarusso RP, Hammill DD: Motor-Free Visual Perception Test: Manual. San Rafael, CA, Academic Therapy Publications, 1972

Connolly AJ, Nactman W, Pritchett EM: KeyMath Diagnostic Arithmetic Test. Circle Pines, MN, American Guidance Service, 1971

Doll EA: Vineland Social Maturity Scale: Manual of Directions, Revised. Circle Pines, MN, American Guidance Service, 1965

Dunn LM, Dunn LM: Peabody Picture Vocabulary Test—Revised: Manual for Forms L and M. Circle Pines, MN, American Guidance Service, 1981

Durrell DD, Cutterson JH: Durrell Analysis of Reading Difficulty, 3rd Edition. San Antonio, TX, Psychological Corporation, 1987

French J: Pictorial Test of Intelligence. Lombard, IL, Riverside Publishing, 1964

Gray WS: Gray Oral Reading Tests. Austin, TX, PRO-ED, 1967

Groth-Marnat G: Handbook of Psychological Assessment. New York, Van Nostrand Reinhold, 1984

Harris DB: Goodenough-Harris Drawing Test Manual. Cleveland, OH, Psychological Corporation, 1963

Hathaway SR, McKinley JC: Minnesota Multiphasic Personality Inventory—2. Minneapolis, University of Minnesota, 1989

Hiskey MS: Hiskey-Nebraska Test of Learning Aptitude. Lincoln, NE, Hiskey, 1966

Jastak S, Wilkinson GS: Wide Range Achievement Test—Revised. Wilmington, DE, Jastak Associates, 1984

Kaufman AS, Kaufman NL: K-ABC: Kaufman Assessment Battery for Children. Circle Pines, MN, American Guidance Service, 1983

Larsen SC, Hammill DD: Test of Written Spelling. Austin, TX, PRO-ED, 1976

Leiter RG: Leiter International Performance Scale: Instruction Manual. Chicago, IL, Stoelting, 1979

Markwardt FC Jr: Peabody Individual Achievement Test, Revised. Circle Pines, MN, American Guidance Service, 1989

McArthur DS, Roberts GE: Roberts Apperception Test for Children: Manual. Los Angeles, CA, Western Psychological Services, 1982

McCarthy DA: Manual for the McCarthy Scales of Children's Abilities. San Antonio, TX, Psychological Corporation, 1972

Morrison JC, McCall WA: Morrison-McCall Spelling Tests. New York, Harcourt Brace & World, 1923

Murray HA: Thematic Apperception Test Manual. Cambridge, MA, Harvard University, 1943

PL 94-142: Education for All Handicapped Children Act, 1975

Raven JC: Progressive Matrices. San Antonio, TX, Psychological Corporation, 1965

Rorschach H: Psychodiagnostics: A Diagnostic Test Based on Perception. Bern, Hans Huber, 1921

Rotter JB, Rafferty JE: Manual: The Rotter Incomplete Sentences Blank. San Antonio, TX, Psychological Corporation, 1950

Shurrager HC, Shurrager PS: Haptic Intelligence Scale for Adult Blind. Chicago, IL, Stoelting, 1964

Slosson RL: Slosson Intelligence Test. East Aurora, NY, Slosson Educational Publications, 1983

Spache GD: Diagnostic Reading Scales, Revised. Monterey, CA, CTB/McGraw-Hill, 1981

Sparrow S, Balla D, Cicchetti D: The Vineland Adaptive Behavior Scale: Interview Edition, Survey Form. Circle Pines, MN, American Guidance Service, 1984

Stutsman R: Guide for Administering the Merrill-Palmer Scale of Mental Tests. New York, Harcourt Brace & World, 1948

Thompson JM, Sones RA: Education Apperception Test. Los Angeles, CA, Western Psychological Services, 1973

Thorndike R, Hagen E, Sattler J: Stanford-Binet Intelligence Scale, 4th Edition. Chicago, IL, Riverside, 1986

Wechsler D: Manual for the Wechsler Preschool and Primary Scale of Intelligence. San Antonio, TX, Psychological Corporation, 1967

Wechsler D: Manual for the Wechsler Intelligence Scale for Children—Revised. New York, Psychological Corporation, 1974

Wechsler D: Wechsler Adult Intelligence Scale—Revised. San Antonio, TX, Psychological Corporation, 1981

Wirt RD, Lachar D, Klinedinst JK, et al: Personality Inventory for Children. Los Angeles, CA, Western Psychological Services, 1977

Woodcock RW: Woodcock Reading Mastery Tests. Circle Pines, MN, American Guidance Service, 1973

Woodcock RW: Woodcock-Johnson Psycho-Educational Battery: Technical Report. Allen, TX, DLM Teaching Resources, 1977

5

Neuropsychological Assessment

Michael G. Tramontana, Ph.D.
Kreig D. Roof, Ph.D.

Child neuropsychology has become the focus of vigorous interest and inquiry. Whereas it once occupied a relatively small and often overlooked place within the general field of neuropsychology, there now are entire volumes devoted exclusively to the topic (e.g., Rourke et al. 1983; Tramontana and Hooper 1988). Among its applications, neuropsychological assessment has become an important component in the diagnosis and evaluation of children and adolescents with psychiatric disorders. This is not only because there is a heightened prevalence of brain dysfunction among psychiatrically disturbed youngsters, but also because, as we shall see, a clear appraisal of a child's neuropsychological assets and liabilities can play an important role in planning psychiatric management and treatment.

In this chapter, we consider neuropsychological assessment from several perspectives. First, we examine the definition and scope of neuropsychological assessment, contrasting it from other kinds of neurodiagnostic procedures as well as from what ordinarily comprises more traditional forms of psychological assessment within children. Next, we discuss various clinical applications of neuropsychological assessment, with particular emphasis on its relevance to child and adolescent psychiatry. Last, we provide an overview and critique of different approaches to neuropsychological assessment, outlining specific methods and procedures for obtaining a comprehensive appraisal of key aspects of neuropsychological functioning.

What Is Neuropsychological Assessment?

Confusion sometimes arises as to what are the distinctive features of neuropsychological assessment and how it differs from simply a general assessment of a child's mental abilities.

Neuropsychological assessment, in contrast to standard cognitive testing of children, involves the use of tests or measures that are "selected, designed, or adapted *to facilitate the conceptualization of a child's performance in terms of known or hypothesized brain-behavior relationships*" (Tramontana and Hooper 1988, p. 29). Sensitivity to childhood brain damage, by itself, is *not* a defining characteristic of neuropsychological tests. Virtually any measure of a child's abilities may be used in making neuropsychological inferences, but some measures are better than others in revealing specific aspects of neuropsychological functioning. It is *this* feature, not simply their sensitivity to brain damage, that is an essential characteristic of neuropsychological tests.

The traditional psychological assessment is not designed to delineate a child's functional strengths and weaknesses as clearly and precisely as can be done in neuropsychological assessment. Although the exact compilation of tests may vary widely, the psychological assessment usually includes measures of intelligence, achievement, and personality functioning (see Chapter 4 for a more thorough overview of psychological testing). With younger children, intelligence testing actually can be fairly sensitive to brain dysfunction, given that decrements in global cognitive capacity often are among the chief manifestations of early childhood brain injury (Boll and Barth 1981; Rourke et al. 1983). This is one reason why intelligence testing is customarily included as a standard component within a comprehensive neuropsychological assessment. However, the neuropsychological assessment goes much further in providing an examination of a broader range of specific skills and abilities such as motor functions, sensory-perceptual abilities, language skills, attention, memory, and so forth. Moreover, regardless of how the two forms of assessment may overlap in the use of tests, there are major differences in how the results are interpreted and conceptualized. In neuropsychological assessment the emphasis is on relating test findings to the neurological features and neurodevelopmental questions pertaining to each child.

Neuropsychological assessment also differs in a number of important respects from other forms of neurodiagnostic evaluation. It may be conceptualized as falling within a continuum of procedures that differ in the extent to which structural-functional elements are the focus of evaluation (Tramontana 1983). This is outlined in Table 5–1. At one end, there are brain imaging procedures such as computed tomography and magnetic resonance imaging in which the focus is on brain structure or morphology. Lesions and other structural irregularities may be visualized quite precisely, although the functional or behavioral implications of these are a matter of clinical inference and extrapolation. Moving further along the continuum, there is another class of procedures represented by the electroencephalogram, positron-emission tomography, and regional cerebral blood flow scanning. Here the focus is on brain function, albeit at a physiological level, analyzed in reference to various brain regions and anatomical sites.

At the other end of the continuum there is neuropsychological assessment. Here too the focus is on function but at an overt, behavioral level. The emphasis is on obtaining a precise delineation of functional capacities using methods specifically developed for that

Table 5–1. Structural-functional continuum of neurodiagnostic procedures

Structural	Physiological	Behavioral
Computed tomography Magnetic resonance imaging	Electroencephalogram Regional cerebral blood flow Positron-emission tomography	Neuropsychological assessment

purpose. The findings may be suggestive of a particular form or localization of brain pathology, but this too would be a matter of clinical speculation—as was true at the opposite end where the results of brain imaging are used to make inferences about behavior. These various procedures can and should be used in a complementary fashion, each contributing a different perspective where questions of brain impairment are involved.

Last, it is important to distinguish neuropsychological assessment from the pediatric neurological examination. The neurological examination serves as a review or screening of basic neurological systems, the results of which may direct the nature and scope of further diagnostic investigations. The format varies, but it typically includes an examination of the child's station and gait, motor and sensory functions, reflex integrity, physical development, and a brief overview of mental status. It differs from neuropsychological assessment in two respects. First, whereas the neurological examination focuses more on lower or more basic brain functions, the neuropsychological assessment provides a much more thorough assessment of *higher* cortical functions. Consequently, the neuropsychological assessment can be more sensitive to various forms of cerebral dysfunction, especially when higher cortical functions are involved. Second, the neuropsychological assessment tends to be more sensitive to *milder* forms of dysfunction, even in the case of lower sensory and motor functions. One of the hallmarks of neuropsychological assessment is the emphasis on the standardization of test procedures and the quantification of test results. Because of this, more subtle levels of dysfunction can be identified that otherwise might be missed in a routine neurological examination. Indeed, normal neurological examinations are common even among children with documented histories of head trauma, encephalitis, or epilepsy (Rutter 1977).

Applications

General Considerations

The neuropsychological assessment of children has evolved to encompass a broad range of applications. In general, these include 1) aiding in the detection of brain dysfunction, 2) specifying the behavioral effects of known brain injury, 3) identifying underlying dimensions of dysfunction in particular handicaps or disabilities, 4) helping to evaluate prognosis and special risks, 5) deriving implications for treatment strategies, and 6) conducting serial assessments of functional change, including response to particular interventions. The precise form and the relative importance of these different applications depend, to some extent, on the particular clinical population under consideration.

Table 5–2 provides some examples of various clinical conditions possibly requiring neuropsychological assessment. By no means is this an exhaustive listing. The examples are broken down into separate categories, with the first one referring to conditions that represent documented neurological disorders. Here, there is no question as to the presence of brain impairment; rather, the question has to do with gaining a precise delineation of its effects. The next category includes examples of various conditions with uncertain central nervous system effects. Just a few of the many possibilities are listed. Associated deficits may be nonexistent or may range anywhere from being mild to profound. Neuropsychological assessment may be especially helpful in detecting milder or more subtle manifestations of cerebral deficit—dysfunction that otherwise might be missed but that nonetheless could be a significant complicating factor in a child's adjustment. The need for neuropsychological assessment in both this and the preceding category is likely to grow. Advances in medical care have brought about a dramatic increase in the survival of children with serious illnesses or injuries. Many of these conditions (or their treatment) can have a potentially adverse impact on the developing brain. Consequently, whereas mortality has decreased, there has been a corresponding increase in morbidity. This has created a greater need for the careful assessment of the extent, pattern, and developmental significance of possible neuropsychological sequelae.

For the last category listed in Table 5–2, developmental disabilities, the aims of assessment are somewhat different. Here, it already may be quite clear that a child is experiencing significant problems in one or more major areas of performance. For example, a child may exhibit a reading disability, deficient attention, or poor language retention. What is not often clear, however, has to do with the precise underlying components of dysfunction that may be contributing to the surface deficit(s). Global functions (e.g., attention) can be differentiated into more specific component processes (e.g., arousal and alertness, selective attention, vigilance, span of apprehension, set shifting, search strategies), each of which are mediated by different neural substrates, are vulnerable to disruption by different etiologies, follow different developmental courses, and possibly are responsive to different types of intervention (Barkley 1988). Likewise, learning disabilities represent a heterogeneous group of disorders that can be differentiated into subtypes according to the particular pattern or profile of component skill deficits (Hooper and Willis 1989; Hynd et al. 1988). When applied in this context, neuropsychological assessment can lend further clarity and precision to the diagnosis process, helping to determine not only whether a function is impaired but precisely *how* it is impaired or what form the deficits can be expected to take.

Table 5–2. Conditions possibly requiring neuropsychological assessment

- Documented neurological disorders
    - Genetic/congenital brain anomalies
    - Seizures
    - Traumatic brain injury
- Conditions with uncertain central nervous system effects
    - Substance abuse
    - Other toxic exposure
    - Malnutrition (including eating disorders)
    - Hypoxic/anoxic/ischemic episodes (including sleep apnea)
    - Possible iatrogenic effects of certain treatments (e.g., intracranial radiation and chemotherapy for cancer)
    - Other assorted conditions including metabolic disorders, infections, and autoimmune disorders
- Developmental disabilities
    - Learning disabilities
    - Language disorders
    - Attention deficits
    - Motor dysfunction

Relevance to Child and Adolescent Psychiatry

There is a heightened prevalence of brain dysfunction among children and adolescents with psychiatric disorders. Exact estimates have varied, depending on the clinical samples studied and the detection criteria used. In any event, the rate is substantially higher than the roughly 2%–5% prevalence rate in the general population, averaging at a rate of one-third or higher when based on more impaired hospitalized samples (Tramontana and Hooper 1989).

Brain dysfunction in childhood carries an increased risk for psychiatric disturbance and morbidity. As was documented in the well-known Isle of Wight epidemiological studies, brain-damaged children show a three to seven times greater risk for psychiatric disorder compared with the 6%–7% risk found in the general population (Rutter et al. 1970). Moreover, the risk is about twice as great than for children with other types of physical handicap (Seidel et al. 1975). The risk increases somewhat as a function of severity of brain impairment and seems to be worse in children with seizures, lower IQ, and other neuropsychological deficits. Among children with traumatic brain injury, the risk is compounded by factors such as psychosocial disadvantage and preexisting behavior problems, but the effects are *additive* not interactive (Brown et al. 1981).

There is a relatively high rate of neuropsychological deficits in children and adolescents with psychiatric disorders, even when cases with known brain damage are excluded (Tramontana et al. 1980). In further examining cases such as these, it was found that neuropsychological abnormality corresponded to differences on various indices of brain structure as assessed through computed tomography scans (Tramontana and Sherrets 1985). The implication was that the neuropsychological assessment was able to detect irregularities that ordinarily would be missed in a routine neurological examination and review of history. Neuropsychological deficits also have been found to be associated with more extensive behavior problems among younger boys with psychiatric disorders; this was not attributable simply to differences in IQ, socioeconomic status, nor whether the deficits could be linked specifically with a history of brain injury (Tramontana et al. 1988). Thus, the presence of neuropsychological deficits may be important in itself, as it evidently comprises an index of increased psychiatric risk or morbidity. Moreover, among hospitalized child and adolescent psychiatric patients, neuropsychological assessment has proved to be better than IQ in predicting academic achievement, whether examined separately or in conjunction with behavioral and demographic factors (Tramontana et al. 1990).

A number of studies have begun to examine whether there are distinctive neuropsychological features or patterns of performance associated with specific forms of child psychopathology. These include studies on autism (e.g., Fein et al. 1985), attention-deficit/hyperactivity disorder (e.g., Passler et al. 1986), and depression (e.g., Wilson and Staton 1984). There are a number of promising leads but few definitive conclusions at this time. The interested reader may wish to refer to Tramontana and Hooper (1989) for a comprehensive review of this line of research.

Turning now to more practical issues, neuropsychological assessment may be viewed as playing an important role not only in differential diagnosis but also with respect to psychiatric management and treatment planning. Some examples of how neuropsychological assessment may be utilized effectively in child and adolescent psychiatry are outlined in Table 5–3. It sometimes may be difficult to recognize when a specific functional deficit is present, especially in children presenting with complex multiproblem clinical pictures. Emotional and behavioral factors may overshadow underlying impediments or disabilities, although these nonetheless may constitute persistent obstacles to successful adjustment. The functional capacities listed in Table 5–3 are especially relevant from a psychiatric perspective and often may require a formal assessment to be delineated clearly. Recognizing where significant deficits exist also may help to clarify why emotional problems may arise or intensify when the child is confronted with certain types of demands. For example, expressive language deficits may contribute to a child's increased anxiety, frustration, avoidance, or withdrawal in particular situations. It is important to distinguish what a child will not do versus what the child *cannot* do or has grown too uncertain to attempt.

Knowing when specific performance deficits are present can help alert treatment staff to situations in which a child's compliance or ability to benefit from certain therapeutic interventions may be seriously undermined. For example, a child with frontal lobe dysfunction often lacks the capacity to anticipate long-range consequences for present actions. Behavior management strategies must take this into account, making sure that feedback and behavioral contingencies are structured within a more immediate time frame. A child with right hemispheric cerebral dysfunction may not provide a reliable subjective report with respect to emotional issues, not necessarily because of resistance or defensiveness, but because of a poor awareness of internal emotional states. Knowing where and how obstacles such as these may be encountered can and should be taken into account when deriving therapeutic strategies, thereby helping to make the treatment planning process more efficient and individualized.

Neuropsychological assessment procedures can be useful in evalu-

Table 5–3. Utility of neuropsychological assessment in child and adolescent psychiatry

- Documenting the presence of deficits in selected functional systems
    - Attention
    - Inhibition
    - Learning and retention
    - Communication skills
    - Planning abilities
- Identifying deficits that may be related to or compounding psychiatric difficulties
    - Increased anxiety
    - Avoidance
    - Frustration
    - Withdrawal
- Helping to distinguish deficit versus defense versus defiance
- Highlighting potential compliance problems and therapeutic pitfalls
- Outlining preferential strategies for therapeutic communication and behavior management
- Helping to evaluate indications for and the effects of certain psychopharmacologic interventions
    - Use of psychostimulants for attention deficits

ating the indications for, and the effects of, certain psychopharmacologic interventions. So far, probably the most common application has been in evaluating medication trials in children with attention-deficit/hyperactivity disorder. Formal, laboratory-type measures of attention and impulse control have been shown to be sensitive to stimulant drug effects and to provide a useful adjunct to parent and teacher ratings of inattentive and overactive behavior (e.g., Barkley et al. 1988).

Approaches to Neuropsychological Assessment

There are many different approaches to neuropsychological assessment. Generally speaking, most of these can be grouped into two main categories: fixed test batteries and eclectic approaches. These are described and contrasted below. The interested reader may wish to refer to Tramontana and Hooper (1988) for a historical overview and a more thorough discussion of the various approaches to assessment in child neuropsychology.

Fixed Test Batteries

In a fixed battery approach, the aim is to provide a comprehensive assessment of brain function using an *invariant* set of validated test procedures. The emphasis is on standardization, with the assumption that individual variability can be captured reasonably well as long as the battery has been designed to tap a sufficiently broad range of abilities. Probably the two best-known examples of fixed test batteries in child neuropsychology are the Halstead-Reitan Neuropsychological Test Battery (HRNTB) (Reitan 1979) and the children's revision of the Luria-Nebraska Neuropsychological Battery (LNNB-CR) (Golden 1987).

Reitan and his colleagues developed two versions of the HRNTB for use with children: the Reitan-Indiana Neuropsychological Test Battery for Children (ages 5–8) and the Halstead Neuropsychological Test Battery for Children (ages 9–14). For convenience, both of these are referred to simply as the HRNTB. A detailed description of the HRNTB can be found in Reitan and Davison (1974). Briefly, the

HRNTB for older children is essentially a downward extension of the adult version of the battery and consists of the following test procedures: lateral dominance examination, aphasia-screening test, category test (168 items), tactual-performance test (six blocks), sensory-perceptual examination, grip strength test, finger oscillation test, trail-making test, speech-sounds perception test (three-choice format), and the Seashore rhythm test. For younger children, the HRNTB consists of modified versions of the older children's tests but with the trail-making test, speech-sounds perception test, and Seashore rhythm test deleted. Six additional tests are included: marching test, color form test, progressive figures test, matching pictures test, target test, and individual performance test. Table 5–4 provides a breakdown of some of the advantages and disadvantages that may be said to characterize the HRNTB.

Golden (1981, 1987) introduced a downward extension of the LNNB for children ranging from ages 8 to 12 years. Tasks that proved to be too difficult for children were eliminated; some new items were added, and other modifications in administration and scoring were made to adapt the battery for use with children. This resulted in a battery consisting of 149 test items (versus 269 in the adult version). Like the adult version of the battery, the LNNB-CR is organized in terms of 11 summary scales: motor, rhythm, tactile, visual, receptive speech, expressive speech, writing, reading, arithmetic, memory, and intellectual processes. Also, like the adult version, these are supplemented by various second-order scales, including the pathognomonic scale (consisting of the 13 items in the battery that provide the best discrimination of brain damage) and the left sensorimotor and right sensorimotor scales (based on items on the motor and tactile scales performed with the contralateral hand). Table 5–5 outlines some of the advantages and disadvantages that may be said to characterize the LNNB-CR.

Overall, it is fair to say that both the HRNTB and LNNB-CR provide a valid and reasonably comprehensive evaluation of brain function in children. The HRNTB clearly has been a dominant approach to child neuropsychological assessment for the last 20 years or so. To many, the LNNB-CR offers an attractive alternative. Probably the chief limitation of both test batteries is that neither one was designed specifically for children. Both of these largely represent downward extensions of test procedures intended originally for adults. This is reflected by the fact that some areas of function, such as attention and learning, receive inadequate coverage, although these clearly are critical aspects of functioning to assess in the developing child. Another limitation is lack of specificity and flexibility associated with all-purpose or omnibus approaches to assessment. Neu-

Table 5–4. General critique of the Halstead-Reitan Neuropsychological Test Battery

Advantages	Disadvantages
Assures a consistently broad-based assessment	Generally does not provide an in-depth analysis of selected aspects of function
Replicability	Inflexibility
Provides a standard data base for comparative studies	Assumes a relatively high degree of patient compliance and no special handicaps
Effectively discriminates between brain-damaged children and control subjects	Little evidence validating its use in localizing childhood brain lesions in the absence of specific motor or sensory signs
Distinguishes children classified globally as learning disabled and has been used in discriminating different subtypes of learning disabilities	Little information on the contruct validity of its individual measures or on the factorial composition of the battery as a whole
	Results overlap substantially with IQ, especially in brain-damaged children
	Weak assessment of certain areas such as language, memory, and attention
	Lengthy administration time
	Testing materials are somewhat cumbersome

ropsychological assessment is becoming increasingly specialized; an assessment strategy that is quite useful in one context might be useless in another. There is a growing appreciation for the need to adapt assessment goals and test procedures according to the clinical questions and specific populations involved.

Table 5–5. General critique of the Luria-Nebraska Neuropsychological Battery, Children's Revision

Advantages	Disadvantages
Assures a consistently broad-based assessment	Generally does not provide an in-depth analysis of selected aspects of function
Replicability	Inflexibility
Provides a standard data base for comparative studies	Assumes a relatively high degree of patient compliance and no special handicaps
Effectively discriminates between brain-damaged children and control subjects	Little evidence validating its use in localizing childhood brain lesions
Distinguishes children classified globally as learning disabled	Although the item format permits the analysis of specific component skills, reliability is jeopardized by the presence of insufficient items
Multifactorial composition, as documented in factor-analytic studies	Weak assessment of certain areas such as attention and frontal lobe functions
Results overlap substantially with IQ, but it appears to add significantly to the discrimination of impairment in children with mild to moderate disabilities	
Relatively quick to administer	
Portability of testing materials	

Eclectic Approaches

This category includes a wide variety of assessment strategies. The one thing that they all have in common is the lack of a strict adherence to a particular set of test devices or procedures. At its worst, this might consist of merely assembling tests and measures in a "hodgepodge" fashion, without a clear rationale or guiding strategy. However, there generally is at least an implicit outline of the relevant neuropsychological constructs that should be assessed. When this is more explicit, the assessment strategy could be referred to as *construct-driven*. Any of a variety of validated tests may be selected to assess each of the functional areas of interest. The psychometric properties of the individual tests (e.g., adequacy of norms), their appropriateness for youngsters of a particular age, and their complementarity when embedded in a battery are usually important factors guiding test selection.

There are a number of advantages with this approach. For one, it preserves the quantitative nature of neuropsychological assessment through the use of well-validated standardized tests. It also permits a balanced and broad-based assessment if the tests are selected according to an explicit conceptual framework. Moreover, there is flexibility with respect to the exact composition of the battery. It can be adapted for different applications and upgraded as new and better tests become available. Potential disadvantages include the fact that varying the composition of a test battery places constraints on its replicability and comparability over time and across settings. Moreover, interpretive problems could arise when evaluating an individual's profile by comparing measures that may differ greatly in terms of normative samples, range of difficulty, and specific test construction.

Let us now illustrate how an eclectic approach to assessment might be organized according to an explicit conceptual framework. Table 5–6 outlines what may be regarded as key constructs in neuropsychological assessment. These represent the major dimensions of functioning that should be incorporated into any comprehensive neuropsychological assessment of a child or adolescent. These define the scope or breadth of assessment, comprising the *horizontal analysis*—so to speak—when examining general neuropsychological functioning. Within each construct or domain of functioning, there also is a *vertical analysis* through which specific component processes are assessed. This is illustrated in Table 5–7. Here one of the key constructs already noted (i.e., language) is highlighted and broken down into a number of components. These define the depth of analysis that might be undertaken in assessing language. The breakdown is flexible and can vary from child to child, depending on practical considerations as well as the extent to which there are concerns regarding particular aspects of language functioning. Specific tests then would be selected to assess the particular skills and component processes of interest. The same general logic would apply across the other key constructs, resulting in an assessment strategy that balances breadth with depth of assessment, consistency with flexibility.

Last, Table 5–8 provides a listing of selected test procedures that may be used in assessing key aspects of neuropsychological functioning. Neither the specific functions listed nor the examples of tests

Table 5–6. Key constructs in neuropsychological assessment

Motor	Attention
Sensory-perception	Memory
Spatial	Problem solving
Language	

Note. A comprehensive evaluation also would include an assessment of intelligence, academic achievement, personality, and adaptive behavior skills.

Table 5–7. Neuropsychological assessment framework

C1	C2	Language	C4	C5 • •	Cx
SC1	SC1	Phonological	SC1	SC1	SC1
SC2	SC2	Speech perception	SC2	SC2	SC2
SC3	SC3	Morphological	SC3	SC3	SC3
SC4	SC4	Semantics	SC4	SC4	SC4
SC5	SC5	Word retrieval	SC5	SC5	SC5
•	•	Comprehension	•	•	•
•	•	Verbal fluency	•	•	•
SCx	SCx	Pragmatics	SCx	SCx	SCx

Note. C = construct. SC = subcomponent.

Table 5–8. Selected test procedures

Domain	Function assessed
Motor	
Finger Oscillation Test	Fine motor speed
Grooved Pegboard	Manual dexterity
Motor Steadiness	Static and resting hand steadiness
Sensory-perceptual	
Tactile Finger Recognition	Simple tactile discrimination
Fingertip Number Writing	Complex tactile discrimination
Speech-Sounds Perception Test	Phonemic discrimination
Seashore Rhythm Test	Nonverbal auditory discrimination
Motor-Free Visual Perception Test	Visual discrimination/closure/memory
Facial Recognition	Complex visual analysis
Language	
Receptive One-Word Picture Vocabulary Test	Word comprehension skills
Expressive One-Word Picture Vocabulary Test	Confrontation naming skills
Verbal Fluency (Conceptual-Phonetic)	Rapid word association
Token Test for Children	Complex verbal comprehension
Spatial	
Developmental Test of Visual-Motor Integration	Graphomotor skills
Embedded Figures Test	Figure-ground discrimination
Rey-Osterrieth Complex Figure Test	Complex visual-perceptual organization
Attention	
Gordon Continuous Performance Test	Vigilance and selective attention
Goldman-Fristoe-Woodcock Selective Listening Test	Focused auditory attention
Matching Familiar Figures Test	Impulse control

continued

Table 5–8. Selected test procedures *(continued)*

Domain	Function assessed
Memory	
Paired Associate Learning	Verbal associate learning
California Verbal Learning Test	List learning
Wide Range Assessment of Memory and Learning	Omnibus memory assessment
Abstraction/problem solving	
Category Test	Conceptual ability, use of feedback
Wisconsin Card Sorting Test	Flexible strategic thinking, ability to maintain/shift mental set

Note. For a more detailed overview and description of neuropsychological test procedures, see Reitan and Davison (1974), Spreen and Strauss (1991), and Tramontana and Hooper (1988).

noted are intended to be exhaustive. Descriptions of these and other neuropsychological test procedures can be found elsewhere (Reitan and Davison 1974; Spreen and Strauss 1991; Tramontana and Hooper 1988). It should be noted that the bulk of test procedures presently available is really suited only for children roughly age 5 years and older. The neuropsychological assessment of younger children, especially infants and toddlers, is a difficult and highly specialized undertaking that only recently has begun to receive more systematic attention (Aylward 1988).

Concluding Remarks

The foregoing discussion should give some idea of the aims, applications, and relevance of neuropsychological assessment—especially as it relates to issues in child and adolescent psychiatry. Various approaches to neuropsychological assessment were contrasted, with the differences amplified for the sake of clarity and accentuation. In practice, there probably are few neuropsychologists who are purists with respect to one approach or another. A melding of approaches is quite common and makes good sense, given that the field is evolving and undergoing dynamic change as new knowledge continues to unfold.

Assessment techniques are becoming increasingly refined, differentiated, and tailored more specifically to particular clinical populations and diagnostic issues. These and other innovations are highlighted and critically evaluated in a multivolume book series devoted exclusively to advances in child neuropsychology (Tramontana and Hooper 1992).

References

Aylward GP: Infant and early childhood assessment, in Assessment Issues in Child Neuropsychology. Edited by Tramontana MG, Hooper SR. New York, Plenum, 1988, pp 225–248

Barkley RA: Attention, in Assessment Issues in Child Neuropsychology. Edited by Tramontana MG, Hooper SR. New York, Plenum, 1988, pp 145–176

Barkley R, Fischer M, Newby RF, et al: Development of a multi-method clinical protocol for assessing stimulant drug responding in ADD children. Journal of Clinical Child Psychology 17:14–24, 1988

Boll TJ, Barth JT: Neuropsychology of brain damage in children, in Handbook of Clinical Neuropsychology. Edited by Filskov SB, Boll TJ. New York, Wiley, 1981, pp 418–452

Brown G, Chadwick O, Shaffer D, et al: A prospective study of children with head injuries, III: psychiatric sequelae. Psychol Med 11:63–78, 1981

Fein D, Waterhouse L, Lucci D, et al: Cognitive subtypes in developmentally disabled children: a pilot study. J Autism Dev Disord 15:77–95, 1985

Golden CJ: The Luria-Nebraska Children's Battery: theory and formulation, in Neuropsychological Assessment and the School-Age Child: Issues and Perspectives. Edited by Hynd GW, Obrzut JE. New York, Grune & Stratton, 1981, pp 277–302

Golden CJ: Manual for the Luria-Nebraska Children's Revision. Los Angeles, CA, Western Psychological Services, 1987

Hooper SR, Willis WG: Learning Disability Subtyping: Neuropsychological Foundations, Conceptual Models, and Issues in Clinical Differentiation. New York, Springer-Verlag, 1989

Hynd GW, Connor RT, Nieves N: Learning disabilities subtypes: perspectives and methodological issues in clinical assessment, in Assessment Issues in Child Neuropsychology. Edited by Tramontana MG, Hooper SR. New York, Plenum, 1988, pp 281–312

Passler M, Isaac W, Hynd GW: Neuropsychological development of behaviors attributed to frontal lobe functioning in children. Developmental Neuropsychology 1:349–370, 1986

Reitan RM: Halstead-Reitan Neuropsychological Test Battery. Tucson, AZ, Neuropsychology Laboratory, University of Arizona, 1979

Reitan RM, Davison LA (eds): Clinical Neuropsychology: Current Status and Applications. New York, Wiley, 1974

Rourke BP, Bakker DJ, Fisk JL, et al: Child Neuropsychology: Introduction to Theory, Research and Practice. New York, Guilford, 1983

Rutter M: Brain damage syndromes in childhood: concepts and findings. J Child Psychol Psychiatry 18:1–21, 1977

Rutter M, Graham P, Yule W: A Neuropsychiatric Study in Childhood (Clinics in Developmental Medicine No 35–36). London, Spastics International Medical Publications/Heinemann Medical Books, 1970

Seidel UP, Chadwick O, Rutter M: Psychological disorders in crippled children: a comparative study of children with and without brain damage. Dev Med Child Neurol 17:563–573, 1975

Spreen O, Strauss E: A Compendium of Neuropsychological Tests: Administration, Norms, and Commentary. New York, Oxford University Press, 1991

Tramontana MG: Neuropsychological evaluation of children and adolescents with psychopathological disorders, in Foundations of Clinical Neuropsychology. Edited by Golden CJ, Vicente PJ. New York, Plenum, 1983, pp 309–340

Tramontana MG, Hooper SR (eds): Assessment Issues in Child Neuropsychology. New York, Plenum, 1988

Tramontana MG, Hooper SR: Neuropsychology of child psychopathology, in Handbook of Clinical Child Neuropsychology. Edited by Reynolds CR, Fletcher-Janzen E. New York, Plenum, 1989, pp 87–106

Tramontana MG, Hooper SR (eds): Advances in Child Neuropsychology, Vol 1. New York, Springer-Verlag, 1992

Tramontana MG, Sherrets SD: Brain impairment in child psychiatric disorders: correspondencies between neuropsychological and CT scan results. Journal of the American Academy of Child Psychiatry 24:590–596, 1985

Tramontana MG, Sherrets SD, Golden CJ: Brain dysfunction in youngsters with psychiatric disorders: application of Selz-Reitan rules for neuropsychological diagnosis. Clinical Neuropsychology 2:118–123, 1980

Tramontana MG, Hooper SR, Nardolillo EM: Behavioral manifestations of neuropsychological impairment in children with psychiatric disorders. Archives of Clinical Neuropsychology 3:369–374, 1988

Tramontana MG, Hooper SR, Curley AD, et al: Determinants of academic achievement in children with psychiatric disorders. J Am Acad Child Adolesc Psychiatry 29:265–268, 1990

Wilson H, Staton RD: Neuropsychological changes in children associated with tricyclic antidepressant therapy. Int J Neurosci 24:307–312, 1984

6

Formulation, Differential Diagnosis, and Treatment Planning

Kenneth S. Robson, M.D.

Formulation

In child and adolescent psychiatric assessments, even more than in general psychiatry, sufficient data to make a definitive diagnosis may only become available with the passage of time. This is the case in part because of the diagnostician's need for extensive exposure to both child and family and for the establishment of trust. Sexual abuse, for example, may be suspected but undocumented for long periods of time. In addition, the nature of childhood and development is such that the evolution of certain pathologic conditions, the transformation of one condition "into" a second, or the disappearance of less grave disorders can require months or years. Furthermore, the plasticity and lack of differentiation in the young child (5 years old and younger) make the discrimination between normal and pathologic behaviors, between "phenotype and genotype," more difficult to assess. Sleep disturbances in 3-year-olds are to be expected; in 10-year-olds they may be part of a major depression or dysthymic disorder. Tantrums in the 2-year-old are normative; in the 12-year-old they can herald the onset of more major mental illness. In many respects, then, diagnosis in child and adolescent psychiatry is a longitudinal process.

Nevertheless, one cannot wait for time to pass. The establishment of a working formulation is essential for therapeutic interventions to begin. The formulation should not be confused with diagnosis and is concerned with 1) life events and chronology, as they relate to the emergence of psychopathology; 2) the pathophysiology of the symptoms, signs, and behaviors in question (see Chapter 1); and 3) the developmental status, leading conflicts, and coping and adaptive mechanisms of the child, using Erikson (1963) and Anna Freud (1963).

The formulation is a kind of road map for the diagnostician and therapist. By pulling together the data gathered in the evaluation, it forces the clinician to integrate findings, generate clinical hypotheses, and plan thoughtfully for interventions. A well-developed formulation should lead to more definitive differential diagnoses as well. In another sense the formulation represents a "distillate" of the data, a concise crystallization of the essential facts, events, and processes at the center of the child's difficulties. In life not too much can go wrong if a child is genuinely loved, in good health, and in reasonably secure reality circumstances. A well-executed formulation should require a paragraph in written reports and 5 minutes in spoken presentations.

Differential Diagnosis

The history of systems of diagnostic classification in child and adolescent psychiatry is of interest in its own right (Group for the Advancement of Psychiatry 1966). The shifting theoretical models of the field can be traced through its nosologies. Each of these systems is out of synchrony with certain clinical syndromes. The Group for the Advancement of Psychiatry classification, although currently out of favor, is clinically useful and emphasizes developmental and pathophysiologic aspects of the child; their monograph is well worth reading, keeping in mind that its primary orientation is psychodynamic. This system deals more effectively than the *Diagnostic and Statistical Manual of Mental Disorders,* Fourth Edition (DSM-IV) (American Psychiatric Association 1994a), in most respects, with less serious developmental disorders, reactive states, and certain character or personality types met with in childhood.

On the other hand, the system now in use (DSM-IV) has powerful descriptive reliability; the orientation is clearly medical. Because of such a perspective, this system tends to be more applicable to the severe disorders of childhood and adolescence that have a structure that is to some degree fixed. Developmental crises and deviations, reactive conditions, and familial dysfunction fit with greater difficulty into DSM-IV, whereas autism, schizophrenia, and affective disorders are well considered. Nevertheless, this multiaxial system approximates the medical model and is vigorously designed and field-tested. *It should be used with every child.* The compact paperbound mini-version of DSM-IV belongs on every diagnostician's desk (American Psychiatric Association 1994b).

Diagnostic categories will relate in varying degrees to the formulation. The exercise of differential diagnosis, however, is essential and invaluable to the clinician. Acknowledging that diagnosis is at best an *approximation,* contains only partial truths and incomplete data, may not point back to etiology or forward to treatment planning, and is at times illusory, it still serves several important ends: 1) clarity and rigor of clinical thinking, 2) problem-oriented treatment planning, 3) standardization for purposes of reporting and research, and 4) compatibility with the medical model and tradition. In addition, there is the issue of third-party reimbursement. With increasing scrutiny by regulatory bodies, fixed limits on hospital and ambulatory levels of payment for clinical services, and the introduction of diagnosis-related groups that establish length of stay in hospitals, the utilization of diagnostic categories (as developed in DSM-IV) is mandatory.

To avoid the often false reassurance of diagnostic labels, the child and adolescent psychiatrist is advised to utilize *both* formulation and differential diagnoses in arriving at a treatment plan. In a sense, the formulation is related more closely to function and the diagnoses to structure. By using both perspectives, more reliably designed interventions will take place. For example, attention-deficit/hyperactivity disorder is a favorite diagnosis in many child psychiatric centers. The criteria for diagnosis of this condition in DSM-IV are unambiguous. Unfortunately, impulsivity, hyperactivity, and attentional difficulties are common to many underlying clinical phenomena, such as anxiety, depression, prepsychotic states, and neurointegrative deficits. Each of these phenomena may require specific therapeutic measures quite different from one another. Furthermore, the roles of familial dysfunction, empathic deficits, and overstimulation in the environment are addressed in the formulation, not the diagnosis, of attention-deficit/hyperactivity disorder. Hence, the wisdom of a combined approach that uses both databases becomes clear.

Treatment Planning

With both formulation and differential diagnoses in mind, the clinician is in a position to design an initial treatment plan. As noted in Chapter 2, the optimal plan in contrast to the possible plan may be discrepant in major ways. In particular, the limitations of the family's (or institution's) psychological *and* fiscal resources will limit the child and adolescent psychiatrist's recommendations and freedom of therapeutic movement. Like politics, treatment planning is the "art of the possible." Although these realities are sometimes (if not often) discouraging, at the same time creative efforts are called into play; necessity can serve as the parent of therapeutic invention. Furthermore, there are few therapeutic outcome studies in child and adolescent psychiatry that would support, with hard data, traditional or specific treatment regimens. Finally, more treatment is not necessarily better treatment. The physician in training will profit from an approach that is characterized by flexibility, curiosity, and a willingness to question traditional modes with a keen and observing eye. With these thoughts in mind, certain principles of therapeutic planning may be outlined:

- The *primary* goal of any therapeutic plan, regardless of the modalities involved, is developmental facilitation of the child.
- The biological family, or parties in loco parentis, must be able to accept minimal essential aspects of this goal; one cannot treat most children or adolescents without significant collaboration from the parties involved, no matter how crucial the need. Hence, the deci-

sion *not* to treat should be appropriately exercised and may, in itself, be therapeutic.

- Financial resources necessary for any treatment plan—whether private, third party, or state/local—must be realistically assessed both before and in the context of planning. Available monies are the "bottom line" of therapeutic strategies.
- The child and adolescent psychiatrist as treatment planner must be willing to assume a variety of roles that include psychotherapist; family worker; consultant to schools, courts, and social service agencies; child advocate in the political systems (e.g., schools, courts, summer camps) surrounding the child; and coordinator and choreographer of all of these.
- Multiple modalities of intervention are generally necessary. The therapeutic needs in any clinical situation *change,* however, with the passage of time, altered developmental status, improvement or deterioration in the child, and the availability of new resources. Regular reassessment of the original plan is essential.

Communicating Diagnostic Information and Treatment Planning

The data from psychiatric evaluations and the treatment plans evolving from them are only as valuable as the skill with which they are conveyed to the key parties involved. Children, and in most instances adolescents, are captive patients who do not refer themselves and cannot be treated without the support of parents, parties in loco parentis, referring nonpsychiatric physicians, and so on. Hence this critical juncture in the clinical process often requires exquisitely sensitive and tactful effort.

Whenever possible, sessions to review diagnostic issues and treatment considerations should include both parents. Children and adolescents can be given a choice to participate in some or all of the meeting, depending on clinical judgment and circumstances. With adolescents it is sometimes advisable to begin treatment *before* conveying further information to parents but to schedule this event at some point in the therapy. With children in foster care or institutional settings, choosing the appropriate participants may be more difficult; knowledge of the power structure and politics of the situation is essential.

Many diagnostic evaluations spontaneously establish both effective alliances with child and family and the need for ongoing treatment. When such is the case, the clinician's task is simply to maintain existing momentum. In other instances, however, parental anxiety, defensiveness, or outright hostility complicates matters, and one walks a kind of therapeutic tightrope. There are no easy guidelines in the latter situation, although bluntness is best avoided unless essential. Further, parents need not hear a DSM-IV diagnosis to feel satisfied that they know the facts. It is always important to stress a child's strengths and assets, as well as parents' commitment to parenting. At the same time, the clinician must convey the nature and quality of a child's difficulties in a manner that is thorough, convincing, and clearly understood. Using parents' own words and perceptions of their child is an appropriate starting point. "Nervous" may be preferred to "anxious," "problems with self-control" to "impulsive," "difficulty telling real from imaginary" to "psychotic" or "poor reality testing." Further, it is probably best to avoid predictions of prognosis or length of treatment unless necessary; these issues will become apparent in time or be more easily discussed when treatment has begun and parents can more readily accept serious disorders.

In conveying to parents the necessity for treatment, it is useful to be concrete. Discussion of *impairments in school functioning, personal relationships, level of unhappiness,* or *symptomatology* helps parents understand the deficits that a child experiences without undue guilt. To the inevitable question "what have we done to cause these problems" it can be helpful to point out that no psychiatric problem is caused by one source of difficulty; that genetic endowment, constitution and temperament, traumatic events, and so on all play a role in the evolution of symptomatology. Finally, in certain situations, it may also be helpful to acknowledge with parents that they have a more difficult child who makes the job of parenting harder; such is often the case. If therapeutic interventions are refused but are, in the clinician's opinion, essential to avoid further deterioration or suicidal risk, directness and firmness are indicated. Confrontation and toughness in the face of necessity are valuable tools appropriate to the child and adolescent psychiatrist's armamentarium.

Written materials deserve careful attention before they are sent on to parents, referral sources (including nonpsychiatric physicians), schools, and courts. A guiding principle is to say *as little* as possible in the *simplest* manner to convey the *essential* information for the party in question to know. Once written materials are sent out they become public information to most or all parties involved. One should not assume that all physician colleagues are psychiatrically sophisticated or sensitive to such issues as timing, terminology, and parental defensiveness. Collaborative editing with colleagues, such as clinical psychologists who have administered test protocols, is important and useful. Finally, in an era where hair-trigger litigation is epidemic, the child and adolescent psychiatrist must consider the legal hazard of written clinical materials about highly sensitive matters, including physical and sexual abuse, rape, abortion, drug abuse, criminal behavior, marital infidelity, and family "secrets." Clinicians are advised to utilize care and tact and *always* to preface sensitive issues with "reported" or "alleged" (e.g., abuse, neglect) in order to protect themselves, their institution, and, in some cases, the child and family members.

References

American Psychiatric Association: Diagnostic and Statistical Manual of Mental Disorders, 4th Edition. Washington, DC, American Psychiatric Association, 1994a

American Psychiatric Association: Quick Reference to the Diagnostic Criteria From DSM-IV. Washington, DC, American Psychiatric Association, 1994b

Erikson EH: Childhood and Society. New York, WW Norton, 1963

Freud A: The concept of developmental lines. Psychoanal Study Child 18:245–265, 1963

Group for the Advancement of Psychiatry: Psychopathological Disorders in Childhood: Theoretical Considerations and a Proposed Classification. New York, Group for the Advancement of Psychiatry, 1966

Section II

Approaches to Treatment

7

Introduction to Treatment

Kenneth S. Robson, M.D.

In Section I of this manual, a model of the pathophysiology of childhood disorders was presented (see Chapter 1). This model emphasizes the role of both internal and external overstimulation through excessive or insufficient, unmodulated levels of arousal-producing contact and empathic failures in parenting in creating a pathogenic environment and developmental deviance. Although far from exhaustive in accounting for pathologic conditions in childhood, this point of view appears to address a significant amount of variance in most clinical conditions and leads to concrete and practical approaches to therapeutic interventions, regardless of modality. Furthermore, although the degree of "fixed" or "structural" psychopathology is difficult to assess in most syndromes and symptom complexes (other than in the catastrophic disorders such as autism and schizophrenia), the model presented here focuses on the modifiable aspects of pathogenic conditions. Percentage-wise, in general, external overstimulation and empathic failures in parenting, through their accessibility to the clinician, offer the most powerful options for therapeutic influence. It follows, from this position, that therapeutic efforts directed at specific current dysfunctions in the parent or parent-surrogate environment are seen as most likely to produce change. Conversely, clinical energies directed toward the intrusive pathologic phenomena in the individual child are viewed as important but less relevant than environmental modifications in successful therapeutic outcomes.

Within the model espoused here, the goals of all forms of treatment remain the same: to modulate internal and external levels of stimulation impinging on the child and to increase empathic levels of caretaking to facilitate development. Hence, the psychoactive agent that reduces agitation, lowers levels of anxiety, or diminishes flooding of the child's ego with depressive affect can play a critical role in helping a child decrease internal levels of overstimulation or excessive vulnerability to external stimuli. Helping parents to relinquish seductive, "orgiastic" models of relatedness, or to avoid loss of impulse control with the child, and to remain related to the child rather than withdrawing in cold, destructive anger are commonly encountered strategies in modulating levels of parental overstimulation. For example, assisting the parent who views excessive masturbation in the prepubertal child as "being oversexed" to see such behavior as a reaction to isolation, depression, and separation concerns can convert unempathic, punitive, parental withdrawal to a comforting, supportive presence. Such shifts have great importance therapeutically. Again, the "crystals" of development require calm or even silence to take shape, and they are fractured by flooding.

The examples cited above convey the central thrust of the therapeutic model being described. Although the underlying concepts are relatively simple, they can be used to organize sensible, well-thought-out, and achievable therapeutic plans. Further, these same concepts provide ongoing evidence, a kind of "therapeutic gyroscope," to the child and adolescent psychiatrist in his or her therapeutic "posture" with child, parents, schools, and courts. This therapeutic schema is illustrated in Figure 7–1. Comparing Figure 7–1 with Figure 1–2 in Chapter 1 will clarify the relationship between the pathophysiology of childhood disorders and corrective treatment strategies. Finally, because careful research into the process and outcome of child therapies is sparse, child and adolescent psychiatry residents are advised to read other thoughtful reviews of this subject (McDermott 1984).

Figure 7–1. Therapeutic interventions in childhood disorders.

MODULATION OF OVERSTIMULATION

Internal (child)

Gain self-control
Reduce impulsiveness
Stabilize regulation of self-esteem
Decrease cathexis and ego-syntonicity of "orgiastic" mode
Reduce vulnerability to anxiety
Reduce depression
Enhance all "ego" skills (e.g., learning, sports, peer relations)
Diminish fears
Strengthen reality testing
Soften harsh and rigid self-criticism
Use of psychoactive agents
Reduce narcissistic "entitlement"
Therapists' "ego-relatedness" with child

External (parents)

Encourage physical modesty
Close bathroom and bedroom doors
Have child sleep in own bed
Avoid harsh, excessive, and frightening physical punishment
Modulate and desexualize physical contact
Increase parental "ego-relatedness"
Increase parental "availability" by modifying depression, anxiety, and schizoid withdrawal
Psychoactive drug treament of appropriate symptoms and conditions
Encourage interactions in play and games that soothe rather than excite
Help child develop the capacity to be alone
Separate from child in appropriate ways
Substitution of alternative environment when necessary (foster care, residential)
Consultation to school environment

INCREASED EMPATHIC CARETAKING

Appreciation of meaning of child's behavior
Appreciation of one's own behavior
Institution of age-appropriate expectations with child
Reduce need for child as "sustaining object"
Help parents recall own childhood
Acceptance of child's development as painful loss
Reduce misperceptions of child's behavior and responses
Enhance parental capacity to identify child's inner affective states
Enhance parental capacity to identify own affective states
Consultation to teachers
Consultation to foster parents, institutional staff
Therapists' empathic relationships with child

FACILITATION OF CHILD'S DEVELOPMENT

Goals and Models of Treatment

Although the larger goal of any therapeutic intervention—facilitation of the child's development—is evident, the process of clearly articulating *specific component goals* can facilitate cost-effective clinical work. Common examples include the following:

- Establishing a working alliance
- Completing diagnostic evaluations
- Starting psychoactive drugs
- Establishing contact with school personnel
- Returning a reluctant child to school
- Resolving a crisis situation
- Manipulating the environment
- Advising lawyers and parents vis-à-vis disruptive custodial arrangements
- Helping parents into individual or marital therapies
- Helping child establish peer relationships
- Making ego-syntonic behaviors ego-alien

Obviously, the nature of therapeutic goals will vary with the passage of time, developmental progress, and changing needs of the child and family. Winnicott's (1967) concept of the "holding environment" is applicable here. The therapist attempts to create an optimal environment, through all available means, within which healthy development can proceed.

Other critical variables over which one has little or no control will play a major role in the design feasibility of treatment interventions. For this reason, the therapist is advised to *prioritize goals* insofar as that is possible. Factors affecting treatment implementation include

- The family's readiness for therapy
- Available money
- Available therapeutic resources
- Therapist and family time constraints

Any or all of these issues can profoundly influence the shape and effectiveness of any intervention.

Finally, the question of which therapy or therapies come into play is subject to significant therapist bias (as well as parent bias). In some training centers or geographic locations certain therapies are traditionally recommended and others are considered less valuable, "second best," or unacceptable. For example, individual, intensive, dynamically oriented long-term work may be seen as optimal, with group therapy and pharmacotherapy seen as undesirable "also rans." Pharmacotherapy may be viewed as the treatment of choice with little or no attention given to family work or school consultation. Short-term work may be considered a "treatment failure." Family therapy is sometimes considered the only treatment of choice.

The child psychiatrist in training will do well to question and avoid such doctrinaire positions. Studies comparing the effectiveness of various modalities of treatment are virtually nonexistent (McDermott 1984). Furthermore, all of these modalities can contribute to progress, and combinations of them frequently accelerate the resolution of pathologic processes and the facilitation of development. Clinical acumen, flexibility, and open-mindedness are valuable assets for the child and adolescent psychiatrist as therapist.

References

McDermott JF (ed): Psychotherapy with children and adolescents (special section). Journal of the American Academy of Child Psychiatry 23:527–568, 1984

Winnicott DW: The location of cultural experience. Int J Psychoanal 48:368–372, 1967

8

Therapeutics I: The Psychotherapies

Kenneth S. Robson, M.D.

In this chapter the major forms of psychotherapeutic intervention are discussed. These modes should not be rigidly construed as separate therapeutic entities. Rather, many treatment plans involve flexible utilization of parent work, family work, individual child therapy, and group therapy either in their own right or in combination with other forms of intervention.

The psychotherapies involve a central role for the relationship between therapist and patients. The strength of this relationship and the manner in which it is used are seen as the agents of change. In fostering change, some or all of the following mechanisms are posited to be significant:

- Support
- Identification with a healthy person
- Provision of a real relationship that replaces a lost or missing one in the child's or family's life, thereby facilitating development
- Insight and reworking of earlier or current psychic trauma
- The learning of new modes of intrapsychic and interpersonal relatedness that enhance self-esteem, autonomy, and coping skills
- Time-out: the creation of a calm, soothing, tolerant, and "ego-related" atmosphere within which to heal and grow

Indications for selecting a particular form of psychotherapy are not available at present; there are too little data comparing outcomes. Bias thrives in such a vacuum. Traditionally, intensive individual and parent therapies evolving out of the child guidance movement and psychoanalysis were thought suitable only for better organized children and families with moderate forms of psychopathology. However, at one point in time, intensive psychotherapy with autistic children was also in vogue. Indeed, certain children with autistic features or schizophrenia appear to benefit from individual psychotherapy. With the onset of the community mental health movement, many more poor and disorganized families and their children were referred to child psychiatric programs, and psychotherapies with these populations can be critically important.

However, because the elaboration of criteria for utilization of the psychotherapies requires further study, the child and adolescent psychiatrist may find the following guidelines helpful:

- All children can benefit from a caring relationship with an adult. Psychotherapy, however, is a scarce, expensive, problem-solving resource. Hence, the nature of the essential problems for child, parents, or family should be clearly identified before referral is made. The need for a friend is not an indication for psychotherapy. Common indications for a child include the following:
    - Treatment of symptoms
    - Enhancement of ego skills (e.g., impulse control, reality testing)
    - Mourning of a loss
    - Resolution of a developmental crisis
    - Clarification of life events (e.g., divorce, sexual abuse)
    - Facilitation of interpersonal skills
    - Acceptance of deviance (e.g., mental retardation, birth defects, psychotic parent)
- Most children, regardless of diagnosis, can profit from some forms of psychotherapeutic intervention. The concept of "good patients" is hazardous.
- Families with better organizational skills for scheduling and regular

attendance can more easily (although not necessarily more usefully) engage in psychotherapies.

- A child's or family's need for psychotherapy, if difficult to implement initially, should not eliminate subsequent introduction of these modes. More definitive discussions of psychotherapeutic modes are available elsewhere (Adams 1982; Barker 1983; Connell 1979; Group for the Advancement of Psychiatry 1982; Haworth 1964; McDermott and Harrison 1977; Rutter and Hersov 1977; Simmons 1981; Slavson and Schiffer 1975).
- The beginning therapist may assume that long-term therapies are more desirable or effective than short-term interventions, regardless of therapeutic modality. Such value judgments are not based on comparative outcome data. Experienced therapists know that brief therapeutic experiences often lead to dramatic results. On the other hand, long-term work may be essential. An unbiased position that views the task of any therapy as doing *as little as necessary* to facilitate the child's development can be a helpful guide.

Parent Work

Whatever therapies the treatment plan for a particular child involves, effective intervention with the parents or parent surrogates is *crucial.* No matter how skilled the therapist or how superior the resources, change will not take place without an adequate alliance with the parents. The child who does not have permission to be in therapy can profit little or none from any form of intervention, including hospitalization or residential treatment. Hence, parent work becomes the cornerstone of all therapies. The child and adolescent psychiatrist in training is oriented toward patients. It is important to keep in mind that parents do not consciously engage the therapist with concerns of their own; they are not and should not be treated as patients. One must relate to them as parents, and the tasks are to enhance their empathic skills and help them modulate levels of stimulation around their child—in short, to render them the "facilitating environment."

From this perspective it follows that, at least initially, even in the face of gross parental psychopathology, the clinician focuses attention on the child's difficulties and the parent's reactions to them. The alliance is made with the "good parent," that aspect of the parent committed to the child's growth and development. The clinician who has children of his or her own easily appreciates the complexity, frustration, ambivalence, and despair that are normal to the tasks of parenting. One can maintain appropriate professional distance and still empathically share this part of personal life.

The role of the parent therapist should be clear. Worried and insecure parents are often willing to turn over their child to the idealized therapist as "perfect parent." The gratification of such a position for the therapist is seductive but not useful; vigilance is important to avoid this pitfall. The parent therapist's function is to strengthen and enhance existing parent skills, not to erode them further. The useful role is as *facilitator* and *collaborator*, not usurper. The powerful resistance to successful child therapy that conscious or unconscious fears of separation pose to parents has been discussed previously. In this vein it can be useful to remind parents that their job is in some respects like no other: The better they perform, the more they relinquish their parental responsibilities as their child develops toward separation and autonomy.

Another recurrent difficulty for the clinician working with parents is the intense reactions to particular kinds of parental attitudes and behaviors. Psychodynamically, these reactions fall under the rubric of "countertransference." Some of the common parental behaviors that can interfere with the child and adolescent psychiatrist's alliance include physical or sexual abuse, other forms of sadism, neglect, and overt rejection. Such behaviors generally reflect the parent's own experiences as a child and are a form of "identification with the aggressor." It is the therapist's task to maintain a nonjudgmental, empathic stance. At the same time, anxiety and denial must not stop the therapist from setting appropriate limits that sometimes include legal interventions. Beginning therapists can confuse sadistic and omnipotent impulses of their own with necessary directness and assertiveness essential for the protection of both child and parent.

In addition to these attitudinal considerations of parent therapy, the practical parameters of time, place, and person are important. In traditional psychotherapy the parents are generally seen once weekly by the social workers who work closely with the child's therapist. This team approach can, however, be cumbersome as it requires intense and regular communication, additional time, and money. In private practice, particularly with preadolescent children, one therapist for parents, child, and family is efficient and effective. The primary indications for co-therapy are for children 12 years or older and in clinical situations that require separation of child and parent "boundaries." However, both of these criteria should be used flexibly because they do not apply in many circumstances.

Some practical guidelines for parent therapy include the following:

- With a child in weekly individual therapy, parent meetings should occur *at least* twice monthly and *optimally* weekly as well.
- Brief meetings with parents, 10–15 minutes, are sometimes utilized to spare parents a second trip to the clinic or office. This practice is extremely limiting and should be discouraged; alternating weekly sessions with child and parents are more likely to produce therapeutic change.
- Co-therapists should meet or speak by telephone at least twice monthly and should meet together with parents in some regularly scheduled fashion.
- Parents should be encouraged to communicate unexpected and important life events (e.g., illness, loss, death of a pet, school crisis, family disturbance) to the child's therapist *before* he or she sees the child. Communication by phone the night before, a note handed to the therapist, or 2–3 minutes in the office before the session begins are usually equally effective.
- Regarding confidentiality, parents should be told that transactions between child and therapist generally remain private. Obviously, in situations of risk or danger to the child, this cannot be the case.

Family Work

The role of family therapeutic efforts in child therapies varies enormously with training, setting, and clinical circumstances. Furthermore, therapy and models range from family therapy as the exclusive mode to more flexible use of family meetings as they seem clinically indicated. At present, rigid or doctrinaire positions do not seem warranted by the available data on therapeutic outcome. Indications for and contraindications to family approaches are unclear and, in the words of one experienced family therapist, are "if it works." The thoughtful clinician will explore the utility of family work from many perspectives because it is powerful and cost-effective. There is probably no therapeutic plan where some family efforts cannot prove useful. Common situations that may call for family therapeutic experience include

- Discussion of "family secrets" revealed by a child or parents in individual therapy
- The need to obtain parental "permission" for a child to speak openly about particular sensitive feelings or events with the therapist
- Intervention in a family crisis
- Mourning of a dead, dying, or absent family member
- Review of custodial arrangements in divorce and separation
- The failure of individual, group, or other therapeutic modalities
- Fiscal constraints

Individual Child Psychotherapy

Several excellent texts on play therapy with children deal with its history as well as theory and technique. Initial criteria regarding suitability for individual child therapy included sufficient intelligence, moderate levels of disturbance, and ego strengths. Such criteria may loosely speak to health but are unnecessarily restrictive and unsupported by existing studies. Furthermore, because the greater part of therapeutic change generally resides in modifying parental functioning as a facilitating environment, the role of the child's therapy per se as a change agent is uncertain or even obscure.

The concept of "individual" child therapy may also be misstated and, at times, antitherapeutic. In general, the psychotherapist is intervening within a family or child/environment system. The target, so to speak, is the *interface* in these relations between the child and the child's world that contributes to overstimulation, parental empathic failure, and developmental deviance. This latter perception of individual psychotherapy cannot so easily isolate work with the child from the whole therapeutic enterprise. Rather than a sequestered, special, "closed" relationship with the child, even in individual child therapy, the *primary goal* becomes improving the facilitating environment.

Nevertheless, there are many uses to which a working alliance with a child can be put in the service of facilitating development. These include a corrective relationship with a caring, empathic but not overstimulating adult. As noted in Figure 7–1 (Chapter 7), and within the context of and "held" by the corrective relationship, specific aspects of the child's behavior, perceptions, symptoms, and interpersonal relations can be modified in psychotherapy. For example:

- The modification of maladaptive behavior patterns, personality styles, and character traits
- Facilitation of movement into a new developmental phase
- Increased affect tolerance
- Improved self-esteem
- Correction of distorted cognitive views of reality events and experiences
- Reduction of inhibition and constriction
- Strengthened coping skills
- More effective interpersonal skills
- Enhanced classroom learning
- Hopefulness in living

Obviously, there are many goals that a therapist may wish to pursue in treating a child. The experienced clinician can often work simultaneously on several developmental tasks. But the beginning child therapist should be rigorous in setting therapeutic priorities; that is, what developmental tasks or lines, what problem areas, if addressed, are likely to facilitate developmental progression.

As noted earlier in this manual, the clinical approach to children and child therapy can feel intimidating, anxiety arousing, and confusing. Sorting out "signal" from "noise" as clinical data emerge can seem impossible. To attempt less, set modest goals, and enjoy one's self with a child are sound starting points. The *essential condition* for the therapeutic process to prosper is to *establish* and *maintain empathic contact with the child.* If the therapist remains aware of the child's emotional state at any point in time, the nature of the therapeutic response becomes self-evident. The content of play and the choice of toys can be seen as clues to the inner affect states and current or past needs of the child. In this way the therapist's choreography and timing mirror those of the empathic parent who senses what is right, how much of it, and when.

The latter point deserves discussion. In one therapeutic session with any child, much may have occurred (the week, night, or hour before) about which the therapist knows little or nothing and will not learn more until later. The child's affect guides the response (e.g., "you seem sad today"). Further, in the course of a session, many shifts of play and behavior will occur. To listen for the affect "driving" these shifts is to disregard distraction and tune in to the simple, central feeling state like the recurrent voice of the French horn in a symphony—it is enough; all else is elaboration.

In the history of child psychotherapy the importance of fantasy and its meanings was an important contribution of psychoanalysis. However, in the practice of contemporary child and adolescent psychiatry where weekly, bimonthly, or less frequent sessions are the rule, the role of fantasy requires reassessment. It is impossible within individual play therapy to sort out reality-based from "imagined" contributions to any play sequence. However, it is generally safer, more accurate, and information revealing initially to consider all play sequences as reality based—as portraying some (traumatic?) aspect of the child's external world. Such an orientation both improves the likelihood of appropriate and helpful therapeutic interventions with the child and guides useful sessions with parents who from shame, anxiety, or unawareness will not be aware of some critically important experience in the child's outside world.

Finally, another consideration is the role of games in individual child therapy. Their primary purpose is to establish and maintain "ego-relatedness" (Winnicott 1967) with the child. As such they should be pleasant experiences for both child and therapist. How the child plays (e.g., intensely, regularly breaking rules, always losing) and what games are important data—but data secondary to the need for establishing and maintaining good contact. In this sense process is more important than content.

In conducting individual psychotherapy with children, the beginning therapist, regardless of the choice of responses to the patient, wishes to be liked by the child or adolescent. This wish is particularly intense in beginning therapists, who tend to be rejection-sensitive with their child and adolescent patients. The child who is aloof, combative, or deliberately hurtful of the therapist's feelings is doing so for some defensive or communicative purpose. Hence, such behaviors should be taken seriously but not too seriously.

Group Therapy

Group psychotherapy in childhood and adolescence is a cost-effective, powerful, and probably underutilized modality of treatment. Troubled interpersonal relationships generally accompany most forms of disturbance in childhood and adolescence. Furthermore, the establishment of good friendships and the strength of group process can rapidly modify intrapsychic problems such as insecurity, low self-esteem, poorly controlled aggression, envy, and difficulty in sharing. Peer pressure appears to be particularly powerful in shaping narcissistic behaviors in children who will relinquish such behaviors often with dramatic speed in a group therapeutic setting. Also, children with special problems (e.g., family dissolution in divorce, serious medical illness, foster care status, mentally ill parents) seem to find ventilation of their concerns more easily in the group context than in individual therapeutic relationships. In adolescence the developmental thrust toward independence may render the group a less intense and regressive environment than one-to-one therapy. Nevertheless, no absolute criteria for selecting individual rather than group therapy in childhood exist, and such decisions probably depend on the training of the referring clinician, the availability of a group therapist, and access to adequate space and play materials.

Because peer groups normally begin to form in the early school-age years (7- to 8-year-olds), therapeutic groups rarely involve children younger than this age. Thereafter, whether in clinics, schools, or institutional settings, groups of four to eight children run by one or two therapists appear to thrive. With children and early adolescents, play and shared activities are more important therapeutic modes than verbal communication. With mid- and late adolescents, of course, talking becomes more useful within the group context. Group psychotherapy should never be seen as a second-class service; it has much to offer (see Chapter 10).

References

Adams PA: A Primer of Child Psychotherapy, 2nd Edition. Boston, MA, Little, Brown, 1982

Barker P: Basic Child Psychiatry, 4th Edition. Baltimore, MD, University Park Press, 1983

Connell HM: Essentials of Child Psychiatry. London, Blackwell Scientific Publications, 1979

Group for the Advancement of Psychiatry: The Process of Child Therapy. New York, Brunner/Mazel, 1982

Haworth MR (ed): Child Psychotherapy. New York, Basic Books, 1964

McDermott JF, Harrison SI (eds): Psychiatric Treatment of the Child. New York, Jason Aronson, 1977

Rutter M, Hersov L: Child Psychiatry: Modern Approaches. London, Blackwell Scientific Publications, 1977

Simmons JE: Psychiatric Examination of Children, 3rd Edition. Philadelphia, PA, Lea & Febiger, 1981

Slavson SR, Schiffer M: Group Psychotherapies for Children. New York, International Universities Press, 1975

Winnicott DW: The location of cultural experience. Int J Psychoanal 48:368–372, 1967

9

Therapeutics II: Family Work

Lee Combrinck-Graham, M.D.

Since a child's family is his or her most important resource, child psychiatrists who are comfortable working with families have a significant advantage in helping their young patients. A child psychiatrist does not need to become a practicing family therapist to gain this advantage, but the psychiatrist does need to "think family" at important junctures of the diagnostic and treatment processes, and does need to have some basic skills in forming working collaborations with parents, identifying some important family processes, and, above all, respecting basic family loyalties.

The benefits of establishing contact with family members include

- Increased investment in the treatment
- Increased compliance with treatment
- Increased understanding of the forces influencing recovery
- Access to family resources
- Assistance with care and protection
- Assistance with accountability and management

These benefits apply to all children and families. Family involvement should occur regardless of the presenting problem in the child. The family does not have to be perceived as central to the etiology of the child's problems in order for them to be productively involved in the treatment. Families' roles in children's problems can be classified as follows:

- The problem is biologically based; the family has no obvious role in its genesis (e.g., autism, Tourette's syndrome, developmental disabilities).
- The child's problem appears to be related to family dysfunction (e.g., behavior disorders).
- Family dysfunction appears to be related to the child's problem (e.g., parent conflict over managing a child).
- The child's problem is an outcome of family dysfunction (e.g., trauma secondary to violence, abuse, neglect).

Treatment teams may mistakenly exclude the family from treatment when the child's problem is thought to be independent of family functioning and when the family is thought to be the cause through exploitation, abuse, or neglect. But even when a child's problem is biologically based, the family's handling of the problem as well as the inclusion of the child in the relationship system can be crucial to the overall success of the management; a family's mishandling of such issues can exaggerate the crippling aspects of children's conditions. Even when family members have harmed a child, emotional ties remain between the child and family members, which should be respected while also taking steps to protect the child. Examples of programs designed to preserve family relationship systems in such cases include providing in-home family work to assist with mastery of the stresses that can lead to violence and neglect; developing foster families as advocates for the primary family relationships of their foster children; and maintaining family connections during the incarcerations of family members. To repeat, since all children have family relationships, it is important to consider them actively in any child treatment.

The basis for family work is established during the assessment phase, and the work itself continues at intervals during the course of treatment. Critical junctures, which should always involve at least important caretakers, if not the whole family, are those in which major decisions are to be made, for only with the family's full understanding and agreement can there be informed consent. Although one parent (usually the mother) is accepted as the family of consent, the consent of only one concerned and responsible family member can often lead to misunderstandings, undermining of treatment, and ultimately non-compliance or premature termination.

What Is a Family?

For the purposes of family work with children, a family is defined as those members of a child's relationship system who have an immediate and consistent bearing on his or her day-to-day experience. There are some variations on how professionals define this group:

- All members of a nuclear family (mother, father, siblings)
- All related members of a household
- All members of a household (includes boarders and live-in house-keepers)
- All members of a household and close extended family members (includes a divorced or separated parent and caretaking grandparents)
- Any of above plus influential contacts (child-care worker, teacher, welfare worker)
- "Problem-determined system" composed of all who are invested in identifying and solving the child's problem

The only time one parent is considered to be the "family" is in the rare instance when a single parent (usually the mother) and child are living in *isolation* from other relationships. Most single-parent headed households have ongoing, influential relationships with others, including siblings of the child or close friends and relatives of the parent. Talking to a mother is not family work, although it may be a beneficial step for history gathering and information sharing. Work with a mother-child dyad that excludes other significant members of the relationship system may have negative results ranging from slow progress (due to noncooperation by others) to deterioration due to unbalancing of the relationship system. For the purposes of family therapy, other children in the family should be included.

What Is Family Therapy?

Many professionals make a distinction between parent education or training and family therapy. This distinction is based on a definition of family therapy as effecting change in individual experience and behavior through altering the family relationship system. Clearly there are many ways to change people through changing their relationship systems, and education and training actually are included as important family therapy modalities. Family psychoeducation, for example, is now regarded as an essential component in the management of severely and chronically mentally ill and disabled individuals.

Because family therapy is aimed at altering the relationship system, the sine qua non of family therapy is the assessment of the relationship system and design of treatment that considers how the system could change and what impact changes would have on the family members. Family therapy always affects all family members, and just as it is not considered ethical for a family to sacrifice some individuals for the benefit of others, so it is not ethical to plan interventions that will benefit some without assuming responsibility for their effects on others. Refocusing the attention of family members on one individual may result in neglect or harm of another. For example, successful treatment of a child's separation anxiety disorder may be followed by deterioration of the person to whom the child was anxiously attached.

There are many modalities of family therapy. Listed below are a few of the more standard forms:

- Working with an individual who is focused on changing his or her relationships to family members. Called "coaching" and developed by Murray Bowen (1978), this is usually done with competent and highly motivated family members. This approach is not commonly used with children.
- Education or training of family members on how to handle specific

problems. Such psychoeducational approaches qualify as family therapy when they specifically deal with strengthening and empowering the family to cope with particular problems that range from severe mental illness and developmental disabilities to behavior problems.

- Conjoint family therapy with a structural focus. The structural approach is derived from the work of Minuchin (1974). Based on the assumption that family organization is the basis of a healthy relationship system, clarifying and differentiating roles and functions in family relationships—particularly in terms of child care, education, and discipline—are the essential features of this approach.
- Conjoint therapy with a strategic focus. The underlying tenet of the strategic approach is that symptomatic behavior and the family's way of organizing around symptoms serve functions that become habitual and ingrained. Because these functions are also unconscious, strategies need to be devised to entice, surprise, or compel family members to discover different ways of interacting.
- Family of origin work. Family of origin work deals with the myths and legacies that are played out in contemporary family life. By examining and reworking the understanding of family history, one can change current family patterns.
- Psychodynamic family therapy. These approaches use psychodynamic concepts to assess family relationships and work with emotional tone, projective identification, and object relations.

Techniques in family therapy include a palette of practices derived from the spectrum of psychotherapies, including cognitive-behavioral, insight and understanding, play, psychodrama, art, movement, and even Outward Bound and wilderness experiences.

This overview of family therapy should prepare a child psychiatrist to respect the involvement of families in their children's treatment and to assist with ongoing family therapy.

Family Involvement in the Assessment Phase

At the very least, a child psychiatrist should sit with the whole family on one occasion during the assessment phase. For many, this session will be in addition to those spent with the parents and the child alone.

Important considerations in this initial contact with the family include

- Timing
- Who should be involved
- What is to be accomplished

Timing

There are different views about when is the best time to have the whole family in. Some therapists prefer to begin with seeing the child, alone, especially if the child is preadolescent or adolescent. Most prefer to meet with the parents first to gain a description of the presenting problem and gather necessary history. If assessment begins with either the child or the parents, the family and the child should be prepared for a whole family session sometime before the assessment phase is over. If the whole family is not involved in some way during the early phases of assessment and treatment, it is very difficult to get them to come in later.

Some therapists believe that it is important to meet first with the whole family. This timing allows for family members to meet the therapist and tell their story before any confidential information has been exchanged or exclusive relationships have been formed. This first view of the problems, in context, can shape the formulation and treatment of the child's problems in a way that uniquely accounts for the relationships and resources of this particular child and family. Those who argue for this timing further observe that the opportunity to tell their stories to the therapist in the initial contact can best avert the feeling on the part of the child that the therapist is in league with the parents and that the parents have imparted information to the therapist in a private session, information that the child does not know and might be humiliating or embarrassing. It also averts the hands-off feeling of parents whose child has been or will be seen individually, and who may reveal family secrets to this, as yet unknown, outsider. Finally, seeing the family, first, stimulates family members to think about themselves and their operations in ways that may invite them to make some changes.

Who Should Be Involved

Ideally, all members of the child's household should be involved, including siblings (even babies) and grandparents. It is also useful to include important figures in a child's life who do not live in the home (e.g., a grandmother who is a major caretaker). There is some logic, too, in including the referring person, if he or she is familiar with the child and not a family member. An example would be the child's teacher or child-care worker.

It is not necessary to include a lot of extra people, but it is necessary to have a sufficient definition of "family" and invite individuals close to the child so that patterns of caretaking, competence, and aggravation may be observed. As already stated, involvement of one parent is not "family involvement" and is not sufficient for this family assessment session. Children have two parents, and even if they are not living in the same household, some effort to have both parents attend should be made. Furthermore, if the household is headed by a single parent, the supportive adults, partners, parents, or good friends should be invited. Siblings should not be exempted from family sessions even if they do not have any problems or because the session interferes with their schedules. Families should be encouraged to bring everyone, not because they are causing or aggravating the problem, but because they care about each other, and they might help. Most family members who are reticent to come and expose themselves to blame will come if they are asked to help out.

Families are usually cooperative and will bring requested family members to the session, especially if the psychiatrist is able to be flexible about scheduling the session to make it as convenient as possible. However, there are many families who are reluctant to bring people and bring up many excuses not to. A nonproductive struggle for control can develop if the psychiatrist does not negotiate collaboratively about who should attend. The phrasing can be something like this: "I want to meet with your whole family, because when one person is experiencing difficulties, everyone feels it and worries. Usually everyone wants to help, too. Could you tell me who lives at home with you and your child?" As the list of household members is produced, the psychiatrist should indicate that it would be good for each member to attend. If there are questions about why, or protests, these can be discussed briefly. After the household members have been discussed, the next question is about other important people in the child's life who should be there. The psychiatrist may mention some examples, such as the caretaking grandparent or the noncustodial parent. If these are argued, it may be best to ask when would be a good time to involve them, rather than insisting on their attendance at this one, first session.

A special effort should be made to include the child's father—in the whole family session, if the father is living in the household or closely involved, and in a separate session including the father and his children without the mother, if the parents are separated and have an acrimonious relationship. Mothers often bear an excessive burden for their children's difficulties, and fathers usually have important contributions to make to their children's well-being that are frequently not utilized. To include the father may be as simple as asking, or it may require major readjustment of schedule and talking to him directly, rather than asking either the child or the mother to persuade him to come in.

After the best preparations, however, sometimes the expected people do not come in. Early in the family therapy movement, the therapists would not see the family unless everyone was there. Now, however, it is considered to be best to see them at the appointed time, regardless of how many people were left out. A fruitful discussion of why it has not been possible to have the expected attendance can be very illuminating, and another session can be scheduled.

What Is to Be Accomplished

The foremost goal for this session is for the child psychiatrist and the family to become acquainted. Secondary goals include achieving a mutual understanding of the problem and achieving a level of collaboration for the upcoming work.

This session should be very simply organized and conducted according to the following procedure:

- Introductions
- Joining
- Inquiring about the problem
- Concluding with a shared view of the family

Each member of the family is *introduced,* usually by a parent, although some ask the identified child patient to introduce his or her family.

Joining is a social phase that grows naturally out of introductions. One technique is to restate the name of each family member who has been introduced and to ask something specific and personal about him or her. For the children, their ages, their grades in school, their favorite activities, something about their friends, and a comment about their appearance (e.g., a pretty dress, a "cool" haircut) are appropriate. For adults, occupation and general level of health and functioning are appropriate. The interviewer can be very responsive and involved in playful interchanges at this point and, if comfortable, can give some responsive information about his or her own experiences or something indicating that he or she can connect with each individual in the family.

If family members describe experiences that are unfamiliar to the interviewer, this is an opportunity to express genuine curiosity. For example, one of the parents may have an occupation that is unfamiliar. The therapist may ask questions to learn more about it and then may say to the assembled family, something like, "I never knew what that was before. You learn something new every day," or "Did you kids know that's what your mom does at work? This is the first time I really understood what that kind of job entails."

This social conversation is for the purpose of establishing some commonalities, not for the purpose of gathering a detailed history or cataloging the family's pathology. The overall message of this section is "You are a family, like other families; you are respectable, and based on what you are telling me, I understand you, and you can understand how I understand you."

When *inquiring about the problem,* it is best to start with a question like, "Who can tell me why you are all here today?" This question may be addressed to everyone, and the first to answer gets the floor first. Or the question may be posed to a particular individual, first. Some choose the identified child; others may ask one of the parents. Who might be selected may be determined by how things have gone in the joining phase. It may be clear that parents are authorities in the family, and it would be inappropriate to address a child first. Or it may be clear that among the siblings there is a spokesperson who might be approached first.

The picture of the problem may have as many facets as there are people to describe it. Thus it is important to hear each family member's views. Even the smallest children may express opinions, and although a very young child may not seem to be on topic, often his or her concerns do contribute a flavor to the family function and concerns.

In addition to the content of people's observations, the interviewer should also be interested in the process. One aspect of the process of interest is the tolerance of family members for each other's expression. Is the family respectful? Do people interrupt each other, argue, or try to correct each other? Another interesting aspect of process is the difference in perspective. Information about relationship system organization is provided by differences in presentation. For example, there may be great difference between a mother's experience and a father's experience of how serious the problem is. A mother may claim that her child is ill; a father may dismiss the symptoms as faking. An older sibling may observe that his brother's upsetting behavior is no different from his own, at that age. A third aspect of process can be the invitation to the family to show the interviewer what they mean. This can be through a simple conversation about something, or a full-scale enactment demonstrating a crucial scene. "I notice that you and your father see this situation differently," the interviewer might say. "Talk to your dad, now, and see whether you can get him to understand your point of view." Or, "Since you seem to have your biggest arguments at dinner, I wonder if you could just show me how it is. Can you pretend that this is a dinner table, and show me where everyone sits, and how these conversations turn into arguments?"

After the family members have been introduced, have been acknowledged and joined with as individuals, and have presented their points of view about the family and its difficulties, it is important for the interviewer to give them some *feedback* about his or her observations. The interviewer should not leave the interview without doing this, because it leaves the family wondering what the interviewer thinks and concluding the worst.

Feedback should be provided in a form that picks up themes in the family so that it can be shared by the family. The interviewer's statement might begin with "I see, this is a family. . . ." Some examples are: "I see this is a family with a lot of different opinions." "I see this is a family that likes to argue." "I see this is a family with a lot of closeness." "I see this is a family that is very concerned about John." For one family with lots of children who were constantly interrupting each other, the therapist concluded, after hearing a confusing story about the laundry, "I see this is a family that has trouble getting their socks in the right drawers."

These statements are nonjudgmental, descriptive, and acceptable to the family. If their response is bewildered, it is probably either not accurate or the concept was too complicated. Generally a family will respond to a summing up that connects. Someone may say, "Yeah, you're right." Someone else may elaborate, correct, offer a detail. And so on. The interviewer will know that a connection has been made.

At this point the interviewer may get businesslike and suggest that the family make some commitments to work on the issues agreed on. Or the interviewer may end the session, allowing the family to reflect further on what they have experienced in the session. One senior family therapist, Carl Whitaker (Whitaker and Malone 1953), likes to leave the family full of the experience of their session. He instructs them not to talk about what went on in the session for at least 24 hours, to prolong the reflection.

When to Do Family Therapy

Family therapy is sometimes considered a modality of treatment and sometimes considered a treatment orientation. For the usual child psychiatrist trained in individual and biological approaches, family therapy is seen as a modality. For the child psychiatrist trained to work with children in context, family systems is a primary orientation to treatment. In the second instance the child psychiatrist will be a skilled family therapist. This chapter is oriented to the child psychiatrist in the first category.

It has already been suggested that the families of virtually all children who present for treatment should be seen and evaluated and some attempt made to have ongoing collaboration with them. In most cases, the ongoing collaboration can take place in the form of collateral visits with the parents. These are not treatment sessions per se, but opportunities to answer questions, give progress updates, discuss treatment regimen (such as medication schedules), and offer suggestions about managing difficult areas. Parent visits can be tagged on to a child's individual session, for 15 minutes before or after. Remember, however, that if only one parent brings the child to the session, a special effort must be made from time to time to connect and share information with the other parent as well.

Family work can also be ongoing with individual sessions. Some child psychiatrists prefer to have this work done by another therapist, trained in family therapy. More and more child psychiatrists prefer to integrate these two modalities themselves. Alternating weeks with individual and child is a common approach. Having long (1.5- to 2-hour) sessions divided in half is feasible for some. Having the family therapist see the family while the child psychiatrist sees the child, with the opportunity to meet together at some point, is also done. This latter practice presents the contradiction that the family contains the child; thus a family session without the child is not really a family session!

Family work is always indicated in some form or other. Whether it be occasional consultations with the parents or full family therapy as the primary intervention or something in between depends on a number of factors. The major factor is the theoretical orientation and skill of the therapist. Family-systems–oriented child psychiatrists, for example, involve the whole family in treatment regardless of the problems of the presenting child. Individuals are seen as subsystems of the family and may be worked with on issues and for periods of time that are a part of the overall family treatment strategy. Biological treatments are administered as a part of the family treatment, recognizing that the family's understanding and approbation of the treatment will increase compliance and increase the realistic evaluation of treatment effects. On the other hand, child psychiatrists who work primarily with an individual-psychodynamic orientation usually do not involve the family centrally in the treatment. For these therapists, family involvement may be limited to occasional consultations or treatment sessions with another therapist.

A second factor is how the child's difficulties are understood to relate to family functioning. Although ultimately the formulation of the child's problems also relates to the orientation of the child psychiatrist, it is generally agreed that misbehavior problems without obvious neurobiological disturbance should involve family members, at least parents, rather intensively, because the success of the treatment depends on the family's consistency. Problems such as depression, anxiety, and psychosis may be addressed in individual treatment, with parent involvement in decisions about treatment frequency, location, medication, and ancillary issues. Beyond the identified problems, themselves, however, is the way the problem is understood in context. For example, a depressed child who has had a number of changes in parenting figures through divorce and remarriage may improve on antidepressant medication and therapeutic support, but also needs reassurance about being wanted and having a place in the family. Thus family therapy should be a central aspect of the child's treatment. On the other hand, a child whose depression appears to deepen despite a consistent supportive family may not require extensive family involvement in the treatment.

A third factor in considering the importance of family work is the estimated functioning of the family and their availability to be involved. Many families seem to feel that they should deposit the child with the therapist and have the child "fixed." For some families, getting the child to the therapist is the best they can do, and the therapist needs to work with that. But more often the family does respond when the child psychiatrist tells them that they need to be involved, at least some of the time. Some families are assessed as untapped resources to the child. They are anxious to help, but do not know how. Some may have actually been turned away by a previous therapist and need to be coaxed back into assuming an active role in their child's recovery. Other families are seen as highly dysfunctional, even toxic, to their children. These include families where there is substance abuse, crime, physical abuse, sexual abuse, emotional abuse, and neglect. Although the easiest and immediately safest action may be to extract the child from the family and place the child in a residential center or foster family, this does not often work well in the long run. Children in placement usually have continuing severe problems, many stemming from the original family environmental dysfunction and just as many resulting from attenuating original family relationships and the multiple placements such children usually endure. For this reason, it is far better to work with the family, even though the child may need to be separate from the family for some period for his or her own safety. With a surprising number of such families, family work may result in their ability to stay together, appropriately foster the development of their members, and care for each other. With some others, living together may not be possible, and family work should focus on maintaining relationship ties as well as being realistic about each other's limitations. Individual work with these children must include an emphasis on this realistic orientation to his or her family relationships, and family work must focus on what is feasible in their ongoing interactions.

Critical Junctures to Involve the Family

If family members understand what is troubling the index child and what the therapeutic objectives are, they can enhance the effectiveness of the treatment through day-to-day interactions. Critical junctures to involve the family include

- Diagnostic assessment
- Discussion of issues pertaining to the safety and accountability of the child
- Points of decision (e.g., medication trials, treatment setting, consultations)
- Termination and follow-up

Diagnostic Assessment

The family can participate in the diagnostic assessment of a child in a number of ways that facilitate the family's understanding of the child's special circumstances. The example of a child with a developmental learning disorder can serve as an illustration. The family presents with a child who is doing poorly in school. In an early session, the child psychiatrist can do a "family neurological screening" in which all of the children participate in a neurological examination performing hopping, skipping, tandem walking, throwing, catching, finger differentiation, rapid alternating movements, and so on. During the assessment, differences in skill and performance are commented on. Each family member gains an appreciation for others' areas of strengths and difficulties, and through this appreciation an understanding of areas that may be difficult for the index child. Such sessions, conducted with the appropriate attitude toward differences rather than deficits, clarify for both the child and the family members what may be difficult for him or her.

Another assessment can be made by having everyone in the family draw some of the figures from the Bender-Gestalt Test (Bender 1938) or the Beery Test of Visual Motor Integration (Beery 1982). In this exercise, if the index child has visual-motor integration problems, those problems will be understood through the other family members' experience of the task. In this way, family members may also be able to come up with strategies to assist the child with these specific areas of difficulty, instead of discounting the child as stupid or lazy. Yet another approach to family involvement in assessment can be done in the feedback sessions following a formal testing battery. One approach is to review the testing with the child first, asking how the child thinks the material should be presented to other family members. The psychologist may decide what material is important to report, but get some ideas from the child about how it should be presented. The results are then presented with hands-on illustrations, so that family members can really understand what was the task, what skills the task called on, and what particular strengths and weaknesses their child brought to these situations. This can be done with parents and child, with or without other siblings.

Safety and Accountability

One of the hazards of psychiatric treatment is how family members respond to the one who is being treated. Children and patients who are mentally ill have in common that they usually are considered innocent and not held accountable. This is a curse, because they are also not taken seriously. For example, the preteen who threatens suicide arouses concern, but also should arouse indignation that he or she would contemplate wasting the great gift of life. Children who endanger themselves through impulsive behavior or threaten the safety of others often have their emotional/psychological state so focused on that limits are not set, and they are not held accountable, as others would be. For example, the young adolescent who steals from his parents to buy drugs may be hospitalized because of impulsive drug-seeking behavior while being excused from legal accountability.

It is best for child psychiatrists to have a relationship with the child and the family such that the family is invited to respond appropriately to the child's behavior. When this happens, even severe disturbances can often be handled by the family, because they are empowered to respond with common sense, and because the child is seen as an accountable person, even with the problems that the child is experiencing. An important aspect of this relationship is what is meant by confidentiality. Whatever the child psychiatrist communicates about confidentiality, he or she has to recognize that it is the child's family who has to live with the child, and they must be prepared to deal with aspects of the child's feelings and behavior that impact on day-to-day experience and the child's overall development and safety. Most would agree that if a child expresses suicidal intentions in an individual session, family members must be told. There are other, less critical issues that children impart to therapists, ranging from complaints about siblings to descriptions about what they do not like about visiting with a noncustodial parent. These items can be treated as information and folded into a diagnostic formulation and treatment plan. They can also be addressed as current and immediate opportunities for the child to negotiate solutions. The family can be involved in such a way that the child can raise issues directly with the therapist there to facilitate constructive exploration.

Decision Points

Major decision points about treatment include the initiation and termination of treatment as well as any changes that may occur along the way. The family's involvement in assessment and diagnostic assessment has already been described. If it has been done this way, the family can give fully informed consent to the proposed treatment.

Two possible treatment decisions that should involve the family are initiation of medication and hospitalization. Family involvement in the decision to institute medication results in better compliance and a fuller evaluation of its effects. The family must be consulted about the decision to place a child in a different treatment setting. The parents need clarification of their continued roles in ongoing treatment and responsibility for the child, and the other children need an understanding of why their sibling is in this special treatment environment and what they can expect about their continued relationship. If the family is not appropriately committed to this level of care, the treatment team may have too much responsibility for the child, and family relationships may be permanently damaged.

Termination and Follow-Up

Some say that family therapy is never terminated, that the family therapist can be more like a family doctor, in that treatment may be episodic and the family may maintain a long-term relationship, using the therapist for counsel on minor as well as major life decisions. But in today's fast-moving world, often families and therapists do not remain in the same community long enough for this type of relationship to evolve and be maintained. Treatment may end with the departure of either child or therapist, or it may come to a conclusion after the treatment goals have been accomplished. In either instance, the child psychiatrist needs to recognize that he or she has become a part of the family's life and that ending the relationship with the child is also ending a role within the family. Involving the family in termination allows not only for the good-byes to be said, but also to prepare for life without the therapist; how can they keep the benefits of the therapy experience alive for the child and for themselves?

Summary

Family work has great importance in child and adolescent psychiatry. The child psychiatrist may not be a highly trained family therapist, but the child psychiatrist must recognize the critical role of the family in his or her patient's life and the critical role of the family in the success of treatment. Family work must be done to effect the constructive influence of the family in caring for their children.

References

Beery KE: Visual Motor Integration. Chicago, IL, Follett Educational Corporation, 1982

Bender LA: A Visual Motor Gestalt and Its Clinical Uses. New York, American Orthopsychiatric Association, 1938

Bowen M: Family Therapy in Clinical Practice. New York, Jason Aronson, 1978

Minuchin S: Families and Family Therapy. Cambridge, MA, Harvard University Press, 1974

Whitaker CA, Malone TP: The Roots of Psychotherapy. New York, Blakiston, 1953

10

Therapeutics III: Group Therapy

Alberto C. Serrano, M.D.
Robert I. Berkowitz, M.D.

Group psychotherapy emerged as a significant treatment modality in the 1940s as a way to treat several patients meeting together at the same time. The goals and techniques used depend on the type of patient diagnosis or problems, the setting, and the theoretical orientation of the therapist.

The unique features of the group approach allow both the relationship with the therapist and the relationships among the group members to be agents of change. The therapist may observe directly the patient's interactions; the patients' observations of each other and their feedback is also a powerful influence. The features of the group aid in developing cohesiveness among the members, mutual support, and modeling for more adaptive behaviors, which are helpful in developing relationship skills and reducing symptoms.

Slavson (1943) and Ginott (1961), who wrote the first books on children's groups, were earlier contributors who described that group modalities with children and adolescents should be divided between group psychotherapy and other group interventions that can be therapeutic but are primarily designed as recreational groups, psychoeducational groups, discussion groups, or other group applications.

Therapeutic Features of the Group Approach

Although written about adults, Yalom's (1985) classic textbook on group psychotherapy provides an extensive review regarding group theory and practice that we find also useful for those working with children and adolescents. Yalom described features of the group experience that are beneficial and that may be operating regardless of theoretical orientation.

"Installation of Hope"

Installation of hope is important in all forms of therapy and is enhanced in the group experience, especially when the group leader and other members believe in the effectiveness of the treatment. For example, one therapeutic feature of substance-abuse treatment programs is that the leaders are often recovering themselves, providing not only hope to others but modeling success as well.

"Universality"

As many patients feel isolated and alone, the group experience offers support by helping members see that their experiences and feelings are shared by others. Members may feel relief and feel freed up to express their feelings and concerns.

"Imparting Information"

Providing specific information is an integral part of the treatment process in many groups that deal with specific changes. This process can improve the self-esteem of those members providing such support.

"Altruism"

Members of the group learn to support others and provide feedback, which can be important in helping others make significant changes. This process can improve the self-esteem of those members providing such support.

"The Corrective Recapitulation"

Patterns developed in the families of group members are often enacted in the group. Becoming aware of these patterns and developing more adaptive skills often become the work of the group.

"Developing Socializing Techniques"

The development of social skills is a goal of many therapy groups and may be the focus of some. By encouraging feedback, the group provides essential information about problematic relationship skills. By relating to other group members directly, members are able to practice new skills.

"Imitative Behavior"

Members of the group will model the behavior of the therapist and other members in the group. By observing, a group member may then imitate new behavior, which can be very adaptive.

"Group Cohesiveness"

Group cohesiveness relates to a group in which acceptance, support, and positive relationships develop, so that meaningful work can proceed. It may be that the most therapeutic groups are those that are cohesive in nature.

Technical Issues

Composition of the Group

One of the most important tasks of the group therapist is the selection of group members. Generally, it is important to select children of the same developmental level, such as 9- to 12-year-old children, and a range of pathologies that can be contained in a group format. An experienced group therapist may be able to include more difficult patients in a group. It is always essential to prepare patients and their parents for group participation following a careful assessment. In general, for a patient who is suffering from acute psychosis or who is severely withdrawn or too agitated, a group modality is not indicated until the patient has become more stabilized and able to contain group anxieties.

Placing a patient who is different from other members into a group should be done with caution (e.g., a girl in a group where the rest of the members are boys). In general, group sizes ranging from 6 to 12 members are effective; a co-therapist is recommended particularly for groups larger than 8. Whether the group is "closed" (no new members allowed in after the beginning or after a few initial sessions) or "open" (new memberships added from time to time) as well as the duration of the group should be defined from the start. Which possible members would be appropriate depends, in part, on the goals of the treatment and the experience and orientation of the therapist.

Developmental Considerations

Schamess (1976) described four broad diagnostic categories in the treatment of children:

- Groups for children with preoedipal developmental and personality problems
- Groups for "atypical" ego-damaged children
- Groups of "impulse-ridden" acting-out children
- Groups for neurotic children

Schamess (1976) and Schiedlinger (1988), among others, underlined the need for careful matching of diagnostic criteria with the type of group approach. The technique selected—activity, play, art, psychodrama, movement, or combinations—should be tailored to the developmental and the diagnostic considerations of each child. Although this is also true for adolescent group psychotherapy, most therapists put more emphasis on verbal techniques with this age group.

Where and How Group Therapy Is Offered

Outpatient Therapy Groups

Groups for adolescents with relationship problems, identity difficulties, or low self-esteem are a frequent indication. These groups often deal with developmentally appropriate issues related to social skills, identity, self-esteem, and interpersonal relationships. Some of these patients are in other forms of treatment, combining individual or family therapy, while they work on peer relationships skills directly (Azima and Richmond 1989).

These groups may also have a psychoeducational component, during which issues related to sex education or substance abuse can be dealt with. Developing empathy that allows for open discussion of issues along with confrontation is often not enough after a group has developed cohesiveness, at which time children and particularly adolescents want to understand the nature of their problems. Brandes and Gardner (1991) recommended a "para-analytic" approach that allows the therapist "the freedom to interpret present group dynamics in terms of the past, able to teach, direct, support, reassure, coax, argue and be a real person" (p. 73).

Acute Inpatient Therapy Groups

Most inpatient units for children and adolescents weave their inpatient group therapy into overall "milieu" along with individual and family therapy, both emphasizing the need for safety, increasing self-esteem by improving skills and competency, and may include use of behavior modification or a token economy system to shape more appropriate behavior. The inpatient group therapy meetings generally focus on the "here and now" issues for the group members, including the development of social skills and impulse-control issues. These are typically very short term (3–4 weeks) and open-ended and meet more frequently than outpatient groups (up to five times weekly).

For example, a teenager may have difficulty with acting-out anger, typically by being destructive of property or becoming verbally abusive. The group may help set limits on the acting out in a supportive fashion, while encouraging more open communication, insight, and problem solving.

A common behavior in isolated, oppositional children or children with attention-deficit/hyperactivity disorder is provocative behavior. Often such behavior is a maladaptive way to obtain attention that typically backfires. In a group, such behavior may have limits set on it, while more adaptive peer behavior is encouraged and reinforced. With preadolescent and latency-age children, these groups frequently combine talking with play, psychodrama, movement, or art therapy activities.

School-Based Groups

There is extensive experience pointing at the effectiveness of group counseling in schools for a wide variety of children and adolescents. Berkowitz (1975) discussed the indications for groups for emotionally disturbed, special education, physically or developmentally disabled children. Groups for children with posttraumatic stress disorder, children of divorce, and children with parents that abuse drugs or alcohol have become newer and popular applications. School-based groups are led by educational and by clinical professionals. To be effective and ethical, these groups require a good understanding of school systems to maximize the collaboration between education and mental health. Issues such as selection procedures, crisis management, confidentiality, and other special considerations are well reviewed in the literature (Litvak 1991).

Behavioral Pediatrics Groups

Group therapy is also being used in pediatric settings with children who have specific conditions and are grouped together in homogeneous groups for treatment.

The use of group therapy in children, using a psychoeducational approach with behavior therapy along with nutritional education, has been applied in the treatment of obesity. A group is held simultaneously for the children with a separate one run for their parents. The focus is on specific behavior change procedures, such as reducing overeating, adopting a low-fat diet, and increasing exercise. Evidence suggests that results are effective, perhaps for as long as 10 years following treatment (Brownell et al. 1983; Epstein et al. 1990).

Groups for anorexia nervosa and bulimia nervosa tend to incorporate cognitive-behavioral techniques. Therapists focus on common situations or cues that trigger abnormal eating, such as a stressful event preceding an episode of binge eating. Cognitive distortions also are dealt with in a group context.

Support groups for children and adolescents with cancer, hemophilia, sickle cell, diabetes, or other chronic conditions and for their families are also useful.

Groups for Victims of Abuse

Group treatment is one of the most common forms of treatment of childhood victims, although treatment outcome studies are few. Nelki and Waters (1989) reported that six latency-age girls underwent a nine-session group experience, with improvement of presenting problems; others reported similar benefits in overall functioning (Friedrich et al. 1992; Giaretto 1982).

A semistructured approach is often used, helping the child cope with the victimization, including feelings of shame, guilt, and powerlessness; helping to prevent more abuse (using assertiveness training and role-playing); and enabling the child to cope with future goals. An important objective is to validate the victim and the victimization, debunking the notion that somehow the victim caused the problem. Parallel groups run with parents have been proposed both to support the child as well as to prevent further victimization.

Substance Abuse Groups

A group approach is an integral component of the treatment for substance abuse. These groups tend to focus on early recovery and longer-term recovery (Vinogradov and Yalom 1989). Early recovery groups focus on providing support, encouraging sobriety, encouraging joining of Alcoholics Anonymous and Narcotics Anonymous, practicing the use of alternative behaviors to cope instead of becoming intoxicated, and developing a sober peer culture. Often the denial of chemically dependent persons is best confronted persistently during this phase. The group approach here remains intensive, meeting once or twice daily in inpatient programs and several times a week for outpatient programs.

Usually after several months in treatment, the patient becomes involved in ongoing recovery groups. Members focus on the continued goals of abstinence, often now with a focus on relapse prevention. Some groups incorporate cognitive-behavioral techniques, using role-playing to rehearse coping strategies with high-risk situations of feeling states. Patients during this phase will learn about coping with slips while not falling prone to relapse. In addition, a focus at this time is on further developing social skills and relationships (Rachman and Heller 1976).

Some Thoughts About Training

The training of the group therapist consists both of course work related to group therapy and of experience in leading groups under supervision. Some of the important techniques are briefly described.

The group therapist generally focuses on *working in the present* or the "here and now." The group members are encouraged to relate directly with each other as they learn to practice more adaptive relationship skills. Thus the goal of the therapist may be to direct children with conduct difficulties to work as a team, sharing and cooperating to complete an art project, as they learn to cope with frustration in more adaptive ways.

A thorough understanding about *group dynamics* is important for the therapist. A group will develop its own leaders as well as subgroups that may be either therapeutic or destructive to the goals of the group. For example, a child, because of poor social skills, may be excluded or scapegoated by other members of the group. A goal for the therapist is to make this apparent to all the members of the group so that therapeutic goals may be worked on.

The therapist will encourage the use of *consensual validation* (Vinogradov and Yalom 1989), by which a group member may compare his or her views with those of other members of the group. This may provide much peer support for a group member or encouragement to change one's ways. For example, one rebellious adolescent was able to see that some adults occasionally can be supportive of kids when other members of the group disagreed with his particularly negative view of the group leader. Further, he was also encouraged by the other group members to become aware of his angry way of approaching adults who in fact were often trying to support him. Specific procedures that pertain to the patient population will also need to be thoroughly understood by the therapist. For example, a therapist for a group of child abuse victims obviously must also be knowledgeable about child abuse, symptoms of posttraumatic stress disorder, and typical reactions of friends or family members in order to facilitate group discussion of these issues.

In Closing

Group psychotherapy for children and adolescents is an effective treatment modality. When adequate training and supervision are not available, clinicians tend to shy away from this approach. Recent emphasis on briefer and cost-effective therapies is bringing renewed interest in group psychotherapy (Reister and Kraft 1986).

References

Azima FJC, Richmond LH (eds): Adolescent Group Psychotherapy (American Group Psychotherapy Association, Monograph No 4). Madison, CT, International Universities Press, 1989

Berkowitz IH (ed): When Schools Care: Creative Use of Groups in Secondary Schools. New York, Brunner/Mazel, 1975

Brandes NS, Gardner ML (eds): Group Therapy for the Adolescent. Northvale, NJ, Jason Aronson, 1991

Brownell KD, Kelman JH, Stunkard AJ: Treatment of obese children with and without their parents: change in weight and blood pressure. Pediatrics 71:515–523, 1983

Epstein LH, Valoski A, Wing RR, et al: Ten-year follow-up of behavioral, family-based treatment for obese children. JAMA 264:2519–2523, 1990

Friedrich WN, Luecke WJ, Beilke RL, et al: Psychotherapy outcome of sexually abused boys: an agency study. Journal of Interpersonal Violence 7:396–409, 1992

Giaretto H: Integrated Treatment of Child Sexual Abuse: A Treatment and Training Manual. Palo Alto, CA, Science & Behavior Books, 1982

Ginott C: Group Psychotherapy With Children. New York, McGraw-Hill, 1961

Litvak JJ: School based group psychotherapy with adolescents: establishing an effective group program. Journal of Child and Adolescent Group Therapy 1:167–176, 1991

Nelki JS, Waters J: A group for sexually abused young children: unraveling the web. Child Abuse Negl 13:369–377, 1989

Rachman AW, Heller ME: Peer group psychotherapy with adolescent drug abusers. Int J Group Psychother 26:373–384, 1976

Reister AE, Kraft IA (eds): Child Group Psychotherapy: Future Tense (American Group Psychotherapy Association, Monograph No 3). Madison, CT, International Universities Press, 1986

Schamess G: Group treatment modalities for latency age children. Int J Group Psychother 26:455–474, 1976

Schiedlinger S: Focus on Group Psychotherapy: Group Psychotherapy With Children and Adolescents. New York, International Universities Press, 1988

Slavson SR: An Introduction to Group Therapy. New York, Commonwealth Fund, 1943

Vinogradov S, Yalom ID: A Concise Guide to Group Psychotherapy. Washington, DC, American Psychiatric Press, 1989

Yalom ID: The Theory and Practice of Group Psychotherapy, 3rd Edition. New York, Basic Books, 1985

11

Therapeutics IV: Milieu and Behavior Therapies

Robert A. Lobis, M.D.

The rationale for addressing milieu and behavior therapies in the same chapter rests on their common basis: that is, the use of behavioral principles such as reinforcement and extinction to shape or reshape actions. These approaches to treatment involve the practical application of learning theory. The practice of contemporary child and adolescent psychiatry requires familiarity and comfort with these paradigms; familiarity with their limitations and the impossibility of "quick fixes" to complex situations is necessary.

Milieu Therapy

Milieu treatment is the use of a complex, comprehensive structured environment to achieve therapeutic goals. Therapeutic milieus were initially developed in the late 1940s and the 1950s in residential schools through the pioneering work of Bruno Bettelheim (1967) and Fritz Redl (1966), among others. Based on psychoanalytic theories of psychopathology, the early therapeutic milieus sought to foster normative personality development in environments where consistent relationships with skilled staff over time built a sense of security and trust in children with psychiatric disorders and, through a variety of corrective emotional experiences, altered maladaptive patterns of functioning. The early residential schools tended to treat homogeneous populations of children and adolescents who primarily had either pervasive developmental disorders or severe conduct disorders. Today milieu treatment is an essential modality not only in residential schools, but in inpatient psychiatric units for children and adolescents and partial hospitalization programs as well. Today, heterogeneous patient populations are treated in complex, highly structured environments that utilize elements of psychodynamic individual, group, and family psychotherapy as well as psychoeducational and behavior treatment approaches.

Goals of Milieu Treatment

The goals of milieu treatment are largely a function of the type of facility in which treatment is delivered. Inpatient milieu treatment is geared to a short-term length of stay of 1–6 weeks and high patient acuity. Its goals are crisis intervention and stabilization, diagnostic assessment, the development of a long-term treatment plan, initiation of treatment, and preparation to carry on treatment in a less restrictive environment. Day-hospital or partial hospital treatment can be either intermediate (up to 1 year) or long term (greater than 1 year). Here, the milieu is geared to identifying and modifying major maladaptive behavior problems. Because the children and adolescents in day treatment are living at home (although many day-treatment patients may be living in foster homes or group homes), identification and modification of patterns of family dysfunction are also among the goals of treatment, and the design of the treatment milieu should include active family participation. Residential treatment provides long-term milieu treatment. Although it is increasingly common to have family involvement in residential treatment, as studies have shown that most children return home after residential treatment, most residential programs provide a milieu that serves as a replacement for the child's family. The milieu is geared to fostering the development of adaptive and coping skills, which include impulse control, affect tolerance and modulation, interpersonal skills, academic and vocational competencies, and problem-solving skills. The goals of longer-term milieu treatment are the internalization of autonomous patterns of adaptive functioning—that is, the ability consistently to demonstrate adaptive behaviors in the absence of staff supervision, the development of a capacity to form mutually gratifying interpersonal relationships, and the development of stable self-esteem.

General Principles of Milieu Management

Regardless of the nature of the facility or the length of treatment, certain general principles apply to all therapeutic milieus:

- Treatment is delivered by a multidisciplinary team.
- The milieu is highly structured.
- There is an integrated array of treatment modalities—psychodynamic, cognitive-behavioral, biological.
- The treatment focus is simultaneously individual, group, and family oriented.
- The peer group will be the most powerful agent for change and growth if harnessed and channeled appropriately. (Conversely, unharnessed or ineffectively channeled peer group processes will invariably lead to disruptive acting out, regressive behavior, aggravation of existing psychopathology, and antitherapeutic outcomes.)
- Moment-to-moment unplanned daily encounters in the milieu among patients and between patients and staff provide valuable diagnostic information and essential grist for the psychotherapeutic mill. This is Fritz Redl's (1966) concept of the "life space interview." A life space interview is conducted by any member of the staff who intervenes with a child as close in space and time as possible when a significant event occurs in the milieu and provides psychotherapeutic input based on accurate understanding of the child then and there.

Organization of Treatment Teams

Milieu treatment teams vary in their organization. Some are hierarchically organized, and the functions of team members are specialized, often along traditional lines. For example, the child and adolescent psychiatrist performs the psychiatric evaluation, medical workup, and medication management; the psychologist does testing; the social worker does the psychosocial assessment and family work; the nurse develops the daily behavioral care plan; and the counselors or psychiatric technicians provide the limit-setting and life space interventions. This type of organization is most common in inpatient hospital milieus where division of labor and specialization may be the most efficient way to achieve the goals and objectives of a short-term hospitalization. Other milieu treatment teams may be organized in a more egalitarian model in which all clinical staff serve as primary therapists for some children, performing any or all of the above functions with the assistance of other members of the treatment team. Regardless of the model employed, the administrative and functional organization of the milieu must be unambiguous, agreed-to by all members of the staff, and clear to the patients and their families. Regardless, too, of the model employed, each child should have one staff member with whom he or she has a primary relationship, and each case must have one staff member who is primarily responsible for managing the treatment. Ideally, the primary therapist and the case manager should be one in the same; however, this is often not possible, nor is it necessarily essential for an adequate treatment outcome.

Although the basic philosophies and general therapeutic principles of milieu treatment may be applicable to all of the children who are patients in it, milieu treatment is not generic treatment. An individualized treatment plan, based on thorough diagnostic assessment, must be developed for each child, and the structure of the milieu must be such that it facilitates individual diagnosis and treatment. This can be best done through a *problem-oriented approach* to assessment and treatment planning. For each child, in addition to DSM-IV (American Psychiatric Association 1994) multiaxial diagnoses, a problem list of target symptoms and maladaptive behaviors is developed. For each problem a goal is set. Goals may be long or short term, and achievement of certain goals serve as end points for various phases of a child's treatment. For each goal there will be a series of objectives to be attained. These objectives should be concrete, specific, and, if possible, measurable. For example, one goal for a child with a disruptive behavior disorder might be "develop cooperative behavior." Concrete objectives might include "follow staff directions," "fewer than three time-outs per day," "waits his turn in games," and "verbalizes anger instead of hitting."

Levels System

The most common way in which the process of diagnostic assessment, treatment planning, and treatment implementation by problems, goals, and objectives is structured into a therapeutic milieu is via a levels system. Patients progress through the levels system by cooperating with their evaluation, learning and obeying the basic rules of the program, identifying problems, setting goals, and attaining objectives. Problem identification and goal setting become the major focus of many individual group and family therapy sessions. Attainment of specific objectives becomes the way in which patients progress through the levels system. The levels system provides incentives for patients to cooperate with their evaluation and treatment through a series of decreasing restrictions and increasing rewards, privileges, and responsibilities. Performance is generally rated with a point system, and earning a certain number of points becomes the way in which children maintain their level or move up to the next higher level. Points are given for following program rules, displaying socially appropriate behaviors, and working on individual problems and toward individual goals. Attitude as well as performance can be rated. Rating should be not only by program staff but also by peers and by self-rating so as to promote positive peer group cohesion and individual responsibility. A levels system thus provides a context for making children aware of their problem behaviors, affords numerous opportunities for problem definition, and allows for clear unambiguous feedback from staff and peers.

Rules

The rules of the therapeutic milieu are important not only for maintaining order but for enunciating basic treatment goals. Program rules should be framed in positive language so as to emphasize the prosocial, nonpunitive nature of the milieu. Common examples of cardinal rules are

- Safety for oneself and others
- Caring for oneself and others
- Honesty with oneself and others
- Respect for oneself and others
- Responsibility for oneself and others

Beyond such fundamental rules there need to be standards of acceptable behavior that set clear behavioral expectations and consequences for misbehavior. Therapeutic milieu rules need to deal with aggressive and abusive behaviors, instigating and noncompliant behaviors, property destruction, sexual acting out, drug use, care of the environment, bedtimes, passes, and activities of daily living.

Behavior Management

The structured therapeutic milieu found in most inpatient, day-treatment, and residential programs today employs a variety of behavioral techniques as well as psychodynamic psychotherapeutic ones. Levels systems, point systems, token economies, star charts, time-out, and other techniques aimed at shaping adaptive behaviors are applications of operant conditioning. In addition, therapy groups and individual interventions frequently employ cognitive therapy methodology. Cognitive therapy attempts to change maladaptive behavior and dysphoric or negative feelings by changing thinking patterns. Children are encouraged to control themselves by "stopping, looking, and listening." They are actively instructed in nonaggressive self-assertion and problem solving. Events are reframed by staff in more positive language; maladaptive basic assumptions and beliefs are challenged; and more adaptive alternatives are proposed.

Reinforcers that provide incentives for adaptive behaviors and active involvement in treatment must be chosen carefully. Reinforcers must be appropriate to patients' developmental ages and must be socioeconomically and culturally appropriate. Most importantly, reinforcers must be valued by the program staff, since reinforcers ultimately have value in the context of the relationships developed in the milieu and the milieu's culture. Ideally, reinforcers should be only positive; however, many patients with conduct disorders from dysfunctional families will initially only understand and respond to negative (i.e., punitive) reinforcers. A good therapeutic milieu utilizes a mix of positive and negative reinforcers; proper balance is essential or the program will be perceived as either too punitive or too permissive. Positive reinforcers include 1) tangible rewards such as food or age-appropriate prizes (toys, games, T-shirts, posters) that may be earned or purchased via a point system or token economy; 2) special time with a chosen staff member; 3) special activities which may be individual (e.g., use of video games) or group rewards (outings, use of a special lounge or workshop); 4) additional special privileges (e.g., bedtimes, visitors, special possessions, additional telephone time); and 5) special status in the milieu (officer of patient government, mentor to new patients).

Reinforcers can provide incentives for not only individual progress in treatment but group progress by adherence to norms of responsibility, cooperation, and maintenance of a positive peer culture in the milieu. Negative reinforcers include loss of privileges, dropping a level, community service, and makeup tasks (such as worksheets that teach constructive alternatives to the misbehaviors that occasioned the negative reinforcement). Time-out as well as various degrees of restriction (to hall or unit, to room, to a "quiet room") are also frequently used as negative reinforcers to attempt to decrease the occurrence of maladaptive behaviors. To be effective, reinforcers must be applied immediately, consistently, and in a nonpunitive manner. The reason for the application of the restriction or loss of status must be clearly stated to the patient, and there should be adequate time devoted to processing the experience with the patient once the patient is calm and in control so that positive alternative behaviors may be learned. Because many patients in residential, day-treatment, and inpatient milieus are impulse-ridden youth with long-standing, severe disruptive behavior disorders, time-out procedures and restrictions are utilized frequently. It is best if they are carried out by staff with an air of firm reasonableness and dispassionate authority; staff should, at all times, model self-control and well-modulated affect.

It is essential that the rules governing the milieu, the levels system, and the behavior management system employed in the milieu be thoroughly explained in advance to the patients and to their parents. It is important that staff gain parents' understanding and support. When this does not happen, the patient may play his or her family against the staff, thereby undermining the treatment. When parents have an alliance with the milieu staff, they often will spontaneously adopt many of the elements of the program's behavior management system at home. Many day programs specifically structure such roles for parents to extend the impact of the milieu. Parent groups also focus on teaching limit setting and instruct parents in the proper use of time-out procedures. Involving parents in administering the milieu behavioral system is a very effective structural family intervention that often has long-lasting beneficial effects on dysfunctional families.

Group Therapy

The therapeutic milieu may be viewed as a continuous complex group process that is subdivided into specific formal groups as well as many informal but no less important interactions. Formal groups will vary as to degree of structure, direction, focus, and composition. Therapy groups will tend to be more traditional (i.e., open ended and non-directive) in longer-term programs. They will be more focused on problems and goals and more directive in short-term programs. Most milieus include specialized groups dealing, for example, with substance abuse, sexual abuse, or divorce. Some groups may take a pronounced educational approach. Activities groups are extremely useful in mobilizing important issues and dealing concretely with such problem areas as trust, cooperation, delay of gratification, planning, and problem solving. A broad range of activities groups would include physical activities such as athletics, movement therapy, adventure-based activities, and art and music therapy. All milieus should have regular community meetings where all patients and staff address the day-to-day state of the milieu and acknowledge the comings and goings of patients and staff. Much therapeutic milieu activity in groups and individual encounters consists of *social skills training*. Social skills training is a composite of cognitive-behavioral and didactic techniques that teach children how to behave in a variety of social situations, how to make friends, how to play, how to carry on a conversation, how to be assertive, and how to manage stress. Role-playing, modeling procedures, and instructional techniques may all be employed in social skills training.

Individual Therapy

Individual psychotherapy, which historically was isolated from the daily workings of treatment milieus, is much more helpful when it is integrated with overall milieu treatment and addresses the specific problems, goals, and objectives of the child's treatment plan. The individual therapist's intimate knowledge of the child's day-to-day behavior in the milieu allows the therapist to link these behaviors to the child's inner feeling states and motivations. Working in this way, the individual therapist and the child can identify patterns, repetitions, themes, and the projections and displacements of intrapsychic conflict into the milieu.

Family Therapy

The interplay between the milieu life and family life likewise has great psychotherapeutic potential. Knowledge of the child's role in the family system sheds light on the child's behavior in the milieu. Conversely, the pattern of maladaptive relationships that the child creates in the milieu sheds light on dysfunctional relationships in the family system, which might not otherwise be revealed in the family therapy sessions. Families should be actively involved with the milieu throughout all stages of the treatment process. During the assessment phase, family problems and family goals and objectives should be developed concurrently with individual ones. Families should be involved in the treatment planning process, and their support of the treatment plan should be viewed as essential for successful treatment outcome. This includes discharge planning, which should begin at the time of a child's admission to the program. In addition to family therapy or family counseling, parent groups, multifamily groups, and family activities are useful components of milieu treatment.

Education

School is another essential part of the therapeutic milieu. An educational assessment should be part of each child's comprehensive initial evaluation. Impaired academic functioning is one of the most sensitive indicators of psychopathology in children and adolescents. Moreover, there is a high incidence of undiagnosed learning disorders in the population admitted to inpatient, day-treatment, and residential programs. School has great therapeutic usefulness in fostering cognitive controls over behavior disorders, as well as helping to develop a variety of coping, adaptive, and social skills. There is a synergy between academic progress and therapeutic progress. Academic achievement in the supportive, understanding atmosphere of the therapeutic milieu increases the child's sense of confidence and mastery, thereby enhancing the child's self-esteem.

Staff Considerations

The organization, development, and maintenance of the staff of the treatment program is a vitally important aspect of the therapeutic milieu. A milieu, no matter how well developed its program and experienced its staff, will not be therapeutic unless morale is high and communication and teamwork are good. A program must have leadership that has authority as well as responsibility for directing the program. Staff roles and job descriptions must be clear. Communication, written and verbal, should be oriented around the specifics of each child's treatment plan. Regularly scheduled rounds, team meetings, case conferences, and staff meetings should be programmed into the milieu. Rounds are for daily chores, dealing with acute events, and managing the milieu-as-a-whole. Team meetings are for pulling together diagnostic assessments, developing the individual child's treatment plan, and reviewing the progress of treatment in depth. (It is often useful to have the child and occasionally the family participate in team meetings.) Case conferences are important for staff development. They may focus on especially interesting or difficult cases and provide an opportunity for input from invited consultants from outside the program. Staff meetings deal with issues of staff morale and its effect on the milieu, institutional issues and their effects on the milieu, and staff countertransferences to difficult patients or families. Although staff meetings deal with staff feelings and dynamics, they are not and should not be run as therapy groups. Staff meetings may also be used for program development and revision, although sometimes separate meetings, committees, or task forces are created for this purpose.

Behavior and Cognitive Therapy

Children and adolescents commonly manifest the signs and symptoms of psychiatric disorder in overt behavior. Therefore, the assessment and modification of behavior plays a major role in the treatment of clinical dysfunction. A fundamental assumption underlying the behavioral and cognitive therapeutic approaches is that most behavior develops and is maintained according to the principles of learning. Within the field of child behavior therapy, a dominant conceptual point of view is a "social learning" theory of behavior, which highlights the importance of both cognitive and environmental influences and their reciprocal interaction. Many disorders in children and adolescents are directly related to the psychosocial adjustment and functioning of their parents. Behavior therapy conducted in isolation often fails to achieve clinically meaningful results because it excludes the role of parental or familial dysfunction. Therefore, it is generally recommended that behavioral interventions be combined with some form of family therapy in the treatment of disorders such as disruptive behavior disorders, eating disorders, separation anxiety disorders, and any other conditions where a problem behavior or symptom is both amenable to behavioral techniques and has functional significance within the identified patient's family system.

Behavioral and cognitive treatments are applied in many different settings outside the child and adolescent psychiatrist's office, including the home, school, hospital, and residential facility. Although some types of behavior therapy involve seeing children and adolescents in individual sessions, it is more common for therapists to work with and through those who are responsible for the care, education, and management of children—that is, parents, teachers, and institutional staff. This is desirable and often necessary because treatment is usually more effective in the child's everyday environment than in the therapist's office. Behavior problems are often situation specific and can best be treated in those situations where they are occurring. Furthermore, those who care for the child often unwittingly perpetuate problem behaviors, so that changing the behaviors of those in contact with the child is often a prerequisite for effective treatment.

Evaluating Behavior Problems

- Obtain specific examples of the child's or adolescent's recurring problematic behaviors. The use of rating scales such as the Child Behavior Checklist (Achenback and Edelbrock 1983) or the Conners Teacher and Parent Questionnaires (Conners 1989) is often helpful.
- Identify antecedents and consequences to the specific behaviors to determine precipitants and to ascertain whether parents are inadvertently reinforcing the behaviors that they wish to control or abolish.
- Ask parents what they think is responsible for the child's problem behavior. This yields useful information about the parents' cognitions regarding the child.
- Assess the child's level of awareness, level of understanding of his or her problem behaviors, and extent to which the child feels responsible and willing to change these behaviors.

Treatment Approaches

Behavior therapy and cognitive therapy focus on observable behavior. These approaches do not concern themselves with remote or underlying "causes" of behavior, but rather focus on environmental contingencies immediately antecedent to the behavior. A second important feature of behavioral and cognitive approaches is the setting of clear and precise treatment goals. Third, treatment is action oriented and directive, following from the assumption that action rather than insight is the primary mechanism for change. Psychodynamic interpretation is rarely used.

Behavioral techniques designed to strengthen, develop, or maintain behavior are based on *classical and operant conditioning*. The fundamental principle here is reinforcement of those behaviors that the therapy aims to promote. With *positive reinforcement* a reinforcer or reward is given after the occurrence of the desired behavior. With a *negative reinforcement*, the reinforcer involves the removal of some negative stimulus after the behavior occurs. Positive and negative reinforcement differ from punishment because their purpose is to increase the likelihood that a particular behavior will occur. Punishment, on the other hand, is employed to reduce the incidence of a particular behavior. Reinforcers may be either tangible items such as food, money, prizes, or privileges, or intangible such as praise, encouragement, and other social reinforcers. Reinforcers that signal that tangible reinforcement is forthcoming are called "conditioned reinforcers."

Behavioral programs that use conditioned reinforcers systematically are generally known as *token economies*. *Modeling*, another technique designed to increase the occurrence of certain behaviors, involves having the child or adolescent observe a model engage in a particular behavior for the purpose of having the child reproduce that behavior. In *social skills training* and *cognitive skills training*, skills are taught through a combination of positive reinforcement, modeling, coaching, instruction, role-playing, and behavioral rehearsal. *Problem-solving techniques* focus on teaching children certain cognitive mediational skills that help them to regulate their behaviors in various situations. Children are taught to use self-statements to identify their problems, generate alternative solutions, decide on one particular solution, evaluate the outcome of their choice, and provide themselves with positive self-reinforcement.

Behavioral techniques designed to reduce or eliminate behavior include *extinction* processes, where reinforcement is withheld after a particular response so as to reduce the frequency of its occurrence, and *differential reinforcement*, in which a child is reinforced for not displaying the problem behavior during a specified time or is reinforced for displaying an appropriate behavior that is incompatible with the problem behavior.

Punishment is often used with the assumption that the introduction of an aversive stimulus such as scolding, spanking, or removal of privileges will extinguish unwanted behaviors. Punishment has many disadvantages. It tends to suppress behavior temporarily rather than actually change it. It may produce serious and unwanted side effects such as the promotion of fear responses, the strengthening of avoidant behaviors, paradoxical reinforcement, and strengthening of the undesirable target behaviors through the negative attention that a child receives during punishment and the learning of undesirable behaviors that are modeled for the child by the punisher such as aggressive physical or verbal behavior and disrespect for the rights of others. The most common punishment procedure used with a minimum of unwanted side effects is time-out. Here a lack of opportunity to obtain reinforcers and social isolation are used to extinguish behavior. In token economies, payment for misbehavior through loss of tokens or points is a common technique aimed at eliminating unwanted behaviors.

Desensitization refers to a group of behavioral techniques based on classical conditioning principles that are used to reduce children's fears. In systematic desensitization a child first works with a therapist to establish a hierarchy of fears about the anxiety-provoking stimulus. Once the fear hierarchy is established the child is helped to feel relaxed by talking to the therapist or a parent, playing quietly, eating a favorite food, or learning muscle relaxation. Relaxation is encouraged because it is incompatible with anxiety responses. Once the child is relaxed the therapist asks the child to imagine the least distressing scene in the fear hierarchy and to indicate if the scene remains distressing. If the scene continues to elicit anxiety, the child is instructed to relax again and then the procedure is repeated until the same scene no longer elicits anxiety on three successive presentations. The therapist repeats this procedure with each successive item in the fear hierarchy until the child no longer reports being distressed by the feared stimulus. In vivo desensitization techniques involve the child's undergoing exposure training to a fear hierarchy in the actual situations producing anxiety rather than through imagined scenes.

Because problem behaviors are often developed and sustained in the home by maladaptive parent-child interactions, procedures that train parents to alter their children's behavior at home are an important part of the behavior therapy armamentarium. In *parent management training* parents are trained to observe, identify, and define problem behaviors in new ways. For example, parents may give in to a child's temper tantrums out of a wish to stop this negative behavior. They may be surprised to learn that this actually increases the likelihood that such behaviors will recur in the future. In parent management training parents are taught to reward appropriate behaviors with attention, praise, tokens, or points and to punish problem behaviors with time-out, loss of privileges, or loss of points. Parents are directed to try their skills initially on relatively simple behaviors where they are likely to be successful. This helps parents to reestablish an atmosphere of parental authority at home. As they become more proficient, parents can address more severely problematic behaviors.

Cognitive therapy techniques, when used in combination with behavior therapy, are powerful tools in the treatment of child and adolescent psychiatric disorders. This approach is now commonly called cognitive-behavior therapy. It assumes that children with disruptive behavior disorders suffer from a deficiency or inability to apply cognitive skills appropriately. Such children tend to generate fewer alternative solutions to interpersonal problems, tend to overlook the intermediate steps between impulses and outcomes, tend to see fewer consequences to their behaviors, tend to fail to recognize the causes of other people's behaviors, and tend to be less sensitive to interpersonal conflicts arising from the behaviors of themselves and others. Accordingly, cognitive-behavior therapy attempts to develop cognitive skills that address these deficiencies, such as alternative solution thinking and means-ends thinking, which develop awareness of the steps required to achieve particular goals as well as sensitivity to interpersonal problems. So-called internalizing types of psychiatric disorders such as depressive and anxiety disorders are assumed to result from cognitive distortions rather than inadequate cognitive development. Such cognitive distortions include errors in thinking, misperceptions, and mistaken assumptions or attribution. In approaching cognitive therapy with children and adolescents, due attention must be paid to their level of cognitive and affective development. Three cognitive-behavior treatment approaches commonly used with children and adolescents are problem-solving training, verbal self-instruction training, and attribution retraining.

Problem-solving training may focus solely on the child or may include the child's parents. It may be applied in individual or group formats. Problem-solving training is useful for helping aggressive and impulsive children as well as hyperactive children. In problem-solving training the first step is to teach children age-appropriate cognitive techniques for inhibiting their aggressive or impulsive behaviors. These include such things as the "turtle response" for young children where they are taught to draw in their arms and legs and lower their head "like a turtle," or the "stop, look, and listen" response for older children. The next step is to teach the child relaxation techniques to decrease the stress and urgency of the situation. Then problem-solving skills are taught via modeling, role-playing, or didactic instruction. These three steps are coupled with the process of behavioral goal setting and rewards for attaining the targeted goals.

In *verbal self-instruction training* children are taught self-directed statements that they use to guide themselves through a problem-solving process. Self-instruction training teaches children a thinking strategy that may be utilized in a variety of settings. Therapists may either provide children with appropriate self-statements or help them to develop their own. By repeating to themselves simple relevant instructions, children may improve their abilities to stay on-task, to refrain from becoming assaultive, to label feeling states, to persist in tasks and thereby improve frustration intolerance, to maintain adequate self-esteem through self-praise and self-forgiveness, and to exercise specific problem-solving strategies. Verbal self-instruction training is useful for hyperactive, impulsive, and aggressive children.

Attribution retraining targets the explanations children have of problematic behaviors and events. Children may incorrectly attribute externally determined events to internal causes (e.g., "my parents are getting a divorce because I am bad") and vice versa (e.g., "your telling me to go to my seat made me punch the wall"), or attributions may be inaccurate and self-derogatory (e.g., "I failed because I'm no good"). Children are trained to learn more appropriate or more adaptive explanations (e.g., "failure means you should try harder," or "failure means you need a different strategy"). Attribution retraining assumes that having more appropriate explanations of problem behaviors will lead children to perform better.

Behavior and Cognitive-Behavior Treatment of Specific Disorders of Children and Adolescents

As indicated above, cognitive-behavior techniques are widely employed primarily in the treatment of disruptive disorders in children and adolescents. Current approaches to disruptive disorders generally consist of combinations of reinforcement paradigms, cognitive-behavior strategies (especially problem-solving training and self-instruction training), and parent training and family therapy.

Anxiety disorders, including separation anxiety disorder and phobic disorders as well as *obsessive-compulsive disorders,* may also be treated with cognitive-behavior techniques. Extinction and systematic desensitization paradigms are employed to decondition anxiety responses. Relaxation training is also frequently used for children and adolescents with anxiety disorders. Verbal self-instruction training and attribution retraining are useful in the treatment of obsessive-compulsive disorders.

In the cognitive-behavior treatment of *depression,* self-instruction training is especially useful. Children may be taught to monitor negative self-attributions, to evaluate the appropriateness of these attributions, and then to self-reinforce alternative positive self-attributions. Teaching children to set realistic goals, to refrain from punitive self-statements, and to utilize positive self-statements is also helpful.

Behavioral techniques are commonly used in the treatment of *pervasive developmental disorders* (PDD) and *mental retardation.* Contingency reinforcement is used to increase the frequency of developmentally and socially appropriate behaviors. The choice of reinforcers for PDD children can be difficult because many things that children typically like are of no interest to them. With PDD children many social reinforcers (e.g., hugs) may be experienced as aversive and therefore may actually decrease the frequency of the desired behavior. As a rule it is advantageous to utilize the most developmentally advanced and socially interactive reinforcers possible. Food is always useful as a reinforcer. Severely autistic children, if all else fails, may be allowed brief periods of self-stimulatory behavior as reinforcers for communicative speech acquisition. In contrast to PDD children, mentally retarded children respond readily to a wide variety of material and social reinforcers. Prompting and behavior-shaping techniques attempt to teach, model, encourage, and combine small pieces of behavior, leading to the establishment of more sustained and complex socially interactive behaviors. Extinction approaches and time-out are not very effective with PDD children but are useful in altering the behavior of mentally retarded children. Other "punitive" behavioral techniques should not be considered for any behaviors other than severe self-injury.

Cognitive-behavior techniques are also commonly used for treating eating disorders. In the treatment of *anorexia nervosa,* contingent reinforcement is used for gaining and maintaining normal weight and for maintaining normal eating habits. Restriction or increased allowance of physical activity is an especially powerful reinforcer for anorexic patients. Generally, comprehensive protocols or structured programs are used, and privileges, hospital admission, or discharge are tied to the attainment of certain specified behavioral goals. Anorexic patients frequently have many cognitive distortions regarding their bodies and food. They tend to overuse dichotomous, all-or-nothing thinking, magical thinking, egocentric thinking, overestimation, and overgeneralization. Anorexic patients almost always have serious deficits in self-esteem and self-concept and are therefore especially suitable candidates for cognitive therapy. For patients with *bulimia nervosa,* behavior therapy protocols are focused on bingeing and purging behaviors rather than on weight per se. Self-monitoring is a widely used technique in which patients keep a careful diary of their eating behaviors. Education regarding the metabolic and physiologic consequences of bulimia nervosa, structured eating plans, and contingency reinforcement to reward following the plan and to discourage bingeing and purging are all commonly employed techniques. Cognitive therapeutic approaches address the same cognitive distortions as with anorexic patients and use the same basic cognitive therapy techniques.

Cognitive-behavior techniques used in the treatment of *tic disorders* include self-monitoring, contingent reinforcement, and relaxation training.

The behavior treatment of *enuresis* is a highly effective yet frequently overlooked approach. Alarm systems for nocturnal enuresis are especially effective. With newer systems a few drops of urine will complete an electrical circuit and trigger an alarm. The alarm causes the child to contract the external bladder sphincter. Increased sensitivity to nocturnal bladder contractions and increased inhibitions of the micturition reflex are conditioned generally within several weeks. If treatment is continued during 3 successive weeks of dry nights, there is a 70% long-term cure rate. It is striking to note that despite this dramatic success rate, only 3% of enuretic children have this treatment prescribed. Positive reinforcement behavior therapy combined with educational and supportive therapy has been reported to yield significant improvement in two-thirds of *encopretic children*.

References

Achenback TM, Edelbrock C: Manual for the Child Behavior Checklist and Revised Child Behavior Profile. Burlington, VT, University Associates in Psychiatry, 1983

American Psychiatric Association: Diagnostic and Statistical Manual of Mental Disorders, 4th Edition. Washington, DC, American Psychiatric Association, 1994

Bettelheim B: The Empty Fortress: Infantile Autism and the Birth of the Self. New York, Free Press, 1967

Conners CK: Conners' Rating Scales. North Tonawanda, NY, Multi-Health Systems, 1989

Redl F: When We Deal With Children. New York, Free Press, 1966

Suggested Reading

Milieu Therapy

Adler J: Fundamentals of Group Child Care. Cambridge, MA, Ballinger, 1981

American Psychiatric Association: Treatments of Psychiatric Disorders: A Task Force Report of the American Psychiatric Association. Washington, DC, American Psychiatric Association, 1989

Lymn R, Prentice-Dunn S, Gagel S: Residential and Inpatient Treatment of Children and Adolescents. New York, Plenum, 1989
Schulman, J, Irwin M: Psychiatric Hospitalization of Children. Springfield, IL, Charles C Thomas, 1982

Behavior Therapy

Braswell L, Kendall P: Cognitive-behavioral methods with children, in Handbook of Cognitive-Behavioral Therapies. Edited by Dobson K. New York, Guilford, 1988, pp 167–213
Kazdin A: Advances in child behavior therapy, in Basic Handbook of Child Psychiatry, Vol 5. Edited by Noshpitz JD. New York, Basic Books, 1987, pp 405–413
Vitulano L, Tebes J: Child and adolescent behavior therapy, in Child and Adolescent Psychiatry. Edited by Lewis M. Baltimore, MD, Williams & Wilkins, 1991, pp 812–831

12

Therapeutics V: Treatment of Severely Disturbed Children and Adolescents

V. Susan Villani, M.D.

Treatment of the severely disturbed child is one of the most challenging aspects of child and adolescent psychiatry. It requires the child psychiatrist to be knowledgeable in all areas of the field; to be able to integrate information about the child into a comprehensive, yet focused treatment plan; and to serve actively as an advocate for the child in the face of ever-dwindling resources and funding. Although there is clearly science involved, particularly with the increased application of psychopharmacology to children, treating severely disturbed children and adolescents is an artful process that often occurs over a span of years and requires considerable dedication on the part of clinicians, family, and school.

The hallmark of severe disturbance is the interference into all aspects of the child's life, from home, to school, to peers. This is not isolated to any one diagnosis and can occur with all diagnoses. Some diagnoses, however, are more commonly represented in the severely disturbed population, and certain early childhood symptoms make one more concerned that severe disturbance is on the horizon. The more common diagnoses include autism, pervasive developmental disorder, childhood schizophrenia, affective disorders, and conduct disorders. The early childhood symptoms include marked language delays, persistent aggression toward others, self-injurious behaviors, and inappropriate sexual behavior. Often attention-deficit/hyperactivity disorder is diagnosed early and is extreme in nature. This may persist and coexist with other diagnoses, complicating management and treatment. An additional group of children at extreme risk for severe disturbance are those who suffer chronic sustained physical or sexual abuse. These children often present with an array of symptomatology that is frequently difficult to categorize using DSM-IV (American Psychiatric Association 1994) classification. Pine's (1982) description of the "borderline child" and more recently Terr's (1991) work describing a schema for understanding trauma in childhood are particularly useful in this regard. Also, comorbid diagnoses of attention-deficit/hyperactivity disorder, learning disabilities, or mild neurologic impairment increase the child's vulnerability to abuse, and decrease the subsequent resiliency to such trauma.

From a different vantage point, the Child and Adolescent Service System Program (CASSP), a division of the National Institute of Mental Health, has defined nationally those children and adolescents at risk to become seriously mentally ill or severely emotionally disturbed, as a result of either environmental or biological factors or both (Table 12–1). Their grouping includes, but is not limited to, those youth who are homeless, either as a family unit or alone; those living with parent(s) who are unable to provide adequate care and nurturing, including drug-addicted parents; those who have been victims of violence; those who abuse drugs; those who are infected with the human immunodeficiency virus; and those who have a family history

Table 12–1. Children at risk for serious mental illness

Homeless children	Children who abuse drugs
Children of drug-addicted parents	HIV-infected children
Children who are victims of violence	Children with family history of psychiatric illness

Note. HIV = human immunodeficiency virus.

of psychiatric illness. The CASSP project work has led to greater emphasis on working with children and adolescents within the context of home; customizing treatment planning and problem management, building on the strengths of the child, the family, and the culture; and taking full advantage of resources within the community. Many children who come to the attention of child psychiatrists through psychiatric emergencies of a severe and compelling nature are often well known to agencies and organizations within their communities. Helping to develop, and to be involved with in an ongoing way, the delivery of care to this population earlier is under the increasing purview of the child psychiatrist.

Planning for the Severely Disturbed Child

The outpatient assessment of the severely disturbed child differs from that of the less disturbed child in both scope and depth (Table 12–2). In addition to performing the usual interviews of family and child, acquiring information from schools, pediatrician, and community agencies is essential. Thorough psychological testing, including neuropsychological testing, can be extremely useful, yet is time-consuming and often hard to perform with children, who by the very nature of their problems are often unable to cooperate for long periods of time. Home visits, and extended assessment through multiple home visits, are now utilized to circumvent the need for more costly interventions such as hospitalization.

Although some severely disturbed children can be assessed as outpatients, frequently there is a need to contain the child safely within a hospital to diagnose and plan for treatment. In addition to providing safety, the inpatient evaluation allows a more complete

Table 12–2. Assessment of the severely disturbed child

Interviews of child	Psychological testing/neuropsychological testing
Family interviews	Home visits/extended home visits
School history	Hospital assessment/milieu assessment
Pediatric history	Psychopharmacology evaluation
Community agency history	

picture of the child's functioning to emerge through observations of the child within the context of the therapeutic milieu. With the advent of health maintenance organizations, managed care, and other cost-containment measures, inpatient hospitalization should be reserved for only the most troubled and dangerous, but still clearly is necessary when issues of safety to self or others are of concern. In terms of risk management, child psychiatrists must keep this in mind when other assessment and treatment techniques have failed, and the child continues to be dangerous or the child's functioning is deteriorating. One must be prepared to explain in detail to third-party payers why the child cannot be safely managed as an outpatient, and exactly what the risks of doing so are.

Hospitalization may also be beneficial when there is a need to assess psychopharmacologic interventions. Careful trials of medications, and often combinations of medications, need to be pursued. Lithium in younger children and medications to manage anxiety and hyperactivity, such as clonidine and methylphenidate, may be helpful and warrant clinical trials. The unstable and inconsistent home environment of many severely disturbed children can make outpatient medication trials virtually impossible to administer safely, much less to determine efficacy accurately. Given that medications can render the child more able to function in a less restrictive setting, one must make every attempt to resolve clearly the role that medication, or even unusual combinations of medications, can play for the child.

Once the child is thoroughly assessed, a crucial part of planning includes deciding whether treatment can occur with the child in a home setting, or whether the disturbance is of such magnitude to warrant placement in an intensive treatment setting (Table 12–3). If the child can be safely maintained at home, in a foster home, or in a specialized foster home, treatment services are planned using the concept of "wrapping the services around the child." This may include provision of special school services, home-based family treatment with a team that actually enters the home for frequent sessions, respite services for families, or day treatment for the child in combination with family in-home services. The clear emphasis is on doing whatever is necessary for the child to be able to be safely maintained at home. Maintenance cannot, however, be the only goal of such interventions.

Table 12–3. Levels of intervention for severely disturbed children

- Child at home
  - Outpatient treatment once or twice a week
  - Special school services
- Child at home
  - Day-hospital treatment
- Child at home with home-based treatment
- Child at home with home-based treatment plus outpatient treatment, day-hospital treatment, and/or special school services
- Foster home
  - Foster home or specialized foster home with services as above
- Group home, combined with outpatient treatment and/or special school services
- Residential treatment facility
  - School on grounds
  - School off grounds
  - Facility staff secure
  - Facility locked
- Hospital-based treatment
  - Unlocked hospital
  - Locked hospital (maximum security)

A keen clinical eye must be watchful for signs of subtle behavioral deterioration, lack of developmental progress, or failure to progress with learning in school. The clinician will need to document clearly and specifically what the risks of not pursuing the next level of treatment are and to predict the cost to the system.

If in-home treatment is unsuccessful, treatment out of the home should be chosen carefully. The types of residential placements available can vary from locale to locale, but usually consist of the options listed below.

Hospital-Based Treatment

There are very few hospitals that provide long-term psychiatric treatment for children. The few that remain are reserved for the most disturbed children whose management 24 hours a day requires monitoring by nurses and physicians. This includes the chronically suicidal or homicidal child, the child with severe self-mutilating behavior, the child with either frequent or extreme violent episodes, the child with severe anorexia nervosa, or the child with coexisting medical illness whose psychological condition interferes with the medical management. Diabetic children, asthmatic children, and children with seizure disorders can warrant this level of intensive intervention. Given the cost of hospital treatment, there is considerable pressure to move the child as quickly as possible to a less restrictive setting. Careful documentation, with clearly articulated treatment goals, is essential if the child's stay is to be paid for by third-party insurance. In some states, the public sector serves as a safety net for this population when all other payment has been exhausted. Increasingly, public sector hospitals are reimbursed by Medicaid dollars, and the scrutiny about utilization is becoming equal to that in the private sector. It can be quite difficult to treat the child when there are considerable external pressures to move the child to a less costly and less restrictive setting. For children who have had frequent disruptions and instability of their living situations in their past, and for those children vulnerable to regression around treatment interruptions, this can be particularly troublesome. To the extent that those treating and those paying can come to an agreement regarding what is to be accomplished during hospitalization as well as the projected length of stay necessary at the treatment planning stage, the child's treatment can move along more smoothly. Clinical case conferences with consultants outside of the treatment team can serve to facilitate treatment and ensure payers that focused treatment is occurring.

Residential Treatment Centers

Residential treatment centers provide the child with 24-hours-a-day structured treatment, without the full range of medical services present in a hospital. The degree of security and intensity of services can vary considerably from locked residential treatment centers to centers that are residential schools. Staffing consists of child-care workers, social workers, teachers, a few psychologists, and usually a consulting child psychiatrist. Some programs also employ a psychiatric nurse and occupational and recreational therapists. Most frequently, educational services are provided on the grounds of the center to decrease the stress often associated with transitions and to provide a consistent, all-encompassing milieu. When school is "off grounds," the program intensity is diluted. Yet if school has been a relative strength for the child or adolescent, then this kind of mainstreaming can be beneficial. Similarly, the mix of individual therapy, group therapy, and family therapy varies from setting to setting. Staff composition and clinical sophistication, in combination with program design, are the crucial components of any residential treatment center. As hospital treatment becomes less and less of an option, residential treatment centers are treating the children that used to be treated in a hospital setting. Unfortunately, many staffs are not adequately trained to deal with the demands of severely disturbed children. The role of the child psychiatrist as consultant, around specific cases and around programmatic issues, is of increasing importance.

Group Homes

Group homes provide residence for children who cannot live at home for either behavioral or emotional reasons, yet who do not warrant intensive on-site treatment. Group homes are usually operated by social service funding and are not generally part of the mental health care system. The basic premise of group care is that severely disturbed children who have suffered emotional trauma within the context of a family cannot tolerate the intimacy of family living. These children frequently have histories of multiple unsuccessful foster care placements. The clinical sophistication of staff at group homes is generally less than that in residential treatment facilities. Similarly, school can be either on grounds or off, with more frequent use of schools within the community. Just as residential treatment facilities are treating a more disturbed population than in the past, those children in group homes are also more challenging. The role of the child psychiatrist as consultant can be of great importance in this setting as well.

Practical Aspects of Specific Placement Choice

Once the level of treatment necessary has been determined, the arduous process of actually obtaining it must begin. The child psychiatrist must join with parent(s) or guardian to advocate strongly for the child. The placements described, with the exception of the hospital, are not generally covered by insurance. For the most part, treatment facilities are funded through public monies from social service agencies, mental health departments, or public school systems. Occasionally, intensive treatment settings are reimbursed by Medicaid. This is relevant for residents of states that have what is an optional benefit for coverage of psychiatric disabilities for the under-21 age group. Similarly, PL 94-142 (1975), which mandates all local schools to provide an education for every child from ages 3 to 21 years, regardless of emotional or physical handicaps, is implemented differently by each state. Child psychiatrists must be well informed about how public monies in their state are spent. Although some states have a single agency that serves children, others have social service, mental health, and juvenile justice agencies. The system for how cases are managed is also variable. There is an increasing emphasis on case management by agencies as a way to contain costs and to move the child through the system efficiently. Many case management systems, however, have cases managers with limited knowledge of clinical issues. Although the case manager may be well intentioned, if his or her understanding of the clinical issues is inadequate for the case in question, it may be prudent to involve the case manager's supervisor. Reports written to obtain funding must clearly and explicitly state not only why the child needs the treatment, but what is likely to happen without it and what the greater cost to the system will be.

Once funding is obtained, the process of actually looking at placements begins. The following issues should be addressed in investigating particular settings:

- Does the program specialize in treating a specific kind of disorder?
- Does the program have a clearly articulated treatment philosophy, and how is this applied to the day-to-day program?
- How long has the program been in existence?
- How are families involved?
- What is the professional composition of the staff?
- What will be the child's daily routine?

- What happens on weekends, holidays, and in the summer?
- How is the program funded, and is the funding source stable?

The referral process can be quite lengthy, making the need to anticipate placement early important. This may translate, for example, to beginning planning for a child's next school year in March of the preceding year. The child and parent(s) or guardian should visit all potential programs with attention to the factors outlined above, as well as to their degree of comfort with the setting, decor, and interactions with staff. The child psychiatrist should help the parents and child to develop their list of questions, thus empowering them as consumers of service. When possible, the child psychiatrist should visit also, and at the very least have extensive discussions with the child and parents or guardian about their impressions. It is extremely difficult for a placement to be therapeutic if this initial entry phase is not successful.

Principles and Pitfalls of Treating Severely Disturbed Children

Understanding the principles of therapeutic child milieu treatment is essential to treatment of severely disturbed children. Children are extremely environmentally sensitive such that a chaotic, disorganized environment can have a marked deleterious effect, and similarly, a calm, well-structured environment can cause an out-of-control child to become much less of a management problem. Helping the child to develop inner controls, strategies for coping with stress, and a better understanding of how to manage routine activities of daily living are common milieu treatment goals. The older literature by Aichorn (1939), Redl (1951), and Bettelheim and Sanders (1979) is worthwhile reading for all child psychiatrists. More recently, articles by Cotton (1989) and her book *Lessons From the Lion's Den* (Cotton 1993) build on the earlier writings and provide the cornerstone of understanding for all residential and hospital milieu treatment. Familiarity with the literature is particularly important for the child psychiatrist who consults to residential treatment settings or group homes.

Treatment effectiveness depends on the integration of milieu treatment with group, family, and individual treatment and school interventions. The treatment team consists of representatives from each of these modalities and from any others that might be used in a particular setting. The team must meet frequently to share information, review progress made toward various treatment goals, and update the operant treatment plan. There is often a delicate balance between the treatment plan that is individualized for the child and the need for consistent behavioral management on the milieu. It is important that the treatment team has leadership that can bring together the clinical thinking of all parties into a cohesive and focused plan. Unfocused plans are a common pitfall as treaters are apt to become lost in jargon that misses the reason the child is in the treatment setting (Table 12–4). Harper's (1989) work on focal treatment planning describes many examples of "fuzzy" treatment thinking and how it can be clarified to be more useful for the child.

Another pitfall of treatment is an incomplete formulation of the case. Perhaps the most common element to be overlooked in treatment planning is the impact of learning disabilities. Many severely disturbed children have significant learning disabilities that have a dramatic impact on their daily functioning. They may look like their age mates, but be unable to process verbal commands, or be totally mystified by visual material. Lewis et al.'s (1989) work on juvenile

Table 12–4. Pitfalls of treatment

- Pitfalls related to the treatment plan
  - Failure to integrate the milieu management into the plan
  - Unfocused plan/"fuzzy goals"
  - Incomplete case formulation
    - Underrecognition of learning disabilities
    - Undisclosed abuse
- Pitfalls related to the treatment team
  - Lack of leadership of the team
  - Overattachment or "adoption process"
  - Disruption of treaters
  - Inability of the team to plan for next setting

murderers highlights the striking combination of early childhood abuse and organic deficits contributing to learning disabilities. All staff who deal with the child must be aware of the child's deficits and how to address them in simple, understandable terms.

Treatment can also be stymied by undisclosed or partially disclosed information. This frequently happens in cases of sexual abuse when the child fears retribution from the abuser. Children frequently need to be in a safe environment that gives permission for them to talk for a considerable period of time (weeks to months) before they begin to describe what has happened to them. Multiple brief hospitalizations, failed therapies, or failed placements that have utilized primarily behavioral interventions should alert one to safely contain the child for a longer period with attention toward underlying, undisclosed abuse. Once the revelation of the abuse occurs, the case can become further entangled legally. Unfortunately, the court process moves slowly, without attention to the effects of delays on the involved child or children. Treating children during this time is fraught with difficulties. It is best done by a therapist who can make a commitment to treat the child through the conclusion of the legal proceedings and who is willing and able to be a strong advocate for the child's best interests.

There are also problems that occur as a function of length of treatment. Staff at hospitals and treatment facilities frequently become overly attached to children in a process described by Palmer et al. (1983) as the "adoption process." This is accompanied by a devaluation and overattribution of the child's problems to the family by treaters. Treatment teams must be wary of this process and work constantly to keep the family involved with the child. This problem can be made worse when the treatment setting is far away from the child's family. Parents need encouragement and empathy to remain connected with such children under these potentially adverse conditions.

Another factor that one must consider is that staff within treatment settings change. Just as a child is becoming attached to certain primary caregivers, they may move on to different employment. Similarly, when individual treatment is disrupted, the child may suffer behavioral regression characterized by increased symptomatology. Although changes are unavoidable, as much consistency as possible should be the goal. The child psychiatrist who becomes involved with the child—as therapist, prescriber of medication, or consultant—should be as clear as possible about the extent of the commitment. Both child and family or guardian should be given this information so as not to raise false hopes or expectations.

The need for lengthy treatment can also mean that the child may grow too old for a particular treatment setting. Planning for the next placement and ensuring a smooth transition require considerable work by the treatment team. There is a somewhat natural tendency for the team to want to see its work completed and thus hold onto the treatment of the child waiting valiantly for some identified change to occur. Consultation to the treatment may be necessary to help the treaters to see that the child's work will not be completed by them, but that they have made a valuable contribution to the child's life. Letting go, so that the next treatment setting can continue the work, requires the team members to deal with their own countertransference to the child and family.

One must remember that the primary goals of treatment are to facilitate development and to render the child able to function in a less restrictive setting. Such "healthier" functioning, however, must be integrated into the child's psyche. If it is merely obtained through behavioral manipulation, or training, then the child will be unable to sustain the changes once outside of the treatment setting, and symptoms will reemerge. Attempts to challenge the child's progress by decreasing structure, either by giving passes home or by increasing privileges within the treatment setting, are important steps toward the assessment of progress.

The long-term outcome for children with severe disturbance is guarded. Much depends not only on the quality of the treatment received during childhood, but on later life events. For many children, life will remain stressful and troubled, and the need for either ongoing treatment or episodic periods of treatment should be expected. The chronic nature of severe disturbance in childhood is not easily accepted by either the public or the insurers. Child psychiatrists must continue to play an active role in educating the public and shaping mental health care delivery systems, if this population is to receive the care it so desperately needs and deserves.

There is, also, a clear and pressing need for more outcome studies that elucidate what is helpful for children. The complexities of this kind of research are many, yet without such studies, it becomes difficult to justify expenditure of precious health care dollars. It is likely that the move toward cost containment will continue to create challenges as treatments become shorter, and the work with severely disturbed persons moves to clinicians with less training and expertise.

References

Aichorn A: Wayward Youth. New York, Viking, 1939

American Psychiatric Association: Diagnostic and Statistical Manual of Mental Disorders, 4th Edition. Washington, DC, American Psychiatric Association, 1994

Bettelheim B, Sanders J: Milieu therapy: the orthogenic school model, in Basic Handbook of Child Psychiatry, Vol 3: Therapeutic Interventions. Edited by Noshpitz JD, Harrison SI. New York, Basic Books, 1979

Cotton NS: The development-clinical rationale for the use of seclusion in the psychiatric treatment of children. Am J Orthopsychiatry 59:442–450, 1989

Cotton NS: Lessons From the Lion's Den: Therapeutic Management for Children in Psychiatric Hospitals and Treatment Centers. San Francisco, CA, Jossey-Bass, 1993

Harper G: Focal treatment planning. J Am Acad Child Adolesc Psychiatry 28:31–37, 1989

Lewis DO, Lovely R, Yeager C, et al: Toward a theory of the genesis of violence: a follow-up study of delinquents. J Am Acad Child Adolesc Psychiatry 28:431–436, 1989

Palmer A, Harper G, Rivinus T: The adoption process in the inpatient treatment of children and adolescents. Journal of the American Academy of Child Psychiatry 22:286–293, 1983

Pine F: A working nosology of borderline syndromes in children, in The Borderline Child. Edited by Robson KS. New York, McGraw-Hill, 1982, pp 83–100

PL 94-142: Education for All Handicapped Children Act, 1975

Redl F: Children Who Hate. Glencoe, IL, Free Press, 1951

Terr LC: Childhood traumas: an outline and overview. Am J Psychiatry 148:10–20, 1991

13

Therapeutics VI: Hypnosis

Joae G. Brooks, M.D.

Hypnosis can be an adjunct to therapy or, occasionally, a primary therapeutic tool with children with certain psychiatric disorders. It has been successfully used for anxiety, phobias, enuresis, encopresis, urinary retention, mutism, stuttering, hair pulling, nail biting, tics, obsessive-compulsive symptoms, school refusal, eczema, asthma, vomiting, psychogenic pain and pain from physical causes, headaches, conversion reactions, learning disability, nightmares, and difficulty falling asleep. It is helpful in the management of anxiety and pain in young burn and cancer patients, in children undergoing surgery and dental procedures, and in adolescent girls about to have their first pelvic examinations (Andolseek 1980; Elkins and Carter 1981; Gardner 1977, 1978; Kuttner 1989; LaClave and Blix 1989; Lewis 1991; Moore 1981; Olness and Gardner 1988; Podoll 1981; B. S. Sokel et al. 1990; S. Sokel et al. 1990; Webster and O'Grady 1991; Williams and Singh 1976).

Several studies discuss the use of hypnosis in children to improve their ability to solve problems and increase their self-esteem and to alleviate behavior and sleep disorders (Olness and Gardner 1988;

Webster and O'Grady 1991; Valente 1990). Compliance with treatment is reported to improve in noncompliant diabetic adolescents (Ratner et al. 1990). Children receiving chemotherapy for cancer coped better with their symptoms and the side effects of treatment and showed increased perception of their own competence when taught self-hypnosis (Hockenberry-Eaton and Cotanch 1989). Night terrors have been alleviated by hypnosis (Kamer 1989). Posttraumatic stress disorder resulting from sexual abuse of children has been helped by hypnosis (Spiegel 1989). Headache in children can be managed by this technique (Hobbie 1989). Hypnosis has been reported to be useful in the treatment of multiple personality disorder in children (Vincent and Pickering 1988).

Hypnosis can increase compliance and cooperation, decrease fear, and give the child a feeling of mastery and control. Children are hypnotized more easily than adults because they are more imaginative and able to fantasize readily, and they tend to be more trusting.

Hypnosis brings about an altered state of consciousness where the mind's focus is narrowed to certain specific stimuli. Thus what the therapist suggests to the child during hypnosis has greater influence. Initially the child should be given some kind of choice concerning what is about to happen. The child may choose which member of the family shall be present when the procedure is carried out. If there is a favorite stuffed animal, the child can be asked if it should go through the procedure first or if he or she wants to do it on the animal afterward. Being permitted to make a decision helps children feel that their feelings and wishes are important and that they have some control over the situation. Children are eager to hear and take hold of ideas that they think will alleviate their fear or pain.

The first step in hypnosis with a child is to secure the understanding and cooperation of the professionals involved and the parents (Andolseek 1980). The therapist must be patient and reassuring with the child. There are various techniques to induce a trance (Olness and Gardner 1988; Webster and O'Grady 1991). It can be accomplished by eye fixation; the child is asked to look at a certain object (e.g., the therapist's thumb or a spot on the child's or therapist's hand). The child can be told that as he or she looks at the spot or object that his or her eyes will feel like closing and that the child will feel relaxed and comfortable. The favorite place technique is where the child is asked to imagine being in a favorite place, asked a few questions about that place, and told that he or she feels pleasant and relaxed. The television technique is where the child is asked to imagine a big blank television screen and then to turn it on and imagine him- or herself in it. The therapist suggests ways to the child of overcoming the problem and seeing that happen on the television screen and feeling positive feelings and a sense of achievement.

Deepening hypnosis can be done by suggesting a downward movement (e.g., going down an escalator or a flight of stairs) or by having the child count slowly. The child is told that he or she feels more and more relaxed or that with every breath the child is relaxing deeper and deeper (Webster and O'Grady 1991). Suggestions of being in a beautiful garden or hearing nice music or lying on soft grass and looking at clouds above are effective. The child can be told there is a heavy book or rock in his or her hand and that the hand and arm are getting lower and lower. The therapist can tell the child that his or her doll or teddy bear is getting sleepier and sleepier or that the child feels like a floppy doll (Olness and Gardner 1988).

Hypnotherapy, carried out when the child is relaxed, consists of suggestions of ways to deal with the child's problem. Children can be taught self-hypnosis. Children can be told that they can control how they feel and are taught how to relax, told that they feel good now, and that they can make this relaxed, good feeling happen (Moore 1981). To reduce anxiety in the operating room, the child is told that the big light above is like the sun and that it feels warm and good like being at the beach (Andolseek 1980).

Examples of hypnotherapy are asking a hypnotized child with eczema to imagine a soft, cool cloud and scooping it up in her hands and gently patting it on her skin. The child is told that her skin feels much better and the creams will keep the itching and soreness away. A child with a tic can be told that now he knows how to get relaxed so the tic won't happen. A child who is fearful is helped to imagine putting on a suit of armor and then no words can upset or hurt or be scary anymore (Webster and O'Grady 1991). Pain can be diminished or banished by having the child imagine painting the afflicted body part with a special numbing medicine. The suggestion is made that the child will be able to relax deeper and deeper, and the pain will drift away and instead there will be comfortable feelings (Olness and Gardner 1988).

Enuresis can be helped by suggesting to the relaxed child that when the pressure feeling is in the bladder the child will wake up and walk to the bathroom and urinate. Thumb sucking (and nail biting) can be helped by telling the hypnotized child that when the thumb is in the mouth it will taste bitter and the child will want it out (Webster and O'Grady 1991).

There has been some success with the use of hypnosis in drug-using adolescents. The youth is taught to relax and told that he or she is beginning to feel very pleasant feelings, much more pleasurable than feelings from the drug. It is suggested then that the adolescent can learn self-hypnosis and be able to experience these feelings whenever he or she wants. The ability to concentrate or to be able to remember and think and write can all be brought about by hypnotic suggestion in young patients with problems concentrating or having test anxiety.

Conversion symptoms can be alleviated by hypnosis. The child is told after induction that sometimes if someone is very upset or frightened that person may not be able to see (or speak or walk and so on) but by learning to relax those upset feelings can go away and the person can see (speak, walk, and so on) again (Webster and O'Grady 1991).

Young children can be helped by hypnotic techniques. Anxiety in a small child can be reduced by asking the child to carry out a simple, repetitive task like putting pegs into holes or lining up blocks or toy animals or figures (Moore 1981).

Posthypnotic suggestions can maintain improvement. It is often necessary to conduct several sessions spaced every 2–3 days or weekly to eradicate symptoms and increase the child's confidence in this new way of having control over anxiety and previous symptoms.

Hypnosis is not likely to be helpful in habit disorders if the child is not motivated to change (Gardner 1978). The child may be deriving too much secondary gain or pleasure to give the habit up. Hypnosis should not be used for symptom removal if it binds severe anxiety or wards off depression, although symptom substitution has not been found to be a problem (Gardner 1978).

References

Andolseek K: Use of hypnosis with children. J Fam Pract 10:503–507, 1980

Elkins GR, Carter BD: Use of a science fiction-based imagery technique in child hypnosis. Am J Clin Hypn 23:274–277, 1981

Gardner GG: Hypnosis with infants and preschool children. Am J Clin Hypn 19:158–162, 1977

Gardner GG: Hypnotherapy in the management of childhood habit disorders. J Pediatr 92:835–840, 1978

Hobbie C: Relaxation techniques for children and young people. Journal of Pediatric Health Care 3:83–87, 1989

Hockenberry-Eaton MJ, Cotanch PH: Evaluation of children's perceived self-competence during treatment for cancer. Journal of Pediatric Oncology Nursing 6:55–62, 1989

Kamer RL: The treatment of childhood night terrors through the use of hypnosis. Int J Clin Exp Hypn 37:283–284, 1989

Kuttner L: Management of young children's acute pain and anxiety during invasive medical procedures. Pediatrician 16:39–44, 1989

LaClave LJ, Blix S: Hypnosis in the management of symptoms in a young girl with malignant astrocytoma. Int J Clin Exp Hypn 37:6–14, 1989

Lewis M: Child and Adolescent Psychiatry. Baltimore, MD, Williams & Wilkins, 1991

Moore CL: Hypnosis: an adjunct to pediatric consultation. Am J Clin Hypn 23:211–216, 1981

Olness K, Gardner GG: Hypnosis and Hypnotherapy With Children. Philadelphia, PA, Grune & Stratton, 1988

Podoll E: The use and misuse of hypnosis in children. Journal of the American Society of Psychosomatic Dentistry and Medicine 28:57–69, 1981

Ratner H, Gross L, Casas J, et al: A hypnotherapeutic approach to the improvement of compliance in adolescent diabetics. Am J Clin Hypn 32:154–159, 1990

Sokel BS, Devane SP, Bentovia A, et al: Self hypnotherapeutic treatment of habitual reflex vomiting. Arch Dis Child 65:626–627, 1990

Sokel S, Lansdown R, Kent A: The development of a hypnotherapy service for children. Journal of Child Care, Health and Development 16:227–233, 1990

Spiegel D: Hypnosis in the treatment of victims of sexual abuse. Psychiatr Clin North Am 12:295–305, 1989

Valente SM: Clinical hypnosis with school-age children. Arch Psychiatr Nurs 4:131–136, 1990

Vincent M, Pickering MR: Multiple personality disorder in childhood. Can J Psychiatry 33:524–529, 1988

Webster WC, O'Grady DJ: Clinical Hypnosis With Children. New York, Brunner/Mazel, 1991

Williams DT, Singh M: Hypnosis as a facilitating therapeutic adjunct in child psychiatry. Journal of the American Academy of Child Psychiatry 15:326–342, 1976

14

Therapeutics VII: Pharmacotherapy

Barbara J. Coffey, M.D.

Psychopharmacologic agents have been used to treat childhood disturbances for many years, but only recently has the era of modern scientific pediatric psychopharmacology begun.

General Principles of Drug Therapy for Children and Adolescents

The present-day child and adolescent psychiatrist or pediatrician can choose from all of the categories of psychotropic agents available to the general psychiatrist or adult practitioner. Knowledge of the basic principles of psychotropic drug use, the workup for their use in childhood, the basic categories of medications available, and their indications and side effect profiles is crucial for up-to-date child and adolescent clinicians.

General Overview of Indications

Developments in basic science and improvements in research methodology have advanced pediatric psychopharmacology in the past decade. As a result, indications for the use of psychopharmacologic agents in childhood and adolescence have increased. Medications, like all forms of therapy in child and adolescent psychiatry, are to be used to promote optimal development and maturation, or to assist in the removal of obstacles for development to proceed onward in an adaptive fashion. In most cases, pharmacotherapy represents one component of a total treatment plan for the child, from the biopsychosocial perspective. Quite frequently, medication can be used to help make the disturbed child more responsive to other forms of therapy. Established indications are discussed in the section on specific agents. General indications for pharmacotherapy include the following categories of disturbance:

- Childhood and adolescent psychosis and pervasive developmental disorder
- Severe behavioral disturbance accompanying mental retardation or child psychiatric emergencies
- Tourette's syndrome
- Enuresis
- Attention-deficit/hyperactivity disorder (ADHD)
- Obsessive-compulsive disorder
- Major depression
- Manic-depressive illness
- Separation anxiety disorder
- Overanxious disorder
- Panic disorder
- Posttraumatic stress disorder
- Sleep disorders

General Guidelines to Pharmacotherapy in Childhood and Adolescence

Comprehensive diagnostic assessment and systematic formulation of each individual case remain the cornerstone of treatment planning in child and adolescent psychiatry.

The biopsychosocial model remains sound as a guiding principle for case formulation. DSM-IV (American Psychiatric Association

1994) has contributed to improved reliability and validity in childhood and adolescent psychiatric diagnosis. The multiaxial system has been particularly useful in child and adolescent work. Children are complicated and often have multiple, coexisting problems, and their context within families must be taken into account.

The multiaxial diagnostic system lends itself to the *target symptom* approach, a general guideline in child and adolescent pharmacotherapy. Although diagnosis serves as a foundation for indications for pharmacotherapy and for medication selection, target symptoms will determine specific medication choice. Target symptoms (or signs) are individual clinical occurrences that are not necessarily specific to diagnostic category; constellations of target symptoms contribute to the diagnostic picture. Target symptoms are potentially medication responsive and include motor overactivity, movement disorders, anxiety, enuresis, sleep disturbance, and others.

Maturational issues must be taken into account when dealing with children and adolescents. Children differ significantly from adults in their *pharmacokinetic capacities.* Children have relatively large liver size in proportion to body weight when compared with adults, and after about a year of age reach adult glomerular filtration rates. Therefore, they seem to function metabolically more efficiently with regard to medication handling. Often children tend to need higher doses relative to body weight when compared with adults (Jatlow 1987).

In addition, evidence suggests that children tend to have less adipose tissue and less protein binding, when compared with adults, and may have more drug available for bioactivity and, potentially, side effects (Rapoport and Mikkelsen 1978).

Growth and development are associated with changes in organ size and proportion and in tissue mass, particularly water and adipose tissue. These changes may have significant effects on medication handling. Adolescents approach adults in their metabolic and pharmacokinetic parameters.

In addition, it is likely that children differ significantly from adults in their *central nervous system (CNS) capacities.* Neurotransmitter development takes place sequentially and at differing rates during childhood; for example, dopamine and norepinephrine pathways and functions probably develop earlier in life than do serotonin capacities

(Coyle 1987). Hormonal changes during adolescence are also likely to affect CNS responsivity. Finally, cognitive development is proceeding rapidly during early childhood, and medication effects on cognition must be a potential factor at all times.

The child's *place in his or her family* context is an essential component of treatment planning. Frequently, children and adolescents are not self-referred for psychiatric intervention; nor are they always willing patients. Typically the child's behavior or emotional state is disturbing to someone else in the environment, usually an adult such as a parent or teacher. Parental attitudes toward the use of medication are crucial. Parents are a necessary source of information about the child's functioning and response to medication. Parents, and at times teachers, need to be considered therapeutic allies in a course of pharmacotherapy for a child; they need to be informed about the reasons for use of medication, the expected response, and likely adverse effects. A child with an unreliable or uncooperative parent who cannot agree to, observe, administer, and monitor the medication may not be treatable with pharmacotherapy. Parental attitudes of uncertainty, anxiety, doubt, or antagonism can obviously affect *compliance.*

The *child himself or herself* is a crucial figure in the decision to use pharmacotherapy. Every child, including the very young, should have an opportunity to ask questions, express ideas, and discuss the decision to use medication. All children have fantasies and beliefs about their particular situation: what the problem is, why it developed, what is needed, and what medication can or cannot do. The use of "pills" or "drugs" to modify behavior or alleviate mental states is likely to be quite emotionally charged for the child. The *meaning* of the medication for each child should be discussed individually; anxiety or worries about how it will affect the child need to be taken up at the outset.

Issues of *informed consent* are another guiding principle. Since many of the pharmacotherapeutic agents used in child and adolescent psychiatry are not formally approved for use in advertising by the Food and Drug Administration (FDA), a detailed discussion between physician and parents or legal guardians must take place when the decision to treat a child with medication is made. In general, clinicians should first use standard treatments including nonpharmacotherapeutic approaches and drugs formally approved by the FDA for advertising for this indication if possible. Benefits versus risks of medication, like any treatment, must be assessed and discussed with the parent or legal guardian. Clinically accepted, but nonlabeled (FDA-approved) medications may be used with detailed discussion (Green 1991b). These medications, and those used outside the age limits recommended by the FDA, may increase liability risk.

Informed consent can be obtained when the patient (if adolescent) or parent or guardian is mentally competent and understands the nature of the condition being treated, the nature of the proposed treatment, and its potential risks and consequences. Natural history of the condition if untreated and alternatives should be discussed (Nurcombe 1991). Documentation of the discussion should be noted in the record. Records should also indicate that the patient and parent or guardian had an opportunity to ask questions during the discussion.

Baseline Assessment and Premedication Workup

All child and adolescent patients who are candidates for psychopharmacologic agents should undergo a thorough medical and psychiatric evaluation at baseline. The clinical workup should include a comprehensive psychiatric evaluation, including

- Chief complaint(s) and target symptoms.
- Present illness.
- Psychiatric history and treatment(s).
- Family history including three-generation genogram; medical and/or psychiatric illness, alcoholism, causes of death, and ages at death should be noted. A medication history for family members with psychiatric illness should be obtained, with responses to medication noted.
- Developmental history, school history, and social-interpersonal history.
- Complete medical history of the child including illnesses, hospitalizations and/or surgery, and allergies.
- Medication history for the child including previous response to medications, dosages, and duration of trials.
- Mental status examination (see Chapter 2).

- Auxiliary data such as psychometric testing can be helpful.
- Biopsychosocial formulation, differential diagnosis on multiple axes of DSM-IV, working diagnosis, and target symptoms.

In addition to a comprehensive psychiatric evaluation, a *complete physical examination* prior to starting medication is of paramount importance. First, for differential diagnostic purposes, physical assessment is necessary to rule out organic sources of the child's disturbance such as temporal lobe seizures or hyperthyroidism. Second, all pharmacotherapeutic agents can have physical effects on the child such as alterations in blood pressure, pulse, or weight. Height, weight, blood pressure, and pulse should be noted at baseline.

A screening *neurological examination* should be performed on all patients who are candidates for psychotropic agents, noting overall developmental level, gross and fine motor coordination, cranial nerve functions, sensory-perceptual apparatus, and gait. Before medication is started, note should be made as to the presence or absence of unusual movements, tics, or stereotypic behaviors. These are commonly seen in psychotic youngsters and need to be distinguished from medication-related dyskinesias (Campbell et al. 1983) (see section on systematic rating instruments).

Children with special problems such as heart conditions or seizure disorders may need consultation with a specialist prior to initiation of pharmacotherapy.

A *minimal laboratory workup* for all children who are candidates for medication includes the following:

- Complete blood count (CBC) and differential blood count
- Urinalysis
- Blood urea nitrogen (BUN), creatinine, electrolytes
- Vital signs and growth parameters including height, weight, pulse, and blood pressure
- Pregnancy test where appropriate, in sexually active female adolescents
- Toxic screen where appropriate, in substance users
- Lead blood level in the child who presents with hyperactivity

For children who are candidates for *tricyclic antidepressants,* the following are useful baseline parameters:

- Thyroid function tests: triiodothyronine (T3), thyroxine (T4), T4I, thyroid-stimulating hormone (TSH)
- SMA-12 (chemistry screen), including liver function tests (LFTs): protein, albumin, bilirubin (direct and indirect), alkaline phosphatase, serum glutamic-oxaloacetic transaminase (SGOT), serum glutamic-pyruvic transaminase (SGPT), lactic dehydrogenase (LDH), creatine phosphokinase (CPK)
- Electrocardiogram (ECG) (see section on specific agents)
- Electroencephalogram (EEG), necessary in the child with preexisting seizure disorder, family history of seizures, or abnormal EEG

For children who are candidates for *neuroleptics* (antipsychotics):

- SMA-12 including LFTs
- Abnormal Involuntary Movement Scale (AIMS) (U.S. Department of Human Services, Alcohol and Drug Abuse and Mental Health Administration 1974)

For children who are candidates for *stimulants*:

- Add Conners' (1973) checklist for ADHD before; it can be repeated after medication. Both parents and teacher can fill out the checklist for 5–7 days prior to medication therapy for baseline, then after the child has reached therapeutic range. This can be useful quantitative data in determining medication response.

For children who are candidates for *lithium carbonate*:

- SMA-12 including calcium
- Thyroid function tests as for tricyclics
- Creatinine clearance helpful, but not mandatory, if urinalysis, BUN, and creatinine have been obtained
- ECG

Specialized tests that are studied in general psychiatry, such as the dexamethasone suppression test, urinary catecholamines, sleep architecture studies, and hypothalamic-pituitary axis stimulation tests, have not been clarified for routine clinical use in this age group, despite some evidence that they may have some value as research tools.

Systematic Rating Instruments

Systematic baseline assessment is necessary for all child and adolescent candidates for medication. The use of structured interviews and rating instruments can be useful as an adjunct in the clinical pharmacotherapeutic setting.

Scales such as the Conners' checklist, AIMS, the Child Behavior Checklist (Achenback and Edelbrock 1983), and the Children's Depression Inventory (Kovacs 1981) have an established place in research studies and can be applied in the clinical setting (Conners and Barkley 1985). Although not all scales have been found to be statistically drug responsive, some can be used for "before and after" comparisons in a single case study format. These can be particularly useful when multiple informants' assessments of the child are being taken into account.

Careful record keeping is a must. Note in the record should be made of

- Target symptoms that are being treated with medication, in a problem-oriented list
- Rationale for medication selection
- Initial dosage and medication plan
- Increases of dosages and response
- Documentation of discussion with parent(s) and child regarding informed consent issues
- Presence of any adverse reactions including expected side effects or any unexpected allergic or idiosyncratic reactions
- Rationale for changing or discontinuing medications

Getting Started

Appropriate *medication selection* requires comprehensive information about the child and the child's history and current functioning. As the categories of medication available for use in children and adolescents have increased considerably in the past decade, the clinician is confronted with a multitude of choices. Medication selection should always proceed with efficaciousness and safety as the guiding principles; in general, the most well-established and least toxic agent should be tried first. If, after an adequate trial, the medication has not ameliorated the symptomatology, another medication or category of medications can be tried. The physician should be knowledgeable about and have familiarity with one or two agents and their indications, dosage ranges, and side effect profiles in each general category.

Pharmacotherapeutic Maintenance and Monitoring

Children and adolescents usually need to be seen at regular and frequent intervals during the initiation of pharmacotherapy, at least once a week. Close communication is necessary with the parent during this time as well. Parents should be encouraged to call the doctor if any questions arise about medication. Good communication between doctor and family facilitates optimal response.

Dosage regulation requires time and experience. Plasma levels of some drugs can be readily obtained, and therapeutic ranges similar to those of adults have been identified, such as with the tricyclic antidepressants and lithium carbonate. In general, except in emergencies, it is best to start with a low dosage and raise by standardized increments at regular intervals until therapeutic effects or range is reached or until the onset of side effects. Often it is necessary to push the dosage up gradually to the point of development of side effects to explore the optimal range. The dosage can then be gradually lowered to find a balance between minimum necessary for therapeutic effect and minimal possibility of side effects.

In the case of the acutely psychotic child with target symptoms of motor overactivity, delusional thinking or hallucinations, and agitation, or the acutely assaultive child in an emergency state, medication can be given more frequently until the child is sedated or calmed. In this situation, oral concentrates can be given every 1–2 hours until a therapeutic effect is achieved (see Chapter 15 on emergencies).

Once the child has been stabilized, usually after several weeks, on a maintenance dosage, a medication maintenance program can begin. Children can generally be seen less frequently, such as monthly, to review therapeutic response and development of side effects. Information from teachers and other clinicians involved in the child's care must be regularly communicated to the prescribing physician.

All children on pharmacotherapy should be considered for yearly medication-free periods to reassess need for medication and to monitor the development of side effects. The duration and timing of the medication-free period will vary with the individual child, type of medication, and clinical situation.

Periodic laboratory screening should be done on a regular basis during the entire duration of pharmacotherapy. It is judicious practice to repeat CBC and differential, urinalysis, and basic chemistry screening at 6 months to a year. Certain specific procedures such as ECG monitoring for tricyclic antidepressants are discussed in the section on specific agents.

In general, it is very useful to record weight and height on a monthly or quarterly basis, as many of these agents can cause weight gain, or in some cases, weight loss. Keeping the National Center for Health Statistics (1978) growth chart can provide the clinician easy access to growth parameters over an extended period of time.

Duration of treatment will depend on the target symptoms, the age of the child, the kind of psychotropic agent, and the unique features of the clinical situation. There are few fixed guidelines as to length of time on the medications, medication holiday programs, and indications for stopping. In general, if a child has not responded to an agent within 4 weeks while in the therapeutic range, it is unlikely he or she will respond at a later date. A rational approach to this situation would be to switch to another drug in the same category or to another category altogether if indicated.

Most children with a therapeutic response to medication will need a 3- to 6-month trial of the agent, depending on the clinical situation. Some will require a longer period of time. In general, no child or adolescent should remain on any agent for more than a year without at least consideration of a medication-free period.

Adverse Effects

Despite their medication handling efficiency, children and adolescents, as compared with adults, are no less at risk and perhaps more at risk in some cases for the development of adverse effects (Table 14–1). This has both physiological and practical significance: the clinician must be acquainted with the side effect profiles of the medication(s) being prescribed and must know how to manage adverse effects should they arise. In addition, children and adolescents are particularly prone to sensitivities about their bodies and how they work, and often get quite frightened or suspicious if a sudden change or dysfunction occurs in the context of pharmacotherapy. Such feelings can interfere with compliance and optimal outcome.

Many of the side effects of neuroleptics, antidepressants, and lithium seen in adult patients can be observed in children and adolescents. Of particular concern are the anticholinergic and cardiovascular side effects of the tricyclic antidepressants and the extrapyramidal side effects (EPS) of the neuroleptics, including dyskinesias (Gualtieri et al. 1980; D. Klein et al. 1980). Withdrawal dyskinesias seem to be more frequent than tardive dyskinesia in young children, but tardive dyskinesia has been observed in this age group.

In general, the best therapy for adverse effects is preventive. The following are guidelines to avoid possible adverse effects:

- Start with a low dose and advance gradually to therapeutic range.
- Use the lowest possible maintenance doses in the therapeutic range once it has been established.
- Try to avoid prescribing more than one drug at a time in a given child. For example, it is best to try lowering the dosage of a neuroleptic slightly for parkinsonism or akathisia if at all possible first, rather than adding an antiparkinsonian agent.
- In most cases, medications should be tapered gradually to discontinue them, both for physiological and psychological purposes. This provides more opportunity for the reestablishment of equilibrium.

Table 14–1. Side effects and their management in children and adolescents

Drug category	Common adverse effects	Clinical management
Neuroleptics (antipsychotics)	**Short-term**	
	Autonomic nervous system	
	• Dry mouth	In general, lower dosage if possible or switch drug if persistent, child may "equilibrate" after several weeks
	• Urinary retention	Bethanechol only if severe and persistent
	• Constipation	Dioctyl sodium sulfosuccinate (Colace) tablets or bisacodyl USP (Dulcolax) suppositories
	• Orthostatic hypotension	Avoid sudden postural changes; dosage reduction if severe
	Extrapyramidal	
	• Acute dystonic reaction	Diphenhydramine or benztropine (im), then switch to oral form
	• Parkinsonism	Anticholinergic/antiparkinsonian medication on an as-needed basis
	• Akathisia	Lower dosage; sometimes anticholinergic can help
	Other	
	• Hypersensitivity/rash	Discontinue drug
	• Drowsiness	Child usually becomes tolerant; if persistent switch to less sedating class
	• Photosensitivity	Avoid sun exposure
	• LFTs	May not have clinical significance; follow-up indicated

	Long-term	
	• Weight gain	Lower dosage; consider switch to another class
	• Dyskinesias (tardive and withdrawal)	Prevention is best; use lowest possible dose for maintenance
Psychostimulants	**Short-term**	
	• Anorexia, nausea, abdominal pain	Reduce dose; give most of dosage in the A.M.; consider switch
	• Insomnia	Move P.M. dose to earlier in the day; reduce dosage; then reintroduce
	• Dysphoria	Consider another stimulant if persistent or tricyclic
	Long-term	
	• Weight loss	Supplement diet, institute drug holidays or change drug
	• Tics/Tourette	Discontinue and probably avoid rechallenge; consider TCA
Tricyclic antidepressants	• Autonomic nervous system	See neuroleptics
	• Cardiovascular (blood pressure, pulse, PR, T-wave changes, ↑ QT_c, and arrhythmias)	Monitor ECGs serially; most changes have little clinical significance in healthy child
	• CNS (seizures)	Discontinue medication gradually, EEG; may need anticonvulsant

continued

Table 14–1. Side effects and their management in children and adolescents *(continued)*

Drug category	Common adverse effects	Clinical management
Anxiolytics and sedative-hypnotics		
Antihistamines	• Oversedation	Decrease total dosage, administer most at bedtime
	• Rash	Discontinue medication
Benzodiazepines	• Disinhibition	Discontinue medication
	• Cognitive decrements	Reduce dosage or discontinue
Lithium	• Gastrointestinal: nausea, vomiting, abdominal pain, diarrhea, metallic taste	Consider dose reduction if persistent
	• CNS: tremor, memory lapses, fatigue	Consider dose reduction if persistent
	• Endocrine: goiter	Discontinue medication and follow with lab studies
	• Renal: polyuria/polydipsia	Monitor BUN, creatinine, electrolytes, and urinalysis on a regular basis (every 2–3 months)
	• Hematologic: leukocytosis	Monitor; may not be of clinical significance

Note. LFTs = liver function tests. TCA = tricyclic antidepressant. ECG = electrocardiogram. CNS = central nervous system. EEG = electroencephalogram. BUN = blood urea nitrogen.

- Avoid giving an agent to a child who has demonstrated previous sensitivity to it such as tics with stimulants or dyskinesias with phenothiazines.

Specific Agents

Neuroleptic (Antipsychotic) Drugs

Neuroleptic medications include the phenothiazines, butyrophenones, thioxanthenes, dibenzoxazepines, dihydroindolones, diphenylbutylpiperidines, and dibenzodiazepines. Formal indications for use of these drugs include target symptoms of 1) childhood and adolescent psychoses and pervasive developmental disorders such as thought disorder, agitation, stereotypies, and social withdrawal; 2) severe behavior disturbance as accompaniment to mental retardation such as self-injurious or assaultive behavior; 3) psychiatric emergencies, including acute homicidal behavior and severe disorganizing anxiety or agitation; and 4) Tourette syndrome. Informal indications include behavior disorders with severe aggression such as conduct disorder.

These medications function as dopamine, alpha-adrenergic, and cholinergic blockers in the CNS and peripheral nervous system. They have antipsychotic actions in adults and in children with such target symptoms as auditory hallucinations and delusions. In addition, these agents can decrease severe agitation and motor overactivity, as well as stereotypic movements and postures, and render an apathetic, socially nonrelated psychotic child more amenable to his or her environment (Campbell and Shapiro 1975). In Tourette syndrome, these medications decrease motor and vocal tics. In general, doses used to treat Tourette syndrome are lower than those used to treat psychotic disturbances.

Overall, neuroleptics tend to be chosen on their side effect profile rather than on clinical effects, which are approximately equal with comparable doses. The low-potency aliphatic and piperidine phenothiazines such as chlorpromazine and thioridazine, respectively, tend to be sedating and more anticholinergic, whereas the high-potency butyrophenones and piperazine phenothiazines such as haloperidol and trifluoperazine tend to be less sedating, but more likely to induce EPS such as akathisia, acute dystonic reactions, and parkinsonism. The thioxanthenes and newer dibenzoxazepines and dihydroindolones tend to be intermediate for anticholinergic effects and EPS (Tables 14–2 and 14–3).

An agitated child with stereotypic behaviors will generally respond more readily to a sedating neuroleptic, whereas an anergic, withdrawn child should probably be treated with a less sedating drug. Sedation effects must be monitored because an oversedated child cannot learn. Cognitive blunting can occur in those treated with neuroleptics at higher doses (Anderson et al. 1984).

Children and adolescents are like their adult counterparts in that they are at risk for development of autonomic nervous system side effects and EPS. EPS associated with neuroleptics include acute dystonic reactions, parkinsonism, akathisia (motor restlessness), neuroleptic malignant syndrome, rabbit syndrome, and tardive dyskinesia (Baldessarini 1990).

There is growing evidence that adolescents and even young children can develop neuroleptic-related dyskinesias. Some studies have indicated that children are more likely to develop withdrawal emergent dyskinesias that are reversible on discontinuation of the medication than tardive dyskinesia or late-appearing dyskinesias; nevertheless, tardive dyskinesia has been reported in young children as well as in adolescents (Gualtieri et al. 1984). Abnormal movements that often present in these disturbed children *prior to* pharmacotherapy must be differentiated from any that develop *after* medication treatment. Baseline and periodic AIMS exams are recommended.

In general, it is good practice to prescribe the *lowest possible* effective dose for maintenance and to take the child off the neuroleptic at least once yearly in the case of chronic psychosis or severe behavioral disturbance associated with mental retardation. In the case of a psychiatric emergency such as acute agitation or assaultive behavior, the child should be taken off medication as quickly as possible following return of psychic, family, and environmental equilibrium.

Antiparkinsonian Agents

The psychopharmacologic treatment of EPS as side effects of neuroleptic therapy in childhood follows guidelines used for adults.

Table 14–2. Neuroleptics (antipsychotics) for use in children over age 6 years

Generic name (trade name)	Indications	Oral dosage range (mg)	Common side effects: Short-term	Common side effects: Long-term
Phenothiazines			Autonomic nervous system: sedation, dry mouth, orthostatic hypotension, urinary retention, blurring of vision	Withdrawal and tardive dyskinesia
Chlorpromazine (Thorazine)[a]	Pervasive developmental disorders and psychoses, acute or chronic; severe behavioral problems associated with mental retardation; psychiatric emergencies; acute agitation	10–300		
Thioridazine (Mellaril)[a]		10–300		Cognitive blunting
Trifluoperazine (Stelazine)		1–20	EPS: acute dystonic reaction, akathisia, parkinsonism	
Fluphenazine (Prolixin)[b]		1–10		Weight gain
Perphenazine (Trilafon)[b]		2–24	Endocrine: prolactin, menstrual irregularities	Same as for phenothiazines
Butyrophenones	Tourette syndrome (Haldol in particular)	1–16		
Haloperidol (Haldol)[a]				
Thioxanthenes	Same as for phenothiazines	1–5	Hypersensitivity: rash, blood dyscrasias, elevated liver function	Same as for phenothiazines
Thiothixene (Navane)[b]		2–20		

continued

Table 14–2. Neuroleptics (antipsychotics) for use in children over age 6 years *(continued)*

Generic name (trade name)	Indications	Oral dosage range (mg)	Common side effects: Short-term	Common side effects: Long-term
Dibenzoxazepines				
Loxapine (Loxitane)[c]	Same as for phenothiazines	5–60	CNS: seizures, behavioral reactions	
Dihydroindolones				
Molindone (Moban)[b]	Same as for phenothiazines	10–50	EPS	
Diphenylbutylpiperidines	Tourette's syndrome			
Pimozide (Orap)[b]		1–10	EPS; ECG changes	
Dibenzodiazepines				
Clozapine (Clozaril)[c]	Treatment-refractory psychosis	25–300	Agranulocytosis; salivation	

Note. EPS = extrapyramidal side effects. CNS = central nervous system. FDA = Food and Drug Administration. ECG = electrocardiogram.
[a]FDA-approved for advertising for use in children under age 6 years.
[b]FDA-approved for advertising for use in children over age 12 years.
[c]FDA-approved for advertising for use in children over age 16 years.

Table 14–3. Recommended neuroleptic (antipsychotic) treatment for children over age 6 years

Suggested treatment regimen for psychosis and pervasive developmental disorders

Chlorpromazine (po tablets or concentrate)

- Start with 0.5–1.0 mg/kg
- Acutely: Give 0.25–1.0 mg every 2–4 hours until therapeutic response or side effects; usually 3 or 4 doses will have therapeutic effect
- Daily maintenance dose range: 2–5 mg/kg

Haloperidol (po tablets or concentrate)

- Start with 0.5 mg
- Acutely: Give 0.01–0.05 mg/kg every 2–4 hours until therapeutic response or side effects; usually 3 or 4 doses will have therapeutic effect
- Daily maintenance dose range: 0.05–0.1 mg/kg

Suggested treatment regimen for Tourette syndrome

Haloperidol

- Start with 0.25 mg for 3–4 days, then increase by 0.25 mg every 5–7 days
- Daily maintenance dose range: usually 1.5–10 mg daily

In general, except for the acute dystonic reactions, it is best to try to decrease neuroleptic dosage before adding an antiparkinsonian agent. If decreasing neuroleptic dosage is not possible or not effective, then antiparkinsonian treatment is indicated.

In general, our practice has been to avoid prophylactic antiparkinsonian medication despite the controversy in the literature. In our experience, choosing a neuroleptic less likely to cause EPS and using lowest possible maintenance dosages lessen the possibility of EPS development. Should the symptoms develop, however, an antiparkinsonian agent can be readily added.

On the other hand, since it is found by some investigators that the greatest risks for acute dystonic reactions occur with males under age 30 treated with high-potency neuroleptics during the first few weeks of treatment, prophylactic use of antiparkinsonian agents for the first few weeks of treatment may be indicated (Neppe and Ward 1989).

Physicians are advised to decide on an individualized basis, taking into account each child and medication. In the case of acute dystonic reaction, treatment with intramuscular diphenhydramine or benztropine mesylate is indicated. The child can then be maintained on oral forms for 2–4 weeks. Any recurrence of EPS symptomatology is an indication for further treatment. Information on dosages can be found in Table 14–4.

Stimulants

The stimulants are some of the most widely prescribed and best-studied psychotropic agents in child and adolescent psychiatry and pediatrics. Methylphenidate, dextroamphetamine, and magnesium pemoline are the agents available for use.

These medications function as general nonspecific stimulators of catecholamine activity in the CNS and peripheral nervous system; they appear to prevent catecholamine reuptake at the synaptic cleft as well as inhibit metabolism and breakdown (Cohen et al. 1983). They are formally indicated in the treatment of ADHD and allow these children to focus their attention more clearly, slow down their motor activity, and become less distractible. Stimulants have had informal use with conduct disorders, which frequently coexist in ADHD, and attention-

Table 14–4. Antiparkinsonian medications for use in children over age 3 years

Generic name	Trade name	Indications	Dosage range (mg)
Diphenhydramine[a]	Benadryl	Acute dystonic reactions	25–50 im
Benztropine mesylate	Cogentin	EPS: parkinsonism, akathisia	1–2 im 1–6 po daily
Trihexyphenidyl	Artane	EPS	2–6 po daily

Note. EPS = extrapyramidal side effects. FDA = Food and Drug Administration.
[a]FDA-approved for advertising for use in children over age 3 years.

deficit disorder, residual type (Gadow et al. 1990). Their effect actually is not paradoxical in that adult males and normal boys also appear to increase concentration and focusing when given a single dose of dextroamphetamine (Rapoport et al. 1980b). Stimulants appear to achieve their effects by short-term improvement of attentional difficulties and concentration; they have been reported to improve performance efficiency, work output, and peer interactions (Pelham et al. 1985). Highly effective in the majority of ADHD patients, they are easy to administer and quite safe.

Because dextroamphetamine and methylphenidate have a relatively short duration of action with peak effects between 1 and 3 hours, they must be administered in divided doses two or three times a day (Dulcan 1990). They are typically given at breakfast and at noontime (or early afternoon). As this may necessitate the child receiving the medication in school, it may sometimes be easier to give it to the child immediately after school as long as it does not interfere with sleep. This may save the child some embarrassment from having to go to the school nurse's office everyday. Pemoline, with a longer duration of action and said to have less side effects, can be given once a day before school (Green 1991a). There are also slow-release forms available for dextroamphetamine and methylphenidate.

Common side effects include nausea, abdominal discomfort, anorexia, and insomnia. There have been some reports of adverse effects on growth parameters that are reversible with discontinuation of the medication, but other evidence has been contradictory (Safer et al. 1972). Several studies have noted decreases in height and weight percentiles over long-term treatment, and reduction in growth velocity (Mattes and Gittelman 1983). However, growth rebound tends to occur after stimulants are discontinued (R. Klein and Mannuzza 1988). A potentially serious side effect is the development of tics or Tourette syndrome in vulnerable children, so that a preexisting tic or family history of tics is in most cases a relative contraindication for use. Stimulants may precipitate psychotic symptomatology, including hallucinosis in children at risk. Methylphenidate seems to be less likely to produce side effects than dextroamphetamine (Cantwell and Carlson 1978). Medication holidays should be considered in most patients to mitigate the potential for side effects. Weekends, school vacations, and summer vacations are optimal times. Some children, however, may not be able to tolerate medication-free periods; these children may need to be maintained on stimulants or undergo dosage reduction.

Fenfluramine is a sympathomimetic amine with stimulant and antiserotonergic properties. It has been studied for the treatment of childhood autism and ADHD. It has not been found to be effective in ADHD but may be helpful in a subgroup of autistic children for target symptoms of hyperactivity and stereotypies (Donnelly et al. 1989; Verglas et al. 1988).

Antidepressants

The use of antidepressants in child and adolescent psychiatry has grown in the past decade; they now appear to be indicated in a variety of conditions. Newer heterocyclic and nontricyclic agents have added to the available choices.

Tricyclic antidepressants are formally established for use in children with enuresis, adolescent depression, and ADHD. In addition, tricyclic antidepressants have been studied for use in conduct disorders, childhood depression, and school refusal based on separation anxiety (Ryan 1990a). Tricyclic antidepressants have also been used in sleep arousal disorders and many other clinical situations. Imipramine, desipramine, and nortriptyline have been most frequently studied (Tables 14–5 and 14–6).

Tricyclic antidepressants may have several different mechanisms of action in the CNS and elsewhere that result in their effectiveness in these several different conditions. In general, the tricyclics prevent reuptake of catecholamines or indoleamines at the receptor level in the CNS and have both adrenergic and anticholinergic activity in the CNS and peripheral nervous system. Enuretic and hyperactive children tend to respond to tricyclics within days of beginning pharmacotherapy, whereas those who are school refusers and depressed children tend to require several weeks to respond.

Studies indicate that imipramine's effectiveness in enuresis is not related to its anticholinergic properties nor to its effects on sleep architecture but perhaps through some direct effects on bladder muscles (Rapoport et al. 1980a).

Table 14–5. Antidepressants for use in children over age 12 years

Generic name (trade name)	Indications	Oral dosage range (mg)	Common side effects	
			Short-term	Long-term
Imipramine (Tofranil)[a]	Enuresis	25–125	Autonomic nervous system: dry mouth, orthostatic hypotension, blurring vision	Same as short-term
Desipramine (Norpramin)	Attention-deficit hyperactivity disorder[b,c]	25–200		
	Major depression[b,c]	100–300	Cardiovascular: alterations in conduction, pulse, blood pressure; prolonged PR, QT_c; arrhythmias	
	Separation anxiety[b] (school refusal)	100–200		
Nortriptyline (Aventyl)[d]	Major depression	50–100	Same as above	
Clomipramine (Anafranil)	Obsessive-compulsive disorder	25–200		
Fluoxetine (Prozac)	Obsessive-compulsive disorder Major depression	10–40	Sedation,gastrointestinal effects, insomnia, activation	Weight changes
Bupropion (Wellbutrin)	Major depression Attention-deficit hyperactivity disorder?	50–150	Central nervous system: lowered seizure threshold	

continued

Table 14–5. Antidepressants for use in children over age 12 years *(continued)*

Generic name (trade name)	Indications	Oral dosage range (mg)	Common side effects	
			Short-term	Long-term
Others				
Amitriptyline (Elavil)	Major depression			
Doxepin (Sinequan)	Major depression			
Maprotiline (Ludiomil)	Major depression			
Amoxapine (Asendin)[e]	Major depression			
Trazodone (Desyrel)[f]	Major depression			

Note. FDA = Food and Drug Administration.
[a]FDA-approved for advertising for use in children over age 6 years for enuresis, over age 12 years for depression.
[b]Also responsive to imipramine.
[c]Blood levels 150–250 ng/ml.
[d]Blood levels: 50–150 ng/ml.
[e]FDA-approved for advertising for use in children over age 16 years.
[f]FDA-approved for advertising for use in children over age 18 years.

Table 14–6. Recommended antidepressant treatment

Suggested treatment regimen for enuresis

- Start with 0.5 mg/kg of imipramine for 2–3 nights
- Increase by 25 mg or 0.5 mg/kg every 2–3 nights until therapeutic response
- Daily maintenance dose range: 0.5–2.5 mg/kg

Suggested treatment regimen for attention-deficit/hyperactivity disorder

- Start with 0.5 mg/kg imipramine or desipramine
- Increase by 25 mg or 0.5 mg/kg every 5–7 days until therapeutic response or side effects
- Daily maintenance dose range: 1–5 mg/kg, probably blood level 150–250 ng/ml

Suggested treatment regimen for childhood major depression

- Start with 0.5 mg/kg imipramine for 2–3 days
- Increase by 0.5 mg/kg every 3–4 days
- Daily maintenance dose range: 3–5 mg/kg or blood level 150–250 ng/ml

---

The mechanism of action in school refusers has not been clearly elucidated at this time. In one placebo-controlled study, 35 school-age children who had failed to return to school through behavioral means returned with imipramine treatment on the average of 159 mg/day (Gittleman-Klein 1975). A more recent study indicated that adolescents with school refusal improve on imipramine (Bernstein et al. 1990). There has been increasing interest in recent years in childhood major depression, and evidence has accumulated that adolescents and even prepubertal children can meet adult research criteria or DSM-IV criteria for major depression.

Studies have shown that some of these children are responsive to tricyclic antidepressant treatment in dose ranges achieving blood levels of 150–250 ng/ml (Puig-Antich 1980).

Some investigators have found that there is no difference in treatment response between antidepressant medication and placebo in some adolescents with major depression. Hormonal influences, neurotransmitter immaturity, and diagnostic confusion are among the hypotheses proposed to account for this lack of robust treatment response (Ryan 1990b).

Desipramine has been studied in the treatment of ADHD (Biederman et al. 1989a). Investigators have found a correlation between clinical response and blood levels in approximately the same range as for the treatment of depression (150–250 mg/ml).

Clomipramine is a newer tricyclic antidepressant with anti-obsessional and serotonergic properties. It has been studied in children and adolescents with obsessive-compulsive disorder and has been found to be more efficacious than placebo (Flament et al. 1985).

Side effects of tricyclic antidepressants are primarily anticholinergic, which tend to be common and transient. In addition, cardiovascular and CNS side effects occur. In vulnerable individuals, with a previous history of seizures, family history of seizures, or history of abnormal EEG, lowering of the seizure threshold could occur.

Cardiovascular side effects are not infrequent but most are not clinically significant. Small but clinically significant elevations in heart rate and blood pressure occur with tricyclics. However, ECG effects with more serious implications are possible, given that the tricyclics have a quinidine-like effect and prolong PR interval and can widen the QT_c interval. There have been four case reports of sudden death of school-age and early adolescent children on desipramine and nortriptyline (Popper and Elliot 1990). These children were apparently on therapeutic dosages of desipramine for treatment of ADHD or depression. Unfortunately, there are no data available as regards medical and cardiovascular history and family history in these cases so that one cannot informatively interpret these catastrophic events.

Until further data are available, it is recommended that children and adolescents who are candidates for tricyclic antidepressants be very carefully evaluated and monitored.

Recommendations for ECG monitoring include the following (Biederman et al. 1989b):

- Careful individual and family history of cardiovascular, neuromuscular, neurological, or other medical problems
- Baseline ECG prior to medication trial

- ECG repeated at 2 mg/kg and with dosage increments up to 5 mg/kg or therapeutic range
- Blood level monitoring with serum levels not to exceed 150–250 ng/ml (depending on lab)
- ECG parameters: pulse < 120; blood pressure < 130/90; $QT_c \leq$ 25% above baseline; PR < .20

Monoamine Oxidase Inhibitors and Nontricyclic Antidepressants

Experience in the United States with monoamine oxidase inhibitors in children and adolescents is extremely limited, particularly in the prepubertal child. Due to their potential for toxicity, these medications are difficult to prescribe for most youngsters. Some adolescents with atypical depressive features or phobias may be candidates (Ryan et al. 1988).

Fluoxetine is a newer antidepressant and antiobsessional agent that blocks serotonin reuptake. It has a long half-life in adults and takes several weeks to reach clinical efficacy. It has been used in open studies to treat childhood and adolescent major depression and obsessive-compulsive disorder with or without Tourette syndrome (Joshi et al. 1991; Riddle et al. 1990).

Bupropion is an aminoketone unrelated to the tricyclics that has antidepressant properties. Not formally approved for patients under 18, it has been studied in the treatment of ADHD (Clay et al. 1988).

Anxiolytics and Sedative-Hypnotics

Despite widespread use in pediatric practice, anxiolytics and sedative-hypnotics have not been well studied in this population. Due to their safety and range of action, these medications have been used for a number of childhood and adolescent conditions such as night terrors, insomnia, anxiety, and hyperactivity.

There are two major classes of medication in this category that are useful in a number of clinical situations: 1) antihistamines such as diphenhydramine and hydroxyzine and 2) benzodiazepines such as diazepam and chlordiazepoxide (Tables 14–7 and 14–8). Experience

Table 14–7. Anxiolytics and sedative-hypnotics for use in children over age 12 years

Generic name (trade name)	Indications	Oral dosage range (mg)	Common side effects: Short-term	Common side effects: Long-term
Antihistamines				
Diphenhydramine (Benadryl)[a]	Bedtime sedation	25–300	Oversedation; hypersensitivity; skin rash; dryness of mucous membranes	
Hydroxyzine (Vistaril or Atarax)[a]	Anxiety states, agitation, bedtime sedation	25–300	Same as above	
Benzodiazepines				
Diazepam (Valium)[a]	Night terrors	1–10	Drowsiness	Cognitive effects?
	Anxiety disorders	2–10	Paradoxical agitation or excitement	Cognitive effects?
Lorazepam (Ativan)	Anxiety: acute or chronic	0.5–6	Sedation	
Chlordiazepoxide (Librium)	Anxiety disorders	10–100	Sedation	
Alprazolam (Xanax)[b]	Separation anxiety; panic	0.25–4	Disinhibition	Withdrawal reactions
Flurazepam (Dalmane)[c]	Bedtime sedation	15–30	Daytime sedation	
Clonazepam (Klonopin)	Anxiety, panic	0.25–3	Daytime sedation	
Other				
Buspirone (BuSpar)	Anxiety disorders	5–30	Sedation; headache; dizzinesss	
Chloral hydrate (Noctec)[a]	Bedtime sedation	500–1,000		

Note. FDA = Food and Drug Administration.
[a]FDA-approved for advertising for use in children under age 6 years.
[b]FDA-approved for advertising for use in children over age 18 years.
[c]FDA-approved for advertising for use in children over age 15 years.

Table 14–8. Recommended anxiolytic and sedative-hypnotic treatment

Suggested treatment regimen for sleep induction (children over age 6 years)

Diphenhydramine or hydroxyzine

- Start with 25–50 mg at bedtime, increase every 5–7 days by 25 mg until therapeutic effect
- Daily maintenance dose range: 25–300 mg at bedtime or 2.0–5.0 mg/kg

Chloral hydrate

- 500–1,000 mg at bedtime

Suggested treatment regimen for pavor nocturnus (night terrors)

Diazepam

- Start at 0.5 mg at bedtime, then increase by 0.5 mg every 2–4 days until therapeutic response
- Daily maintenance dose range: 1–10 mg at bedtime

Suggested treatment regimen for anxiety/agitation

Diphenhydramine or hydroxyzine

- Acute: Start with 25–50 mg, then repeat dose every 2–4 hours until therapeutic effect
- Chronic: Start with 25–50 mg, then increase by 25 mg every 2–3 days
- Daily maintenance dose range: 75–300 mg or up to 5 mg/kg/day

Lorazepam

- Acute: Start with 0.5 mg, then increase by 0.5 mg every 2–4 hours
- Chronic: Start with 0.5 mg daily; then increase by 0.5 mg every 2 or 3 days
- Daily maintenance dose range: 0.5–6 mg

---

with other sedative-hypnotics such as barbiturates and propanediols for anxiolysis is limited in this age group.

The mechanism of action of the antihistamines is thought to be blockade of the central muscarinic action of acetylcholine, and blockade of histamine receptors type 1 (H_1).

The antihistamines are useful for anxiolysis in the nonpsychotic, mild to moderately disturbed population of children and for sedative-hypnotic effects in the preschool through adolescent age groups. Sleep disturbances such as inability to fall asleep due to restlessness, fearfulness, or hyperactivity in the young child are likely to respond to an antihistamine.

Night terrors (pavor nocturnus) is a particular form of sleep disturbance seen in young children during non–rapid eye movement sleep, frequently on arousal from Stage 3 or 4 to lighter sleep stages. Characteristically, the child awakens in a terror, screaming, with signs of physiological arousal; is inconsolable during the episode; and later is amnesic. Diazepam in small doses administered at bedtime for several weeks can be useful for this particular problem.

Benzodiazepines have been found to be generally safe and effective anxiolytics for adult patients. There are few studies of such use in the pediatric population in the United States. Benzodiazepines seem to function as "selective depressants," possibly acting on subcortical structures or specific receptors. There have been some reports of paradoxical reactions or disinhibition to these medications in young patients, such as pathological aggression or excitement; perhaps this has limited their practical use and investigation. Another dilemma for the pediatric practitioner has been the confusion and, until very recently, lack of validated criteria for defining anxiety disorders.

In the nonpsychotic, non-substance-using adolescent population, benzodiazepines can be useful in limited quantities for anxiety that threatens to interfere with daily functioning. Chlordiazepoxide and lorazepam have found some usefulness in this situation. In some adolescents with early and middle insomnia, flurazepam can be used for limited periods of time.

Interest has increased recently in the use of alprazolam in the child and adolescent with separation anxiety or panic disorder symptomatology, paralleling its uses in adults with endogenous anxiety.

Side effects with both of these classes of medication are relatively infrequent, particularly with the antihistamines. Cognitive effects, which have not been systematically assessed, are potentially problematic in use of the benzodiazepines (Coffey 1990).

Buspirone is a new anxiolytic formally approved for use in adults that is a partial 5-HT_{1a} agonist. It does not have muscle relaxant or anticonvulsant properties nor is it likely to cause dependence. There are only two published reports of use in childhood, including a report of use in separation anxiety disorder and in a small number of autistic patients (Kranzler 1988; Realmuto et al. 1989).

Lithium

Experience with lithium in the child and adolescent population has increased in the past decade. Lithium has been clearly found to be effective for treatment of acute mania and prophylaxis for bipolar disorders in the adult population and is formally indicated in children and adolescents with bipolar disorder. In addition, studies suggest that some adolescents and children with certain kinds of behavior disorders can be treated effectively with lithium despite lack of formal indications for use in this age group (Campbell et al. 1984) (Tables 14–9 and 14–10).

It appears that children with periodic or cyclic disturbances of

Table 14–9. Lithium for use in children over age 12 years

Generic name (trade name)	Indications	Oral dosage range (mg)	Common side effects	
			Short-term	**Long-term**
Lithium carbonate (Eskalith or Lithobid)[a]	Bipolar and some recurrent unipolar affective disorders; some behavior disorders with aggressivity; augmentation for refractory major depression	150–1,800 (blood levels: 0.6–1.2 mEq/L	Gastrointestinal: nausea, vomiting, diarrhea, abdominal distress	Weight gain
			CNS: tremor, memory lapses, fatigue	Cognitive blunting
			Renal: polyuria, polydipsia	Tubular changes
			Hematologic: leukocytosis	Endocrine: goiter

Note. CNS = central nervous system. FDA = Food and Drug Administration.
[a]FDA-approved for advertising for use in children over age 12 years.

Table 14–10. Recommended lithium treatment

Suggested treatment regimen for childhood and adolescent bipolar disorders and aggressive behavior (children over age 6 years)

- Start with 150 mg in the A.M., then increase by 150 mg every 3–5 days until blood level is in 0.6–1.5 mEq/L range (some may need higher levels)
- Daily maintenance dose range: 300–2,400 mg daily (0.6–1.2 mEq/L)

behavior and mood, children with such disturbances who have relatives who have been lithium responsive, and children with severely aggressive behavior disorders are potentially lithium responsive (Campbell et al. 1982; DeLong 1977; Youngerman and Canino 1978). Studies are ongoing in this area at present and promise a potentially exciting and useful approach to some of the most difficult patients in the child and adolescent psychiatric population.

The mechanism of action of lithium is not completely clear. Some theories have proposed effects on neurotransmitters, cyclic adenosine monophosphate, or membrane stabilization. Because children and adolescents run the same risks for side effects and toxicities as do their adult counterparts, they must be carefully worked up and monitored. Children and adolescents may need higher doses of lithium than do adults, relative to body weight.

Plasma levels should be obtained to monitor clinical effects on a regular basis. During initiation of treatment, twice-weekly levels are called for, which can be followed by weekly and then approximately monthly levels once equilibrium and steady state have been reached. Levels of 0.6–1.2 mEq/L are in therapeutic range, but some patients may require higher levels to attain therapeutic efficacy. Kidney, endocrine (thyroid, calcium), and cardiac function must be monitored on a regular basis.

Anticonvulsants

Familiarity with anticonvulsant medication is essential for the practicing child and adolescent psychiatrist. Psychiatric symptoms and psychopathology appear to be overrepresented in epileptic patients;

seizures themselves are often accompanied by changes in mood or behavior. Treatment of patients with temporal lobe epilepsy is frequently complicated, requiring collaboration between the child and adolescent psychiatrist and pediatric neurologist.

Seizures can be roughly divided into partial and generalized subtypes:

Partial

- With simple focal symptoms: motor or sensory (no clouding of consciousness)
- With complex symptoms: temporal lobe, psychomotor seizures (clouding of consciousness)

Generalized (clouding of consciousness)

- Tonic-clonic seizures
- Myoclonic, atonic, or akinetic seizures
- Absence or petit mal

Anticonvulsants can be roughly divided into the following groups: hydantoins, barbiturates, carbamazepine, succinimides, benzodiazepines, sodium valproate, and others.

Table 14–11 outlines the specific medications commonly used for different types of seizures, their dosage ranges, and common side effects.

Other Drugs

In recent years, other drugs available to the adult practitioner have been investigated in the pediatric and adolescent population. The beta-adrenergic blocker propranolol has been found useful in some young patients with uncontrollable aggressive behavior, those with lithium-induced tremors, and those with certain anxiety states manifested by physiological symptomatology such as posttraumatic stress disorder (Famularo et al. 1988; Williams et al. 1982). They are contraindicated in diabetic patients, asthmatic patients, and patients with cardiac disease. Their use is still experimental in this age group at this time.

The alpha-agonist clonidine has enjoyed increasing clinical use in

Table 14–11. Anticonvulsant medications for use in children

Generic name (trade name)	Dosage (mg/kg/day)	Therapeutic serum concentration (μg/ml)	Type of seizures	Common side effects
Carbamazepine (Tegretol)	10–20	4–12	All except petit mal and infantile spasms, especially valuable in complex partial seizures	*Dose-related:* drowsiness, ataxia, dysarthria *Other:* gastrointestinal upset, leukopenia, thrombocytopenia, elevation of liver enzymes
Clonazepam (Klonopin)	0.01–0.15	0.015–0.06	Petit mal, minor motor; adjunctive therapy in major motor	*Dose-related:* sedation, dizziness *Other:* behavioral effects including impulsivity, irritability, sleep disturbance, inattentiveness
Clorazepate (Tranxene)	0.3–1.0	0.05–0.075	Adjunctive therapy for generalized and partial seizures, especially complex partial	*Dose-related:* sedation, dizziness *Other:* elevation of liver enzymes, gastrointestinal distress

Ethosuximide	20–40	40–120	Petit mal; adjunctive for refractory seizures	*Dose-related:* sedation *Other:* nausea, vomiting, irritability, sleep disturbance, leukopenia, pancytopenia
Phenobarbital	2–6	20–40	All except petit mal and infantile spasms	*Dose-related:* sedation, ataxia, irritability *Other:* hyperactivity, irritability, depressed affect, hypoglycemia
Phenytoin (Dilantin)	5–10	10–20	All except petit mal and infantile spasms	*Dose-related:* nystagmus, ataxia, irritability *Other:* irritability, depressed affect, gum hypertrophy, hirsutism, tremor, fever, lymphadenopathy, choreoathetosis, thickened facial features
Primidone (Mysoline)	10–20	5–15[a]	All except petit mal and infantile spasms; especially valuable for complex partial and myoclonic	*Dose-related:* sedation, ataxia, irritability *Other:* hyperactivity, irritability, depressed affect, attention-deficit hyperactivity disorder, hypocalcemia

continued

Table 14–11. Anticonvulsant medications for use in children *(continued)*

Generic name (trade name)	Dosage (mg/kg/day)	Therapeutic serum concentration (μg/ml)	Type of seizures	Common side effects
Mephobarbital (Mebaral)	6–12	20–40[b]	All except petit mal and infantile spasms	See phenobarbital
Valproic acid (Depakene)	30–60	50–150	Petit mal and refractory major and minor motor	*Dose-related:* sedation, elevation of liver enzymes *Other:* nausea, vomiting, tremor, transient hair loss, leukopenia, thrombocytopenia, pancreatitis, hepatotoxicity[c]
Phenacemide (Phenurone)	25–40	Not usually measured	All refractory seizures except petit mal and infantile spasms	*Dose-related:* sedation *Other:* personality disorders including suicide attempt, psychosis, depression and aggression; hepatitis, leukopenia, aplastic anemia
Acetazolamide (Diamox)	10–20	Not usually measured	Adjunct in petit mal and major motor	*Dose-related:* sedation, gastric distress *Other:* crystallurea, renal calculus, bone marrow depression, hemolytic anemia, thrombocytopenic[c] purpura, drowsiness, confusion

[a]Primidone is metabolized in part to phenobarital and phenylethylmalonamide; only primidone and phenobarbital are usually measured.
[b]Measured as phenobarbital.
[c]Hypersensitivity and drug allergy may occur with any anticonvulsant.

psychiatry and has been found in some studies to be useful in the treatment of Tourette syndrome. It can be used in combination with haloperidol in low doses or as primary pharmacotherapy. Some evidence indicates that it has been useful in decreasing the motor and verbal tics that characterize the disorder as well as in modifying the behavioral concomitants that often accompany the tics such as attentional problems, hyperactivity, and lability of mood (Leckman et al. 1991).

Several studies in the past decade have featured the use of clonidine for ADHD. Children who appear to be good candidates for the use of clonidine for ADHD are those with highly aroused impulsive characteristics; clonidine ameliorates these symptoms seen in many patients with ADHD but may not be quite as efficacious for the cognitive effects of ADHD such as inattention and distractibility (Hunt et al. 1990).

Opioid antagonists have been studied in the treatment of autistic disorder and Tourette syndrome and in self-injurious behavior in mentally retarded individuals (Campbell et al. 1989; Sokol and Campbell 1988). Naltrexone is a long-acting opiate antagonist that may be useful in a subgroup of autistic patients with elevated opioid peptides. Target symptoms in Campbell et al.'s open study included social withdrawal, stereotypies, and verbal productivity, which improved significantly, and aggressiveness, which did not improve significantly. Sedation was the primary side effect.

Common Drug Interactions in Children and Adolescents

Drug interaction occurs when one agent alters the therapeutic or adverse effects of another agent. Interactions can occur at any phase in a drug treatment plan. Common points of interaction include alterations in

- *Absorption,* such as in the gastrointestinal tract
- *Distribution,* such as competition for binding sites
- *Metabolism,* such as effects on liver enzyme functions

Table 14–12. Common drug interactions in children and adolescents

	Neuroleptics	Stimulants	Antidepressants	Sedative-hypnotics/ anxiolytics	Lithium
Neuroleptics	—	See under neuroleptics	See under neuroleptics; can raise TCA blood levels	See under neuroleptics	Neuroleptics can suppress nausea 2° to lithium toxicity
Stimulants	Thioridazine raises MPH effects in hyperactive patients	—	See under stimulants	See under stimulants	—
Anti-depressants	TCAs potentiate anticholinergic effects; both lower seizure threshold	MPH raises effects of TCAs and raises blood levels; MAOI and stimulants to be avoided	TCA-MAOI combination requires caution	Potentiate anticholinergic effects of MAOI	—
Sedative-hypnotics/ anxiolytics	Neuroleptics potentiate CNS depressants	Stimulants may oppose hypnotic effects	—	—	—
Lithium	Some reports of neuroleptic-haloperidol neurotoxicity	—	—	—	—

Others					
Anticonvulsants	Can raise sedation but not anticonvulsant effect	—	Barbiturates lower TCA blood levels	—	—
Anticoagulants	Phenothiazine lowers effect	MPH potentiates effect of ethyl biscoumacetate	—	Chloral hydrate lowers effects of coumarin preparation	—
Anti-inflammatory agents	—	MPH inhibits action of phenylbutazone	—	—	—
Vasopressors	Neuroleptics block effect of epinephrine and lower blood pressure	—	—	—	—
Antihelminthics	Piperazine and phenothiazines cause seizures	—	—	—	—
Diuretics	Can lower blood pressure	—	—	—	Lowers lithium clearance and raises lithium toxicity

Note. TCA = tricyclic antidepressant. MPH = methylphenidate. MAOI = monoamine oxidase inhibitor. CNS = central nervous system.

- *Excretion*
- *Receptor site* function (Shinn and Shrewsbury 1985)

The best rule of thumb is to try to avoid interactive effects by avoiding polypharmacy whenever possible. However, if at times it becomes necessary to prescribe two or more agents simultaneously, the clinician should be alert to possible interactions.

A few of the more common drug interactions to occur in children and adolescents are listed in Table 14–12.

References

Achenback T, Edelbrock C: Manual for the Child Behavior Checklist and Revised Child Behavior Profile. Burlington, VT, Thomas M Achenback, 1983

American Psychiatric Association: Diagnostic and Statistical Manual of Mental Disorders, 4th Edition. Washington, DC, American Psychiatric Association, 1994

Anderson L, Campbell M, Grega D, et al: Haloperidol in the treatment of infantile autism: effects on learning and behavioral symptoms. Am J Psychiatry 141:1195–1202, 1984

Baldessarini RJ: Drugs and the treatment of psychiatric disorder, in Goodman and Gilman's The Pharmacological Basis of Therapeutics, 8th Edition. Edited by Gilman PI, Rau TW, Nies AS, et al. New York, Pergamon, 1990, pp 383–435

Bernstein GA, Garfinkel BD, Borhardt C: Comparative studies of pharmacotherapy for school refusal. J Am Acad Child Adolesc Psychiatry 29:773–781, 1990

Biederman J, Baldessarini R, Wright V, et al: A double blind-placebo controlled study of desipramine in the treatment of ADD, I: efficacy. J Am Acad Child Adolesc Psychiatry 28:777–784, 1989a

Biederman J, Baldessarini R, Wright V, et al: A double blind-placebo controlled study of desipramine in the treatment of ADD, II: serum drug levels and cardiovascular findings. J Am Acad Child Adolesc Psychiatry 78:903–911, 1989b

Campbell M, Shapiro T: Therapy of psychiatric disorders of childhood, in Manual of Psychiatric Therapeutics. Edited by Shader RI. Boston, MA, Little, Brown, 1975, pp 137–162

Campbell M, Cohen I, Small A: Drugs in aggressive behavior. Journal of the American Academy of Child Psychiatry 21:107–117, 1982

Campbell M, Grega DM, Green WH, et al: Neuroleptic-induced dyskinesias in children. Clin Neuropharmacol 6:207–222, 1983

Campbell M, Small A, Green W, et al: Behavioral efficacy of haloperidol and lithium carbonate: a comparison in hospitalized aggressive children with conduct disorder. Arch Gen Psychiatry 41:650–656, 1984

Campbell M, Overall JE, Small AM, et al: Naltrexone in autistic children: an acute open dose range tolerance trial. J Am Acad Child Adolesc Psychiatry 28:200–206, 1989

Cantwell D, Carlson G: Stimulants, in Pediatric Psychopharmacology: The Use of Behavior Modifying Drugs in Childhood. Edited by Werry J. New York, Brunner/Mazel, 1978, pp 171–207

Clay TH, Gualtieri CT, Evans RW, et al: Clinical and neuropsychological effects of the novel antidepressant bupropion. Psychopharmacol Bull 24:143–148, 1988

Coffey B: Anxiolytics: traditional and new drugs. Journal of Child and Adolescent Psychopharmacology 1:57–83, 1990

Cohen D, Shaywitz B, Shaywitz S, et al: Pharmacotherapy of attention deficit disorders, in Pediatric Update, Vol 5. Edited by Moss AJ. New York, Elsevier–North Holland, 1983, pp 43–61

Conners CK: Rating scales for use in drug studies with children, in Psychopharmacology Bulletin (Special Issue: Pharmacotherapy With Children), 1974, pp 24–84

Conners CK, Barkley R: Rating scales and checklists for pediatric psychopharmacology. Psychopharmacol Bull 21:809–815, 1985

Coyle J: Biochemical development of the brain: neurotransmitters and child psychiatry, in Psychiatric Pharmacosciences of Children and Adolescents. Edited by Popper C. Washington, DC, American Psychiatric Press, 1987, pp 1–26

DeLong R: Lithium carbonate treatment of select behavior disorders in children suggesting manic-depressive illness. J Pediatr 93:689–699, 1977

Donnelly M, Rapoport J, Potter W, et al: Fenfluramine and dextroamphetamine treatment of childhood hyperactivity. Arch Gen Psychiatry 46:205–212, 1989

Dulcan M: Using psychostimulants to treat behavioral disorders of children and adolescents. Journal of Child and Adolescent Psychopharmacology 1:7–20, 1990

Famularo R, Kinscherff R, Fenton T: Propranolol treatment for childhood post traumatic stress disorder, acute type. Am J Dis Child 142:1244–1247, 1988

Flament M, Rapoport J, Berg C, et al: Clomipramine treatment of childhood obsessive compulsive disorder: a double blind controlled study. Arch Gen Psychiatry 42:977–983, 1985

Gadow K, Nolan E, Sverd J, et al: Methylphenidate in aggressive-hyperactive boys, I: the effects on peer aggression in public school settings. J Am Acad Child Adolesc Psychiatry 29:710–718, 1990

Gittleman-Klein R: Pharmacotherapy and management of pathological separation anxiety. International Journal of Mental Health 4:255–271, 1975

Green W: Amines and central nervous system stimulants, in Child and Adolescent Clinical Psychopharmacology. Edited by Green WH. Baltimore, MD, Williams & Wilkins, 1991a, pp 75–76

Green W: General principles of psychopharmacotherapy with children and adolescents, in Child and Adolescent Clinical Psychopharmacology. Edited by Green WH. Baltimore, MD, Williams & Wilkins, 1991b, pp 7–49

Gualtieri CT, Barnhill J, McGimsey J, et al: Tardive dyskinesia and other movement disorders in children treated with psychotropic drugs. Journal of the American Academy of Child Psychiatry 19:491–510, 1980

Gualtieri CT, Quade D, Hicks R, et al: Tardive dyskinesia and other clinical consequences of neuroleptic treatment in children and adolescents. Am J Psychiatry 141:20–23, 1984

Hunt R, Copper L, O'Connell P: Clonidine in child and adolescent psychiatry. Journal of Child and Adolescent Psychopharmacology 1:87–103, 1990

Jatlow PI: Psychotropic drug disposition during development, in Psychiatric Pharmacosciences of Children and Adolescents. Edited by Popper C. Washington, DC, American Psychiatric Press, 1987, pp 27–44

Joshi PT, Walkup JT, Capozzoli JA, et al: The use of fluoxetine in the treatment of major depressive disorder in children and adolescents. Paper presented at the 36th annual meeting of the American Academy of Child and Adolescent Psychiatry, New York, October 11–15, 1989

Klein D, Gittelman R, Quitkin F, et al: Diagnosis and Drug Treatment of Psychiatric Disorders: Adults and Children, 2nd Edition. Baltimore, MD, Williams & Wilkins, 1980

Klein R, Mannuzza S: Hyperactive boys almost grown up, III: methylphenidate effects on ultimate height. Arch Gen Psychiatry 45:1131–1134, 1988

Kranzler H: Use of buspirone in an adolescent with overanxious disorder. J Am Acad Child Adolesc Psychiatry 43:3388–3392, 1988

Kovacs M: Rating scales to assess depression in school-aged children. Acta Paedopsych 46:305–315, 1980–1981

Leckman J, Hardin M, Riddle M, et al: Clonidine treatment of Gilles de la Tourette syndrome. Arch Gen Psychiatry 48:324–328, 1991

Mattes J, Gittelman R: Growth of hyperactive children on maintenance regimen of methylphenidate. Arch Gen Psychiatry 40:317–321, 1983

National Center for Health Statistics: Growth Chart. Washington, DC, U.S. Department of Human Services, Health Resources Administration, National Center for Health Statistics, Centers for Disease Control, 1978

Neppe VM, Ward NG: The evaluation and management of neuroleptic-induced acute extrapyramidal syndromes, in Innovative Psychopharmacology. Edited by Neppe VM. New York, Raven, 1989, pp 152–176

Nurcombe B: Malpractice, in The Comprehensive Textbook of Child Psychiatry. Edited by Lewis M. Baltimore, MD, Williams & Wilkins, 1991, pp 1127–1139

Pelham W, Bender M, Caddell J, et al: Methylphenidate and children with attention deficit disorder, dose effects on classroom academic and social behavior. Arch Gen Psychiatry 42:948–952, 1985

Popper C, Elliot G: Sudden death and tricyclic antidepressants: clinical considerations for children. Journal of Child and Adolescent Psychopharmacology 2:125–132, 1990

Puig-Antich J: Affective disorders in childhood: a review and perspective. Psychiatr Clin North Am 3:403–424, 1980

Rapoport J, Mikkelsen E: Antidepressants, in Pediatric Psychopharmacology: The Use of Behavior Modifying Drugs in Childhood. Edited by Werry J. New York, Brunner/Mazel, 1978, pp 208–233

Rapoport J, Mikkelsen E, Zaradil A, et al: Childhood enuresis II. Arch Gen Psychiatry 37:1146–1152, 1980a

Rapoport J, Buschbaum M, Weingartner H, et al: Dextroamphetamine: its cognitive and behavioral effects in normal and hyperactive boys and normal men. Arch Gen Psychiatry 37:933–943, 1980b

Realmuto G, August G, Garfinkel B: Clinical effect of buspirone in autistic disorder. J Clin Psychopharmacol 9:122–125, 1989

Riddle M, Hardin M, King R, et al: Fluoxetine treatment of children and adolescents with Tourette's and obsessive compulsive disorders: preliminary clinical experience. J Am Acad Child Adolesc Psychiatry 29:45–48, 1990

Ryan N: Heterocyclic antidepressants in children and adolescents. Journal of Child and Adolescent Psychopharmacology 1:21–31, 1990a

Ryan N: Pharmacotherapy of adolescent major depression: beyond TCA's. Psychopharmacol Bull 26:75–79, 1990b

Ryan N, Puig-Antich J, Rabinovich H, et al: MAOIs in adolescent major depression unresponsive to tricyclic antidepressants. J Am Acad Child Adolesc Psychiatry 217:755–758, 1988

Safer D, Allen R, Barry E, et al: Depression of growth in hyperactive children on stimulant drugs. N Engl J Med 287:217–220, 1972

Shinn A, Shrewsbury R: Evaluation of Drug Interactions, 3rd Edition. St. Louis, MO, CV Mosby, 1985

Sokol M, Campbell M: Novel psychoactive agents in the treatment of developmental disorders, in Psychopharmacology of the Developmental Disabilities. Edited by Aman M, Singh N. New York, Springer-Verlag, 1988, pp 147–167

U.S. Department of Human Services, Alcohol and Drug Abuse and Mental Health Administration: Abnormal Involuntary Movements Scale. Rockville, MD, National Institute of Mental Health, 1974

Verglas G, Banks S, Guyer K: Clinical effects of fenfluramine on children with autism: a review of the research. Journal of Autism and Neurological Disorders 18:297–308, 1988

Williams D, Meyl R, Yudofsky S, et al: The effects of propranolol on uncontrolled rage outbursts in children and adolescents with organic brain dysfunction. Journal of the American Academy of Child Psychiatry 21:129–135, 1982

Youngerman J, Canino I: Lithium carbonate use in children and adolescents. Arch Gen Psychiatry 35:216–224, 1978

15

Emergencies I

Judith E. Robinson, M.D.

When a child is brought to the emergency room for psychiatric consultation, the child's *physical safety* represents the first priority of the consulting psychiatrist. It is the psychiatrist's responsibility to assess the nature of the presenting problem rapidly and to determine what *immediate course of action* needs to be taken. The psychiatrist must decide if the child

- Needs medical intervention by the pediatrician on call
- Requires constant observation for suicidal precautions
- Is at risk for running away from the emergency room
- Is at risk of being taken prematurely from the emergency room by a caretaker

Only when the child's physical safety has been ensured can a systematic evaluation process begin.

A *thorough psychiatric examination* is essential for the successful management of psychiatric emergencies. This provides the child psychiatrist with the data necessary to make a working formulation, an accurate diagnosis, and an appropriate treatment plan. In the emergency room, as in the clinic, a complete evaluation includes the following:

- Presenting problem
- Present illness and precipitating stress
- Psychiatric history
- Family history (with special attention to present stressors and the ability of the family to cope with the child now)
- Family psychiatric history
- Developmental history (as relevant)
- Medical history (as relevant)
- Social history (as relevant)
- Detailed interview with the child and family, including mental status examination

The physical examination should be part of every evaluation. It is essential if the child presents with suspected or confirmed physical or sexual abuse, alcohol or drug intoxication abuse or overdose, abrupt change in behavior, or history of a recent suicide attempt.

Additional information may need to be gathered from sources other than the child or the parents. Such sources often include the child's therapist, social service worker, or pediatrician. Ready access in the emergency room to frequently used telephone numbers facilitates the evaluation.

In evaluating psychiatric emergencies in children, an assessment must also be made of the children's parents or caretakers. Psychiatric symptoms in children often reflect pathology in the parent-child relationship. It is essential to determine if the child is expressing symptoms that reflect a pathological and unsafe family situation. One must be alert to the possibility of physical, sexual, and emotional abuse.

Assessment of parents is also aimed at determining the parents' capacity to support an at-risk child within the home environment. Many children in need of inpatient hospitalization are denied this treatment course by third-party payers. It is of critical importance for the child psychiatrist to evaluate the family's ability to care at home for the at-risk child to keep the child safe and to follow through with ambulatory care.

At times, the situation arises that the psychiatrist does not feel comfortable sending home a child even though third-party payers will not approve hospitalization. An important responsibility of the psychiatrist is to advocate for the safety of the child. It is the psychiatrist's responsibility to communicate unambiguously with a third-party reviewer the necessity of the hospitalization. Should hospitalization not be approved, it is the psychiatrist's responsibility to know the community resources to ensure the child's safety. Often this responsibility includes involving the Department of Social Services, the Department of Mental Health, the hospital administration, or the hospital's legal department. No child should leave the emergency room to an unsafe disposition.

Suicide

Suicidal ideation and behavior are among the most frequent psychiatric emergencies in childhood and adolescence. Successfully completed suicide is virtually nonexistent in children under age 5 years and rare in children ages 6–12, although threats and attempts are not uncommon. In adolescence, the suicide rate is significant and is rapidly on the rise. Over the last three decades, in the 15- to 19-year-old age group, the suicide rate has tripled (Brent et al. 1987). Although more girls than boys demonstrate suicidal behavior, nearly five times more teenage boys commit suicide than do teenage girls (Shaffer et al. 1988). Although drug overdose is by far the most common method used in suicide attempts, it accounts for few completed suicides in teenagers. In the United States, adolescents of both sexes are more likely to commit suicide with firearms, males being more likely than females to use violent weapons. The next most common suicide method used by boys is hanging, whereas for girls it is jumping (Brent et al. 1987).

Any child or adolescent who attempts suicide usually does so as a last resort. Even if the suicidal behavior is seen as a gesture or manipulation and not as a genuine effort to end life, it must *always* be seen as a desperate attempt on the part of the child and must *always* be taken seriously. It is important to remember that although only a minority of those who attempt suicide go on to commit suicide successfully, the rate of completed suicide is considerably higher in this population than in the general population. A suicide gesture is a psychiatric emergency.

Suicidal ideation and suicidal behavior in childhood usually reflect serious and chronic problems within the family. Children who contemplate suicide have frequently had early separation from their parents or inadequate mothering, sometimes including physical or emotional abuse. Many of these children present as depressed, empty, and lonely, with an accompanying sense of themselves as expendable (Pfeffer 1981).

Often the child of latency age or younger may threaten or attempt suicide without understanding the nature of death, its permanence, or its irreversibility. For children at this age, death may mean removal from an unpleasant situation to a happier one; it may also be an attempt to gain love from unresponsive parents or to join a parent or loved one who had died.

In a study of suicidal behavior in children ages 6–12, Pfeffer et al. (1980) found that a child's suicidal potential correlated significantly with a sense of depression, hopelessness, and worthlessness; the wish to die; preoccupation with death; and severe depression and suicidal behavior in parents.

Suicidal adolescents understand the meaning of death. Usually these youngsters are seriously troubled. Many suicidal adolescents present with a history of a major depressive mood disorder, substance abuse, or antisocial behavior. A significant portion of youngsters who successfully complete suicide have first- or second-degree relatives who have attempted or completed suicide. Most children or adolescents who attempt suicide have very low self-esteem. Immediately prior to their attempt there often is a history of arguments, especially with parents or significant others, a history of school problems, trouble with the law, or the breakup of a romantic relationship. In girls there is an association between a history of recent assaults and suicidal behavior (Hoberman and Garfinkel 1988). All of these precipitants further lower self-esteem. The suicide attempt represents the overwhelmed and desperate child's or adolescent's effort, often impulsive, at extrication from a seemingly impossible situation.

Evaluation

The immediate treatment of a suicide attempt is to provide medical lifesaving measures. Only when the patient is out of danger can the formal evaluative process begin.

The suicidal patient should be evaluated in a safe environment and should be seen in a room with no sharp objects and no open windows. At no time should the patient be left alone.

The child psychiatric consultant must establish a working alliance with the child or adolescent. In a nonjudgmental and nonpunitive manner, the consultant must stress the seriousness of the situation and convey genuine concern and desire to help. Ideally the child and family should be interviewed separately, and the child should be helped to understand clearly that his or her feelings are important and will be listened to.

The evaluation should follow the format outlined earlier in this chapter, with special attention to the following:

Presenting problem. It is important to assess

- The *lethality* of the suicide attempt. What method did the patient use; what was the likelihood of success? Was the action planned or impulsive, was rescue imminent? Was a note left? What was the content?
- The *motivation.* Why does the patient want to commit suicide? Is the patient depressed and feeling hopeless? Is the patient angry and wishing to punish someone? Is the patient hoping to show a loved one how much he or she means to them? Is the patient responding to a hallucination? Was the patient's judgment impaired by drugs or alcohol?
- The patient's *concept of death.* Is the patient hoping to find peace and an end to suffering? Is the patient hoping to join a dead relative or loved one? Does the patient understand clearly that death is permanent?
- Current *attitude.* What does it mean to the patient not to have died? Is the patient sad or relieved? Has the patient's perspective changed or is the patient planning to try again?

These data are particularly good indicators of the acute risk of further suicidal behavior.

The precipitating stress. It is important to ask specifically about

- The patient's relationship with parents or caretakers, emphasizing any recent arguments or problems
- Any breakup in a romantic relationship or an important friendship
- Any changes within the family, any illnesses, any losses (or anniversaries of losses)
- Any changes in the patient's own health, including pregnancy and sexually transmitted diseases
- Recognition of gay or lesbian sexual orientation
- Any difficulties in school, any problem with the authorities, any situation in which the parents may soon learn something very negative about the child
- Participation in incest or sexual abuse
- Any other change that may have altered the patient's view of life or of self-worth

Interview with the family. An essential element of the psychiatric evaluation is the interview with the parents or caretakers. A suicide attempt on the part of the child is a *family* problem, and many suicidal children have a history of long-standing family problems. It is important to assess the family's understanding of the child's actions and the family's conscious and unconscious attitude toward the patient and toward the patient's suicide attempt.

It is important to note, however, that a number of studies indicate that neither parents nor teachers are generally accurate judges of depression in children. These individuals tend to underestimate affective disorders as well as substance abuse (Hoberman and Garfinkel 1988).

Continued suicide risk is associated with

- A negative attitude or lack of concern toward the patient
- A minimization of the seriousness and an attempt to see it only as attention-getting behavior

- Family's instability and inability to cope with the child and provide a safe, supportive environment
- The incidence in the family of suicide attempts, and serious depression, because suicide attempts in children correspond significantly with parental suicidal ideation

Mental status examination. It is critical to assess the patient's reality testing, judgment, impulse control, mood, and affect. It is essential to determine if the patient's suicidal ideation is based on a psychiatric disorder such as psychosis (are voices telling the patient to commit suicide?), affective disorder, or intoxication with alcohol or drugs.

After the child and family have been interviewed and pertinent historical information has been gathered, a psychodynamic formulation must be made. This formulation should help to clarify what forces have combined to place this particular child in jeopardy and make his or her life not worth living, and what changes are necessary to shift the equilibrium. The child psychiatrist must determine whether these changes are possible given information on the child and the child's family and situation.

Assessment. Final assessment of the suicidal child should take into account that certain children are statistically at high risk for self-destructive behavior. They include children

- With chronic family problems
- Living outside of a natural family
- With poor relationships and few supports
- With poor school performance
- With family history of suicide attempts
- Whose parents do not like them or whose parents see them as expendable
- With a concomitant psychiatric diagnosis especially of affective disorder or a history of drug or alcohol abuse
- Who understand the meaning of death and who have a true wish to die
- Whose attempt was very lethal
- Who make poor relationships with the evaluator

- Who have made a previous suicide attempt
- Who are depressed and hopeless

Disposition of a Suicidal Child or Adolescent

The primary goal of the psychiatric consultant is to keep the child safe from harm. The question that inevitably arises in the emergency room is whether the child is safe to go home or whether hospitalization is needed. The decision depends on a variety of factors:

- The child's *immediate potential* for continued self-destructive behavior.
- *Concurrent psychopathology* of the child. If the child is psychotic, hypomanic, severely depressed, or intoxicated with drugs or alcohol, the child must be held in the protective environment of the hospital.
- The assessment of the child's *intrapsychic needs,* based on the psychodynamic formulation and the likelihood that these needs can be adequately met. If they cannot be met, in short order, the child must be held in the protective environment.
- The *family's unambivalent desire* for the *child* to *live,* their understanding of the suicidal behavior as an individual as well as a family problem, their ability to mobilize around the child and to assume appropriate parental response for the child. Since most suicidal children have chronic and complicated family problems, parents may not be able to make immediate changes that are necessary, and the child may need psychiatric hospitalization as the initial treatment.
- *Practical limitations* of the family's ability to provide adequately supervised support and keep the patient safe from harm.

If there is any doubt as to whether or not the patient should be sent home from the emergency room, the child should be hospitalized. Within the hospital, protection from physical harm continues to be the primary concern. The suicidal child should be placed in a safe room without sharp objects or access to windows through which the child could exit. Around-the-clock sitters who can observe and protect the child or other suicidal precautions will be required, depending on the setting's structure. For the severely agitated or psychotic child, chemical or physical restraints may be necessary.

In the event that the child is sent home, a follow-up appointment should be made for the next day, and a phone number should be given to a family member for emergency contact.

Aggression

Many children are brought to the emergency room with the presenting problem of aggressive behavior. For younger children, often by the time the psychiatrist sees the child, the presenting behavior has subsided and the evaluation is based largely on historical information. Usually the parent reports several weeks of increasing aggressive behavior, culminating in an event precipitating presentation to the emergency room. Frequent complaints include the child's not listening or the child's striking out physically at parents, at siblings, and even at family pets. The children may or may not display this behavior with others outside of the home environment.

Extreme aggressive behavior in preschool children (who are medically and neurologically intact) is usually reflective of child-parent problems. This is especially true when the parents report the aggressive behavior as directed primarily toward them. Often these are children with whom the parents have an ambivalent attachment; such children are frequently raised with inconsistent limit setting, at times by a parent with unconscious masochistic tendencies. In other instances children may act out their parents' own unconscious hostility. Some children may come from families where aggression and physical acting out, including physical means of discipline, are the norm. In this case, the child's aggressive behavior may reflect both the heightening of aggressive drives and an identification with an aggressive parent.

Aggression seen in older children often reflects unhappiness and insecurity. Aggressive behavior frequently is seen in response to frustration related particularly to problems with peers or family members who are seen as uncaring. Drug or alcohol use may precipitate violent outbursts. Aggressive behavior may also develop in children who have been physically or sexually abused. Often these children have not disclosed the abuse, and the behavioral symptoms are the first manifestation that something is wrong.

In most adolescents, aggressive behavior usually follows a buildup of tension. Often a struggle over control precipitates an episode of rage. Although threats may be made and furniture flung, usually no one is hurt, and by the time the adolescent is seen, the anger has diminished. In most instances, the consultant's task is crisis intervention. After evaluating the situation, listening to both parent and child, the child psychiatrist most frequently suggests some environmental manipulation to ease the tension temporarily. An outpatient referral is made for a more extended evaluation, beyond the scope of emergency consultation. Many of these aggressive children and parents carry diagnoses of depression and sociopathic or borderline character disorder. Some children also have attention-deficit/hyperactivity disorder, conduct disorder, or substance abuse disorders. All of these problems may require long-term treatment.

In some cases, however, aggressive children and adolescents present a more immediately serious and complicated picture in the emergency room. Some of these patients are angry, agitated, and out of control. Assessment of these children can be difficult, and at times the consultant, especially the inexperienced consultant, may feel frightened or overwhelmed. It is important for the consultant to remember that usually the child is also frightened by his or her own loss of control and that the child is looking to the consultant as to a good parent, to help regain control in a nonthreatening, nonhumiliating way. The "uncontrollable" child should be interviewed in a quiet room in the emergency area. If it seems likely that the child will continue to act up, the evaluator should make certain that other staff members are readily available to help contain the child. The consultant must attempt in a calm, yet authoritative way, to evaluate the situation.

The consultant has as one goal to determine whether this behavior is an exacerbation of a chronic pattern for this child, or whether this is a change in behavior reflecting a psychiatric condition, physical illness, intoxication, or a response to trauma such as physical or sexual abuse. Whatever the etiology of the behavior, the clinician's second goal is to understand the patient's problem and to ensure the safety of the patient and others until longer-term treatment can be undertaken.

The psychiatric consultant must ascertain the following:

- Is there something specific that has triggered the patient's upset or outburst? Is that behavior the culmination of a buildup of tension or did this behavior develop de novo?
- Is the patient's anger focused at someone or something in particular or is the aggression poorly organized and undirected?
- Does the child know what would help to make him or her feel better? Is this reasonable and is this possible?
- Has this child caused self-harm or harm to others or is the child likely to do so?
- Does this child's reality testing appear intact?

If the child has had an acute change in behavior, organic causes should be considered before psychiatric diagnosis can be made. Specifically, one should consider a neurological problem such as a temporal lope epilepsy or an organic brain syndrome secondary to infectious, metabolic, oncologic, or toxic process. In terms of psychiatric diagnosis, one should consider hypomania, borderline personality disorder with psychotic decompensation, and schizophrenia, or brief reactive psychosis, possibly secondary to physical or sexual abuse or other trauma.

The consultant must keep in mind that patients with intoxication, organic brain syndrome, or acute psychosis are at particular risk for serious acting out of their aggressive feelings because of their poor impulse control, impaired reality testing, and inadequate judgment. When a diagnosis of an underlying disorder can be made, treatment should be aimed at this underlying disorder.

During the course of evaluation, many agitated patients regain their composure. Some, however, continue to escalate and pose a risk to themselves and to others. Every effort should be made at resolving the situation verbally; at times, however, the patient's behavior requires external controls. Before considering chemical intervention, it must be clear that this is not medically contraindicated. If this is the case, the patient must be physically restrained under observation until the agitation subsides or until medication can be used. Whenever medication is used, it must first be clearly explained to the patient that he or she is going to be given something that will help control aggression and help the patient feel better.

For the moderately agitated and aggressive younger child who is not psychotic, diphenhydramine or hydroxyzine may be useful in reducing the disruptive behavior. Recommended dosage is 25–50 mg orally every 2 hours or until the behavior is diminished or the child is sedated. For acute treatment of children or adolescents with severe agitation or psychotic rage, major tranquilizers are recommended. The dosage regimen is similar to that detailed in the section in this chapter on psychosis; however, for the acutely agitated client, the medication may be pushed to the point of sedation.

Generally, medication should be offered first in the oral form; if this is refused, it should be given in the injectable form. In situations where immediate sedation is required, the intramuscular route is the treatment of choice. If it is given intramuscularly, the dose should be reduced by approximately one-half.

For the child with a psychiatric or medical illness precipitating aggressive behavior, inpatient evaluation is generally recommended. Placement in a facility that can provide a secure environment with 24-hour observation and protection is obviously recommended.

For the child or adolescent who does not have a primary psychiatric or medical illness but who presents with serious aggressive behavior, the initial management in the emergency room is the same as for the patient with an underlying illness. Chemical or physical restraints may be necessary to ensure safety as the evaluation proceeds.

Research on teenagers who have committed serious crimes indicates certain risk factors. Nurcombe (1991) compiled a profile for an adolescent at risk for committing an aggressive act:

- Older male adolescent
- Low socioeconomic status
- History of neurological impairment or learning disability
- History of drug or alcohol abuse
- Tendency to act out anxious or hostile feelings

- Family history of acting-out behavior
- History of neglect or physical or sexual abuse
- History of previous aggressive acts

There is further risk if

- The patient has a strong drive to be violent
- The patient has a history of affective illness or is experiencing command hallucinations.
- The patient has a designated victim with whom the patient has a relationship.
- The patient has suffered a real or perceived narcissistic injury in this relationship.
- The patient has access to a weapon.
- The patient belongs to a subgroup where acting out with aggression is acceptable.

If it is determined that the patient is at risk for continued aggressive acts, a protective milieu may be necessary (Nurcombe 1991).

Homicide

Although it is relatively uncommon, some children, like adults, threaten and go on to commit serious acts of violence including homicide. Young children and preadolescents who murder comprise a heterogeneous group that includes children who accidentally kill in the course of play; those who mean only to hurt the victim; those who wish to kill out of anger, frustration, and hopelessness; those who act out what they have been taught; those who act out the unconscious wishes of others, particularly adults in their lives; and those with severe developmental delays as well as organic, borderline, or psychotic disorders (Petti 1980).

Adolescents constitute the majority of homicidal youngsters. In 1985, 8% of murders in the United States were committed by juveniles under age 18. Homicide is the second leading cause of death for individuals in the 15- to 24-year-old age group and the leading cause of death for young black males in that group (Lewis et al. 1988; Morbidity and Mortality Weekly Report 1990). The psychiatrist in the emergency room is sometimes called on to evaluate the aggressive adolescent who is threatening to kill. To do such an evaluation, it is best to know as much as possible about the characteristics of the juvenile murderer.

Over the last decade, much research has been directed at learning about the biopsychosocial characteristics of the juvenile murderer. A major part of this work was done by Lewis et al. (1988), who have extensively studied incarcerated adolescents and compared juvenile murderers, violent juveniles, and nonviolent juveniles. They highlighted a constellation of vulnerabilities that characterize those who commit murder. These include

- Neurological impairment
- Psychomotor symptoms
- Episodic psychotic symptoms occurring sporadically without the diagnosis of schizophrenia
- History of abuse as a child
- History of severe parental psychopathology and violence

For all of those who murdered, the individual act was not a single act of uncontrollable violence but was part of a history of extensive aggressive acts. In addition, the majority of murderers had a first-degree relative with major mental illness or with a history of psychiatric hospitalizations. Although delinquents who murdered had significantly more neurological impairment, came from a significantly more violent household, and were twice as likely to have been physically abused than "ordinary" violent delinquents, both groups shared many neuropsychiatric and behavioral characteristics. Juveniles who murdered were very different, however, from nonviolent juvenile delinquents. Lewis et al. (1988) postulated that although the nonviolent juvenile delinquent might have any of the characteristics of the violent or homicidal juvenile delinquent, it was the constellation of vulnerabilities in the context of the abusive environment that seemed to facilitate severe aggression.

In addition to the above, further risk factors include (Allen 1981;

Bender 1959; Lewis et al. 1979, 1988; Morbidity and Mortality Weekly Report 1990; Sendi and Blomgren 1975):

- A history of fire setting
- A history of cruelty to animals
- Labile affect
- Orientation toward action
- Ability to see killing as a feasible act
- Membership in a culture or community accepting of violent behavior
- A psychiatric diagnosis
- Intoxication with drugs or alcohol
- Possession of a weapon
- Formulated plan of action
- History of previously having murdered

A psychodynamic understanding of juvenile murderers provides a further framework for the evaluation of the adolescent patient. Literature on murder by children refers to early traumatic events as contributing to severe ego weaknesses and deficits. Often these adolescents with arrested ego development and impaired object relations have difficulty maintaining a stable view of others when confronted with frustration or rejection. Aggressive impulses including murderous narcissistic rage may be unleashed in an attempt to maintain ego integrity.

A substantial number of those who murder kill family members or others well known to them. Usually these victims are people who, in the context of their relationships, provide the future perpetrator with a sense of self-esteem. A threatened loss of the relationship is the precipitant to the homicidal act.

A significant number of these youngsters who go on to kill give clues prior to committing the act. Psychological autopsy reveals many premonitory signs (Malmquist 1971):

- An object loss in a relationship that served to provide the perpetrator with a cohesive sense of self
- A threat to one's sexuality (or a homosexual threat)
- An ensuing shift in mood to hopelessness and often to self-hate

- An increasing restlessness, agitation, and irritability
- A use of drugs to alter feelings and impulses from concomitantly impairing thought processes and diminishing ego controls
- Increasing somatization, hypochondriasis, or recurrent medical problems
- A cry for help that may range from a muted call often not perceived by others to an explicit verbal warning or direct threat
- An emotional crescendo with a loosening of thought processes and a breakdown of ego control over affective discharge

Malmquist (1971) suggested that for homicidal individuals in the face of hopelessness, helplessness, and ego disintegration, aggression is directed away from the self (suicidal ideation) and projected onto the victim (homicidal ideation) in an attempt at survival.

Many individuals threaten "to kill." The majority of them never seriously contemplate murder. Some, however, do go on to commit murder. When an individual presents in the emergency room with homicidal ideation, a psychiatric consultant must consider all of the aforementioned characteristics of juvenile murderers. It is, however, difficult even for the experienced clinician to predict with accuracy which individuals will go on to act on their homicidal threats. If there is any concern in the consultant's mind that there is serious risk of violence if the patient is released from the emergency room, a protective milieu must be considered. Many patients are relieved to be offered such treatment. In the case of the patient who refuses voluntary treatment, the consultant must be familiar with local laws that permit the patient to be detained.

Child Abuse

Although child abuse has existed through the centuries, it is only within the last 25 years that this problem has begun to receive the attention it deserves. Statistics vary greatly concerning the number of children actually abused; a realistic estimation seems to be that each year close to 1 million female adolescents are sexually assaulted and more than 1.5 million children and adolescents are abused by adults responsible for them (Christoffel 1990). The child psychiatric consultant is generally involved with these children as they present in the emergency ward for medical treatment. In cases of flagrant abuse, the consultant may be called after the diagnosis has been made. In cases of more subtle abuse, the child psychiatric consultant may be asked for help in establishing the diagnosis.

Although child abuse includes physical abuse and neglect, sexual abuse and neglect, and emotional abuse and neglect, we deal here primarily with physical abuse. Emergency treatment of sexual abuse is dealt with in Chapter 16.

Physical abuse implies a nonaccidental injury to the child. Many families practice physical punishment, and there is wide cross-cultural variation in forms of such punishment. When this punishment results in an injury that requires medical attention, there is little controversy over concern. All states now have laws requiring that a physician who suspects physical abuse must report it to the appropriate authorities.

The first steps in detecting physical abuse are to recognize that it is a widespread phenomenon and to maintain a high level of suspicion when a child presents with an injury that cannot be explained by the parents to the satisfaction of the physician. Frequently, abusive parents alter their story as they tell it to different physicians or independently give differing histories of the injury, give explanations of the injury that are beyond the developmental capacity of the child, or place blame on the "baby-sitter." History or physical evidence of previous injuries and a delay in seeking medical attention should also raise the question of abuse.

Additionally, certain types of injuries are suggestive of abuse:

- Multiple injuries at various stages of resolution
- Bruises in the pattern of finger marks or strap marks
- Burns from cigarette butts
- Scalding injuries
- Bite marks
- Bald spots (from hair pulling)
- Injuries of the long bones, especially dislocated metaphyses or epiphyses, spiral fractures, or subperiosteal thickening

- Rupture of viscera
- Change in neurological status without explainable medical etiology

If abuse is suspected when the psychiatric consultant evaluates the child and parents, the consultant must remember that in most cases parents do not willfully intend to harm their children; rather, under stress, they have experienced a failure in their capacity to cope. Abusive parents are likely to be immature, with unmet dependency needs of their own. Most have come from unnurturing, unsupportive families. Many have themselves been abused. Most have serious external stressors and poor impulse control.

In many cases the abused child is one who either poses a problem for the parent or places a demand on the parent. Infants and preschool children, nonverbal but demanding, are in the group statistically most likely to be abused. Also at high risk are children with medical problems and children who are mentally retarded, physically handicapped, neurologically impaired, hyperactive, colicky, or difficult to care for. A child to whom the parent has not bonded well is at particular risk.

The diagnosis of abuse depends heavily on a careful history, physical examination, X-ray and laboratory studies, and interview with the parents and child. Ideally, the history of the injury should be obtained separately from the child and the parents. For the most part, young children do not fabricate physical abuse. *Any allegations they make should be taken seriously.*

Physical examination should be directed not only to the presenting injury, but also to the possibility of old injuries. A bone survey is useful in providing additional data. For the child reported to be "an easy bruiser," a coagulation profile may be in order.

The results of history and physical examination should be carefully documented.

A joint interview with the parents and child provides additional data. It is important to assess the child's relationship with the parent. Does the child seem frightened? Is the child unusually quiet in the presence of the parent? Is the child overly solicitous of the parent? Does the parent seem to have unreasonable expectations of the child? Does the child have the role of "parentified" child, caring for the parent and for siblings? If these questions can be answered in the affirmative, then the suspicion increases that abuse has occurred. The final diagnosis of abuse is usually made collaboratively by the pediatrician, the child psychiatrist, and the social worker; often a legal consultant is involved. In many hospitals all suspected abuse cases are reviewed by an advocate group, and a team determination is made.

In the past, it was generally advised that a child with suspected abuse be hospitalized. Hospitalization allowed both for treatment of the injury and protection of the child. Currently, unless there is a medical or psychiatric necessity for confinement, the child is not hospitalized. In all cases of suspected child abuse, it is mandatory throughout the country that the physician file a report with the state protective service agency. The decision to return the child home or to place the child outside of the home is then generally made by the worker from this agency with the recommendation from the hospital staff. If there is any question that returning the child home places the child at risk, then the child must be placed outside of the house.

It is also the physician's responsibility to inform the parents of the diagnosis that has been made. The medical reasons for the diagnosis and the legal requirement to report such cases should be explained. Discussion with the parent should be nonjudgmental. Parents should be told what will happen following the receipt of the report, including subsequent investigation by a social service worker. The clinician should emphasize that reporting of the incident will enable them to receive helpful services. Many parents feel relieved and supported by these approaches. Others appear angry and indignant. Considerable skill may be required on the part of the physician to help parents accept what is being done is out of concern for a child and for them. A physician who can communicate concern for a child and family can do much to pave the way for successful intervention.

Psychosis

Psychosis is relatively uncommon in childhood and adolescence. When it does occur, the psychiatric consultant must determine the etiology of the condition. The major emergency considerations are the differential diagnosis of functional and organic psychoses and the assessment of the concomitant risk of suicidal, homicidal, or other dangerous behaviors.

Functional psychosis is less common in children than adults and is more difficult to diagnose in childhood because it may be less obvious to the untrained observer. While mid- and older adolescents may present with symptoms similar to those of schizophrenic or manic-depressive adults, children and young adolescents characteristically present with a history of gradual deterioration. They often have evidence of progressive social withdrawal, emotional blunting, and a decline in school performance. Their odd behavior has typically been ongoing and is frequently seen by their parents more as a part of their character and less as a part of a psychiatric disorder. When schizophrenia does occur in childhood, it is more often an undifferentiated type than paranoid or catatonic, although older adolescents may have these latter subtypes.

When these children come to the attention of the emergency room psychiatrist, they often present not with a picture of acute schizophrenic decompensation, but with such symptoms as suicidal ideation or behavior, increased agitation and aggression, or extreme anxiety. By focusing on mental status examination, history of present illness, and family history of mental illness, a tentative diagnosis may be made and an appropriate treatment undertaken. Children with acute psychotic decompensation are often a danger to themselves or others and often need emergency treatment in a hospital setting.

In some children with previously undetected "quiet psychoses," extreme stress may potentiate an acute psychotic decompensation. In these instances, the child may exhibit the more characteristic signs of psychosis such as hallucinations, delusions, or frankly bizarre behavior.

Over the last several years, an increasing number of non-schizophrenic children have presented in the emergency room with acute onset of psychotic features including auditory or visual hallucinations, paranoid ideation, and a loosening of thought processes. A significant portion of these children are youngsters with premorbid borderline ego functioning who have experienced sexual abuse (and less frequently physical abuse) and who have consequently deteriorated with psychotic functioning. The classic symptoms of posttraumatic stress disorder may be present, but often are not.

Children with organic psychoses typically present with an acute picture. Their decompensation is usually of recent onset, and there is no history of a precipitating emotional stress. They have no family history of mental illness. They are often agitated, disorganized, and disoriented. Their memory may be impaired. They may be experiencing hallucinations. Frequently, these hallucinations are visual rather than more characteristic auditory hallucinations of schizophrenia (an exception being the auditory hallucinations seen in alcoholic hallucinosis).

Many medical conditions may be associated with acute psychosis. These include neurological, infectious, metabolic, oncologic, and immunologic processes. In addition, acute psychosis can be associated with alcohol or drug intoxication or withdrawal and with vitamin deficiency.

Neurological disorders are among the most common causes of organic psychosis. Meningitis, encephalitis, cerebral vascular accidents, subarachnoid hemorrhages, and subdural hematoma can be associated with acute behavioral changes presenting as acute psychosis. Children with congenital heart disease and leukemia are at special risk for cerebral vascular complications, and their neurological status should be evaluated before their behavioral changes can be attributed to stress from their illness.

Patients with brain tumors occasionally present with symptoms of acute psychosis. Metastases to the central nervous system may also present a psychotic picture. Children with seizure disorders may present with interictal or postictal behavior that can be mistaken for psychotic behavior. Symptoms resembling childhood schizophrenia may be seen in children with early neurodegenerative disease.

Patients with metabolic disorders, especially myxedema, thyrotoxicosis, or Cushing's disease, and less frequently diabetes, may appear to have acute psychosis. Similarly, patients with pulmonary disease resulting in anoxia may also present with psychotic-like symptoms. In these patients, the obvious physical signs and symptoms will suggest organic etiology. Diagnoses can then be confirmed by appropriate laboratory tests.

Porphyria and Wilson's disease may present with psychiatric manifestations before other evidence of the disease is present. Patients with lupus erythematosus can develop symptoms of organic psychosis. Sometimes it is difficult to know if the disease or the treatment for the disease (steroids) is the cause of the psychiatric symptomatology.

Deficiency of nicotinic acid or thiamine may cause symptoms of psychosis. Intoxication with lead may do the same.

Some medications produce central nervous system side effects that resemble psychotic-like symptoms. Anticholinergic agents, such as those found in over-the-counter sleep-inducing preparations, as well as antihistaminic agents are known in toxic amounts to produce psychosis. Overdosage of sedative-hypnotics or abrupt withdrawal of these agents may also result in a psychotic state. A careful drug history is essential for accurate diagnosis and management.

Intoxication with street drugs is particularly problematic in that it may be unclear if the acute psychotic symptomatology is a direct result of the drug use (i.e., a "bad trip"), is a drug-induced psychotic disorder (i.e., drug-induced delusional disorder), is a consequence of withdrawal, is a functional psychotic state precipitated by drug use or a predisposed individual, or is a postdrug "flashback." Psychotic states induced by lysergic acid diethylamide (LSD) or psilocybin may mimic an acute schizophrenic decompensation or a psychotic mood disorder. Amphetamines—in the intoxication state, the prolonged delusional postintoxication state, or a withdrawal state—can mimic a manic episode or paranoid schizophrenia. The withdrawal state also is characterized by symptoms of severe depression, at times with accompanying suicidal ideation. LSD, phencyclidine (PCP), and amphetamine-induced psychoses (in long-time users) can persist for weeks to months after the drugs have been cleared from the system. LSD and PCP are also associated with flashbacks that occur long after the drug use has ended.

Patients who abuse drugs are frequently unable to give an accurate history of what they have taken. Many street drugs are impure or mixed with other drugs unknown to the patient. It is important to be familiar with the physical signs and symptoms associated with intoxication with the various hallucinogenic drugs. Such familiarity helps the consultant in making a working drug diagnosis in the absence of an accurate history and laboratory data (Table 15–1).

A toxic screen may be helpful in determining what drug has been

Table 15–1. Signs and symptoms of substance abuse

Substance	Psychiatric symptoms following intoxication	Physical signs following intoxication
Amphetamines (intoxication)	Talkativeness, restlessness, anxiety, agitation, elation, grandiosity, visual and tactile hallucinations, paranoid ideation.	Dilated pupils responsive to light, elevated blood pressure, tachycardia, diaphoresis, tremulousness, hyperreflexia, stereotyped movement. *If severe:* hypertension, hyperpyrexia, cardiac arrhythmia.
	Psychosis consistent with a delusional disorder can persist for days to months following ingestion in those who have been moderate to heavy drug abusers over long periods of time. Symptoms similar to those of functional psychosis, not intoxication.	
Amphetamines (withdrawal)	Dysphoria, insomnia, or hypersomnia, psychomotor agitation. Possible paranoid or suicidal ideation.	
Cocaine	Similiar to amphetamine intoxication and withdrawal but much shorter duration.	Similar to amphetamine but shorter duration.

continued

Table 15–1. Signs and symptoms of substance abuse *(continued)*

Substance	Psychiatric symptoms following intoxication	Physical signs following intoxication
LSD and mescaline (intoxication)	Apprehension, panic, perceptual distortion (including slowed sense of time and synesthesias), depersonalization, derealization, hallucinations (visual and auditory).	Dilated pupils, tachycardia, sweating, palpitations, blurred vision, tremors, incoordination.
	Hallucinogen delusional disorder or hallucinogen mood disorder may develop after hallucinogen use. The course is variable, ranging from a transient to a long-lasting disorder.	
	Flashbacks (posthallucinogen perceptual disorder) are not unusual. They may persist anywhere from months to years.	
PCP (and ketamine)	Anxiety, euphoria, disorientation, hallucinations (suicidal behavior is not uncommon).	Pupils normal or small, nystagmus (vertical or horizontal), muscular rigidity, grimacing, numbness or decreased sensory perception, hypertension.
	May be associated with waxing and waning of psychiatric symptoms for up to 1 week.	

Sources. American Psychiatric Association (1987), Greenblatt and Shader (1975), and the Medical Letter (1980).

taken. It is important for the consultant to be familiar with the substances that are routinely included in a hospital's toxic screen. If the consultant suspects intoxication with a drug for which routine screening is not done, the consultant may request that the laboratory look specifically for that drug. Certain drugs leave the bloodstream so rapidly that they may be undetectable in a serum toxic screen. PCP, best excreted in an acid urine, may appear only in a serum sample. For this reason, both urine and serum screen should be sent to the laboratory. Since there appears to be a high percentage of false-negative reports from routine screening, the consultant is best advised to rely heavily on history, physical findings, and mental status examination and to use the laboratory results as diagnostic only if they confirm the suspicions.

Once the safety of the patient has been established and the etiology of the psychosis has been determined, treatment decisions must be made. The acute treatment of functional psychosis depends on the presentation of the patient. If the patient presents with a major change in personality or behavior, if the patient is extremely distressed or anxious, or if the patient is hallucinating, delusional, suicidal, or overly aggressive, hospitalization is the initial treatment of choice. In the hospital, the patient must be maintained in a safe, structured, nonstimulating environment with close observation. A room program that actively utilizes the patient's own living space for behavioral control is optimal. Visitors should be restricted. Nursing care should be delivered by a core group of nurses. Reassurance, support, and consistency are the most important therapeutic maneuvers.

For acute psychosis, major tranquilizers are the treatment of choice. Those most commonly used in children are chlorpromazine and haloperidol. These are approved for children over age 3. Table 15–2 details use of these drugs for emergency situations. These doses should be titrated downward for children under age 6. In adults, lorazepam has been shown to be effective in the management of acute catatonia (Greenfeld et al. 1987; Salam et al. 1987). We have used it successfully with catatonic adolescents. In the emergency situation, we recommend 1 mg tid; we have had best results using the intramuscular route initially and, when the patient has improved, switching to the oral route. We have also found it helpful in combination with antipsy-

Table 15–2. Drugs used for emergency treatment of acute psychosis

Drug	Initial dose	Sequential dose
Chlorpromazine (po)	0.5–1.0 mg/kg	0.25–1.0 mg/kg q 2–4 hours until child responds or until side effects contraindicate, up to about four doses.
Chlorpromazine (im)	Reduce initial dose by 50%	If agitation continues, without significant hypotension, dose may be repeated in 1 hour. Adjust upward as needed and as tolerated. Subsequent doses should be at 4- to 6-hour intervals following initial sedation.
Haloperidol	0.5 mg (total dose)	0.01–0.05 mg/kg q 2–4 hours until responsive or side effects are limiting, up to about four doses.

chotics in management of the adolescent patient who is both psychotic and agitated. For this purpose it may be given orally, unless the patient is extremely agitated and needs rapid sedation. It is approved for children over age 12. For younger children, we recommend use of hydroxyzine or diphenhydramine if sedation is required beyond that achieved with a major tranquilizer alone. Care must be taken, however, to avoid cumulative anticholinergic effect, with resultant anticholinergic-induced psychosis.

In the case of organic psychoses, definitive treatment should be directed at the underlying disease. Acute management of the psychotic episode is similar to the management of such an episode in patients with functional psychosis. If agitation is severe, psychotropic intervention may be necessary, but this must be done with consideration of the underlying disease process.

In the instance of drug-induced psychoses, if the patient does know specifically what has been taken, management decisions may be simplified.

For patients who are intoxicated with anticholinergic or antihistaminic drugs, physostigmine provides specific and rapid relief of symptoms; its action, however, is short-lived. Since it also has major side effects of its own, including production of seizures, it must be used with extreme caution. Major tranquilizers are specifically contraindicated. Use of them exacerbates symptomatology.

In the case of cocaine-induced psychotic reactions, the psychosis is generally of such short duration that medication is not necessary. If medication is required, use of a major tranquilizer is recommended. Haloperidol po or im is the treatment of choice.

For amphetamine intoxication, haloperidol is recommended, since it provides adrenergic blockage. Propranolol may also be useful in blocking the amphetamine-induced beta-adrenergic hyperactivity. Acidification of the urine is also helpful, since it shows the half-life of the drug (Jaffe 1989).

In the case of hallucinogen-induced psychosis, there is no specific treatment. Reassurance is the most important therapeutic measure.

When it is not known what medication the patient has ingested, sedation and tranquilization should be attempted only if the patient's agitation or anxiety is quite severe and other measures of management have failed. If medication is necessary, short-acting benzodiazepines such as lorazepam are the drugs of choice; they provide sedation with a minimum of other undesired side effects.

Major tranquilizers and barbiturates are particularly risky when the pharmacology of the underlying intoxication is not known. In patients with anticholinergic intoxication, phenothiazines may precipitate agitation, delirium, and a drop in blood pressure. In patients who have abused PCP, phenothiazines may cause an alpha-blockage, precipitating life-threatening postural hypotension.

Barbiturates can produce depressed respiration and coma. If a major tranquilizer must be used, the smallest possible amount of high-potency drug, such as haloperidol, is recommended. In all instances, the patient must be carefully monitored. In amphetamine-induced psychoses as well as in hallucinogen- and PCP-induced psychoses, psychotic symptoms with concomitant chance of harm to self and others may persist for many days after drug cessation. Hospital admission is often necessary.

Eating Disorders

Patients with eating disorders may present as psychiatric emergencies. Since morbidity and mortality rates in these patients are among the highest for psychiatric disorders, it is essential that the psychiatrist in the emergency room be familiar with signs and symptoms of these disorders and with indications for hospitalization. Further, the risk of suicide in this population is increased.

It is estimated that anorexia nervosa or bulimia nervosa affect 5%–10% of teenage girls and young women (Herzog and Copeland 1987). Although males may also suffer from these disorders, more than 90% of anorexic and bulimic patients are women. These disorders most often begin in teenage years. Both usually begin with a moderate effort to lose weight that escalates to a relentless attempt to achieve thinness. Restrictive anorexia is characterized by a severe reduction in caloric intake. There is a refusal to maintain normal body weight, a loss of more than 25% of original body weight, a disturbance of body image, and an intense fear of becoming fat. Bulimic anorexia nervosa is characterized by a restriction of caloric intake alternating with episodes of binge eating, usually followed by self-induced vomiting or use of laxatives or diuretics. Both syndromes affect multiple organ systems, and both can be fatal.

In the case of the restrictive anorexic patient, the physical complications of concern to the emergency room psychiatrist are, for the most part, those of starvation. These include the inability to maintain body temperature, dehydration, total body sodium and potassium loss, and cardiac arrhythmia due to either electrolyte imbalance or anatomical cardiac changes secondary to starvation.

For the bulimic anorexic patient, physical complications are associated with bingeing and purging and include the risks of acute gastric dilation and rupture, Mallory-Weiss tear, aspiration, and electrolyte disturbance. Diuretic abuse, cathartic abuse, and self-induced vomiting all predispose to serious hypokalemia, which can precipitate fatal arrhythmia. Ipecac abuse can cause direct myocardial dysfunction and precipitate sudden death.

The physician in the emergency room must assess the physical and emotional status of the patient and the risk for death. Indications for hospitalization include

- History of a recent precipitous drop in weight or history of a steady drop in weight over the last several months approaching loss of 25%–30% of body weight
- History of increased bingeing or vomiting or increased use of cathartics or diuretics to a frequency or intensity that seem life endangering
- History of change in mental status with increasing depression or suicidality or emerging psychotic decompensation
- Metabolic disturbance such as serious alteration in vital signs, imbalance of electrolytes (especially low sodium or potassium), elevation of blood urea nitrogen with otherwise normal renal function
- History of chest pain or arrhythmia or presence of an abnormal electrocardiogram

Initial treatment should address the medical or psychiatric indications precipitating the hospitalization. Further treatment should include continued medical management, individual and family psychotherapy, and behavioral treatment for restitution of weight and control of bingeing and purging. Psychopharmacologic intervention may be useful.

References

Allen NH: Homicide prevention and intervention. Suicide Life Threat Behav 11:167–179, 1981

American Psychiatric Association: Diagnostic and Statistical Manual of Mental Disorders, 3rd Edition, Revised. Washington, DC, American Psychiatric Association, 1987

Bender L: Children and adolescents who have killed. Am J Psychiatry 116:510–513, 1959

Brent DA, Perper JA, Allman CJ: Alcohol, firearms, and suicide among youth. JAMA 257:3369–3372, 1987

Christoffel KK: Violent death and injury in U.S. children and adolescents. Am J Dis Child 144:697–706, 1990

Greenblatt DJ, Shader RI: Bad trips, in Manual of Psychiatric Therapeutics. Edited by Shader RI. Boston, MA, Little Brown, 1975, pp 185–193

Greenfeld D, Conrad C, Kincare P, et al: Treatment of catatonia with low-dose lorazepam. Am J Psychiatry 144:1224–1225, 1987

Herzog DB, Copeland PM: Eating disorders. N Engl J Med 313:295–303, 1987

Hoberman HM, Garfinkel BD: Completed suicide in children and adolescents. J Am Acad Child Adolesc Psychiatry 27:689–695, 1988

Jaffe JH: Drug dependence: opioids, nonnarcotics, nicotine (tobacco), and caffeine, in Comprehensive Textbook of Psychiatry/V, 5th Edition, Vol 1. Edited by Kaplan HI, Sadock BJ. Baltimore, MD, Williams & Wilkins, 1989, pp 642–686

Lewis DO, Shanok SS, Pincus JH, et al: Violent juvenile delinquents, psychiatric, neurological, psychological, and abuse factors. Journal of the American Academy of Child Psychiatry 18:307–319, 1979

Lewis DO, Lovely R, Yeager C, et al: Intrinsic and environmental characteristics of juvenile murderers. Journal of the American Academy of Child Psychiatry 27:582–587, 1988

Malmquist C: Premonitory signs of homicidal aggression in juveniles. Am J Psychiatry 121:461–465, 1971

The Medical Letter: Diagnosis and management of reactions to drug abuse. The Medical Letter on Drugs and Therapeutics, Vol 22, No 18, September 5, 1980

Morbidity and Mortality Weekly Report: Homicide among young black males, United States, 1978–1987. Morbidity and Mortality Weekly Report 39:869–873, December 7, 1990

Nurcombe B: Malpractice, in Child and Adolescent Psychiatry: A Comprehensive Textbook. Edited by Lewis M. Baltimore, MD, Williams & Wilkins, 1991, pp 1127–1139

Petti TA: The juvenile murderer, in Child Psychiatry and the Law. Edited by Schetky D, Bendek E. New York, Brunner/Mazel, 1980, pp 194–203

Pfeffer CR: Suicidal behavior of children: a review with implications for research and practice. Am J Psychiatry 138:154–159, 1981

Pfeffer CR, Conte MR, Plutchik R, et al: Suicidal behavior in latency age children. Journal of the American Academy of Child Psychiatry 19:703–710, 1980

Salam S, Pillai A, Beresford T: Lorazepam for psychogenic catatonia. Am J Psychiatry 144:1082–1083, 1987

Sendi I, Blomgren P: A comparative study of the predictive criteria in the predisposition of homicidal adolescents. Am J Psychiatry 132:423–427, 1975

Shaffer D, Gould M, Fisher P, et al: Preventing teenage suicide: a critical review. Journal of the American Academy of Child Psychiatry 27:675–687, 1988

16

Emergencies II: Sexual Abuse and Rape in Childhood

Maria Sauzier, M.D.

Sexual abuse and rape of children, increasingly common emergency room presentations, evoke powerful emotional reactions not only in trainees, but in all professionals. Medicine and psychiatry have only recently begun facing these issues, paralleling societal developments toward endowing children with more rights. Debate continues on the issue of the boundaries between the traditional rights of parents (privacy within the home; parental, and particularly paternal, authority over family members) and society's responsibility to protect children (Bourne and Newberger 1977). A second controversy relates to professional intervention: Who bears the primary responsibility? Is it pediatrics, psychiatry, child protective social service agencies, the police, or district attorneys? Different states are using a variety of solutions to this problem, but most new legislation stresses the need for cooperation between professionals from mental health, protective services, and the judicial system (Massachusetts General Laws 1983).

The goal of this chapter is to give clinicians a basic framework of knowledge encompassing clinical terminology, related legal issues, and some relevant research data, followed by practical guidelines.

Sexual abuse (including incest) and rape are reviewed separately. The focus is on the first phase of intervention, not on later or ongoing treatment. The whole family is seen as the object of intervention. Child victims, perpetrators, and nonabusing mothers, fathers, and siblings are described.

Intervention with and treatment of sexually abused and raped children still present great challenges because they are new frontiers: treatment programs are at the most 15–20 years old. There are at present no long-term outcome studies comparing different intervention strategies. Nevertheless, contemporary clinicians agree that the child who presents with a report of sexual abuse or rape needs more than traditional psychiatric treatment (Sgroi 1982). We thus speak of "intervention." This includes the following:

- Psychiatric evaluation and treatment
- Medical care
- Child protective investigation
- Legal involvement, if appropriate

These facets of intervention need to be described together, just as they need to be interwoven in clinical practice. For the child psychiatrist, treatment of a sexually abused child may offer a unique opportunity to cooperate with child protective and law enforcement systems under very stressful circumstances.

Childhood sexual abuse has been identified as a major stressor leading to long-term psychopathology in the trauma spectrum disorders, which include multiple personality disorder; borderline personality disorder; and somatoform, panic, and anxiety disorders (Herman et al. 1989). Recent research findings point to important effects of sexual abuse on the child's neurophysiologic and hormonal development (e.g., increased stress-related hormones and early puberty) (Putnam 1989). These developments indicate that sexual abuse is a major mental health issue requiring child psychiatrists to become ever more knowledgeable and to get more involved. Guidelines for expert intervention are essential and have been formulated by the American Academy of Child and Adolescent Psychiatry (1990). They are available to the mental health community.

Sexual Abuse

Incidence

Information about sexual abuse comes from case histories (Ferenczi 1933/1955; Katan 1973), small-scale psychological studies (Adams-Tucker 1982; Peters 1976), and large-scale sociologic studies (Finkelhor 1979; Kinsey et al. 1953). After prolonged controversy about sexual abuse as fact or fantasy (Freud 1896/1962; Herman and Hirschman 1981) and widely differing statistics, there is currently a consensus on prevalence for women:

- General population
  - 38% sexual abuse before age 18
  - 16% incest before age 18
  - 4.6% father-daughter incest (Russell 1986)
- Psychiatric population (hospitalized)
  - 59% abuse before age 18 (sexual abuse in 43%) (Bryer et al. 1987)

Prevalence for men is based on far fewer studies, with a great range of results:

- College population
  - 9% (Finkelhor 1979)
  - 30% (Landis 1956)

Tufts–New England Medical Center study. One broad psychological research project—conducted at the New England Medical Center (NEMC), Boston, Massachusetts—used 181 cases of sexual abuse (156 confirmed, 25 unconfirmed) (Gomes-Schwartz et al. 1984, 1985, 1990). In all cases studied, the last abuse or the disclosure of abuse had occurred within the previous 6 months. All families were thus in a state of crisis when referred. Concomitant with data collection was the provision of therapy for the child and the child's family, including the offender. The data gathered are generally accepted to be representative of current occurrence, with one exception: boy victims are underrepresented in this study.

The children seen were between 6 months and 18 years old; 72% were girls. Of the offenders, 94% were male, ranging from teenaged baby-sitters to grandfathers. Only 3% of offenders were total strangers. Incest in the biological sense occurred in 41% of the cases seen. If one includes parental figures, the number rises to 62%. The sexual abuse reported ranged from nontouching or attempted abuse to full intercourse, with some genital contact occurring in 88% of the cases. Only 21% of abuse occurred as one single incident of rape or incest. Most occurred over a period of time, some spanning for more than 5 years, with a frequency varying from several times for the whole time span to more than weekly. Most abuse occurred in places familiar to the child, like the child's home or the perpetrator's home. The families studied were representative of the greater Boston population in terms of race, religion, and socioeconomic status. The only remarkable demographic difference found was a higher predominance of households headed by single mothers. Although this research is not described in detail here, it informs all aspects of this chapter.[1]

Clinical Terminology

The term *sexual abuse* covers a wide range of physical behaviors and psychosocial interactions (Lewis and Sarrel 1969; Summit and Kryso 1978). Distinguishing between terms such as *sexual abuse, sexual misuse, incest,* and *rape* is important, as they describe distinct but overlapping entities. *Common to all is abuse of power and breach of trust.*

Sexual abuse. Sexual abuse covers the widest range of activities in which a child is used for the sexual gratification of an adult. By

---

[1]The research was supported by Grant 80-JN-AX-0001 from the Office of Juvenile Justice and Delinquency Prevention.

definition, a child cannot be a consenting partner to any sexual act with an adult. A child can also be abused by another child if the perpetrator is significantly older than the victim (5 years or more), or uses threats, intimidation, or force to create a power differential (e.g., as exists between a baby-sitter of any age and his or her charges). Consensual show-and-tell and doctor games among peers need to be differentiated from enforced participation.

Sexual abuse is often progressive (e.g., starting as cuddling while watching television, with increasingly direct genital touching). Sexual abuse usually involves secrecy, ranging from "this is our special little secret" to "it would kill your mother to know" or "you'll never see your cat again if you tell."

Sexual misuse. Sexual misuse (Brant and Tisza 1977) occurs when the adult is truly not aware of any sexual gratification he or she may be receiving (e.g., as when a parent continues to treat a genital or anal irritation with checking, washing, and application of ointment originally prescribed but no longer necessary). The child may feel stimulated, confused, deeply ashamed, and intruded on. There is usually no enforced secrecy. Sexual misuse may also occur when a parent suspects abuse and becomes overinvolved in checking or questioning the child.

Incest. Incest in the strict sense occurs when blood relatives interact sexually. The broader and more current definition includes relatives who are not consanguineous (e.g., an uncle by marriage), as well as stepparents, live-in partners of parents, or any adult who is given parental authority in the household.

Sexual abuse and, in particular, incest may thus be complicated by the fact that the child has a complex relationship with the offender that encompasses more than just the abuse. Incest implies individual and family dynamics allowing or even prompting it to occur and requires each family member to adapt to the family pathology. There are thus certain common features found in incestuous families that require therapeutic intervention.

Rape. Rape involves a more overt use of violence and occurs more often in isolated incidents, perpetrated by a stranger or acquaintance.

Legally, rape definitions vary from state to state, but usually involve some sexual penetration. Rape victims are less frequently manipulated or threatened into secrecy. Rape can be incestuous; incest can be rape; and sexual abuse can include episodes of rape.

Ritualistic abuse. Ritualistic abuse, defined as "repetitive and systematic sexual, physical and psychologic abuse of children by adults as part of cults or satanic worship" (Kelley 1989, p. 502), has become the focus of attention more recently. Such abuse more often involves several or many children and is thus more likely to occur in settings where children are available (e.g., day care, nursery schools). The psychological consequences are often profound and lasting.

False allegations. False allegations are rare, but are important to consider. They are particularly difficult to decipher in divorce and custody disputes when one parent becomes the champion of the alleged victim. A national sample showed a low incidence (only 2% of all divorce and custody cases involved any sexual abuse allegation, true or false), but also a disproportionately high expenditure of resources (Thoennes and Tjaden 1990). When they occur, children are often paralyzed by conflicting loyalties and can neither validate nor deny the allegation made on their behalf. Multiple evaluations by multiple experts are common.

Legal Issues

Mandated reporting. The last several years have seen a steady increase in the number of reported cases of sexual abuse of children due to stronger mandated reporting laws, media attention to the problem, and more sophisticated and reliable responses from child protective services. Child psychiatrists should be aware of the legal requirements in their state. In Massachusetts, for example, professionals—including physicians, nurses, therapists, and teachers—are mandated to report *findings* or *suspicions* of abuse to the Department of Social Services (Massachusetts General Laws 1983). False reports made in good faith cannot be held against the reporter. Mandated reporters can be held liable and fined for not reporting.

Confidentiality. Confidentiality issues arise when a child or adult reveals current sexual abuse during ongoing therapy, leading to ethical and therapeutic dilemmas. The mandated reporting of information regarding child abuse overrules the privilege of doctor-patient confidentiality. In accordance with the literature, reporting is strongly recommended (Burgess and Nichols 1978; Sgroi 1982). With only rare exceptions, the clinician should alert parents about the intended report to child protective services, give a rationale, and stress the importance of cooperating with the agency for the benefit of the child.

The maintenance of a therapeutic alliance is most often given as the reason for failing to report, but unresolved countertransference issues are usually involved (Harper and Irvin 1985; Pollak and Levy 1989). The incestuous family is riddled with secrets that empower the abuser at the expense of other family members. The therapist who participates in the secret thus loses effectiveness in the eyes of the child and of the offender. Everyone loses, including the offender, who may want to be stopped by outside intervention.

Even more difficult are those situations in which a child gives clues but does not openly talk about being abused. Here, staying observant, with the child's safety as the primary focus, may be the only course of action.

Mandated reporting of serious cases to the district attorney is a recent development in several states (e.g., Massachusetts), but does not imply automatic prosecution. It does, however, have implications for the format of clinical interviews and medical records, as discussed below. Parameters of confidentiality privileges in criminal cases vary across disciplines and should be reviewed accordingly.

Report writing. This critical component of responding to sexually abused children requires care, precision, and knowledge of the potential pitfalls.

- Remember that all reports may end in court. If poorly written, they may be misused to the detriment of the child.
- Describe, using as little psychiatric jargon as possible; nonpsychiatric professionals need to understand you. "She overreacted to

the dolls" does not mean anything to them.

- Write legibly (or you may be subpoenaed just to explain your emergency room note).
- Do not prejudge and do not use legal definitions; the judge decides if there was rape. Until then, the finding is "status post-alleged rape." Write "alleged offender" unless talking about a convicted child abuser.
- State your sources: "Mrs. T says her husband drinks a six-pack each night", not "Mr. T is an alcoholic."
- Describe the known components of the alleged offense in the victim's words as much as possible. Record idiosyncratic details, expressions of affect, play, and story interruptions.
- When writing a report ordered by the court, describe what you have seen and educate when indicated. Stay brief. The paragraphs most likely to be read are the description of the abuse, your diagnostic impression, and the recommendations. The recommendations should be clear, understandable, and logical extensions of your impressions and diagnosis.

The child in court. Historically, the court system has not been kind to children. Their special needs (e.g., size, attention span, voice volume) were disregarded, and their credibility was intrinsically suspect (Herman and Hirschman 1981). This is slowly being corrected with victim assistance programs, child-sized furniture or booster seats, short sessions with bathroom stops, microphones, and so on. Reducing the number of interviews by different people has been attempted by increasing cooperation between agencies.

More difficult to resolve is the conflict between the right of the defendant to face his or her accuser, and the right of the state to prosecute alleged offenders—relying, in these cases, on witnesses who need to be protected from further harm. With rare exceptions, there is no case if the child cannot tolerate being a witness. Some states are debating broader hearsay exceptions (e.g., allowing the child's statements to a therapist to become evidence) or videotaping laws (taping the disclosure interview once, to be used by all agencies, including defense attorneys and at trial). As is described later, disclosure is a process that can include retractions, minimizations, or exaggerations.

A "bad" videotape can be used against the child. It is thus important to remember that there are no easy answers in this area.

Clinical Issues in Sexual Abuse

Presenting Complaints

Sexual abuse will be considered in a differential diagnosis only if one's consciousness has been raised about the prevalence of such problems. Minimization of the issue of sexual abuse of children is related to the wish to deny its existence and has been supported by traditional theory as well as aided by the paucity of clear clinical indicators. Diagnosing sexual abuse is hindered by the fact that symptoms are usually nonspecific and do not provide clear and unequivocal proof. Physical signs, such as cuts and bruises, are rare (Rimsza and Niggerman 1982). For the most part, sexual abuse of children does not require the use of overt violence (present in 23% in the Tufts-NEMC study) (Gomes-Schwartz et al. 1984). Children can be made to comply with the use of authority, bribes, or misrepresentation of social values. In most cases only a broad picture, including a detailed history of onset of symptoms, and consideration of the developmental age of the child can permit one to draw reasonable conclusions. The following presentations require investigation:

Physical Signs and Symptoms

- Genital or anal tears, bruises, or irritations
- Sexually transmitted diseases (vagina, rectum, urethra, or oropharynx)
- Sperm in genital or anal area
- Pregnancy
- Encopresis as a possible result of anal rape
- Enuresis as a possible symptom or regression, overexcitation, or fear related to sexual abuse
- Psychosomatic symptoms (headaches, stomachaches, sleep and appetite disturbances)

Statements

- A child who states that he or she has been sexually abused has to be listened to with an open mind. In the Tufts-NEMC study, only 7 of the 181 referred children made false allegations (Gomes-Schwartz et al. 1984).
- A parent who states that his or her child has been sexually abused also has to be taken seriously. This is particularly important when a child is preverbal. It is extremely complex, however, when the accusing parent and the alleged offender are battling over custody or visitation. Expert and open-minded attention is needed.

Emotional and Behavioral Symptoms

- Symptom onset at alleged time of abuse and symptoms that are place and person related are more suggestive.
- Most symptoms can be attributed to anxiety and thus misunderstood.
- Most symptoms are age specific rather than abuse specific.

Preschool-Age Children

- Age-inappropriate sexual behavior: knowledge of adult sexual acts; sexual provocativeness; sexual fears; joyless, compulsive masturbation; excessive intrusion on the privacy of adults or peers; abuse of another child by force, threat, bribe, or manipulation; revictimization
- Anxiety symptoms related to particular people, places, or events: fearfulness, somatic symptoms, nightmares, regression, separation problems
- Aggressive behaviors
- Dissociative phenomena, symptoms of posttraumatic stress disorder

Latency-Age Children

- All of the above
- Depression and suicide attempts

- School phobia, truancy
- Acting-out behaviors, cruelty to animals, running away
- Eating disorders

Adolescents

- All of the above
- Dissociative phenomena, including flashbacks, amnesia, fugue states, depersonalization, multiple personality disorder
- Sexualized behaviors, including prostitution and rape (as victim or offender)
- Depression, including shame, self-mutilation, drug abuse, suicide

The Disclosure Process

Victimized children want their abuse to stop, but many know, often far better than we do, what negative consequences will follow disclosure. Their disclosure may thus be purposeful, accidental, or ambivalent. *Purposeful disclosure* is usually made to a parent or another trusted adult. *Accidental disclosure* is usually not overtly wanted by anyone, not even the victim, and may follow medical findings or observation or suspicion of the abuse by someone who then reveals it. Confusion arises when verbal disclosures are called purposeful and nonverbal ones accidental. A small child whose behavior "discloses" sexual abuse may actually be more eager to tell than an adolescent who verbally reveals incest in the heat of an argument. Adding the category of *ambivalent disclosure* (Sauzier 1989) helps clinicians be better prepared for the frequent minimizations or even retractions following disclosures made by latency-age or adolescent victims who disclose verbally before they have really decided to do so.

Revelations during psychotherapy may be purposeful, accidental, or both. Clues are available if the clinician is receptive to them. In the past, these clues were understood to relate to fantasy material and wishes. The task of the clinician in such a situation is a difficult one: to elicit further information without leading the child to feel more stimulated, intruded on, or even revictimized.

Examples of clues include:

- Drawings (focus on genitalia, disguised representations of sexual acts)
- Hypersexual behaviors (seductive or excessively masturbatory)
- References to secrets, secret pacts, special favors, extra meetings with caretakers or teachers

Disclosure of sexual abuse always precipitates a crisis situation for the victim and the victim's family. For the victim, disclosure offers hope for change, but also fear of negative consequences. In cases of incest, the victim has kept the secret to prevent being blamed or shamed or losing the affection of the family (Summit 1983). For the nonoffending parent, usually the mother, the crisis is severe and may impede her ability to make choices that protect and support the victim. For the offender, the first response to the revelation is usually denial, with or without attempts to lead the victim to retract.

Crisis Intervention

The clinician's role needs to be diverse, comprehensive, and flexible, going beyond the classic model of the neutral, insight-oriented therapist. *Teamwork and action are essential.* For clinicians trained in the passive mode, this may present some difficulty.

Responding to a sexually abused child and the child's family requires work on several tracks and does not follow the usual sequence of diagnostic evaluation, formulation, treatment planning, and treatment implementation. The diagnostic sessions go hand in hand with a constant evaluation of the child's safety, which may require action before all the diagnostic work has been done.

Crisis intervention can take 6–8 or even 12 weeks. Long-range plans may include individual psychotherapy for the child, mother, offender, and siblings. Group therapy is very effective for all involved (Goodwin and Talwar 1989). Children and adolescents tend to stay in treatment longer if their mother is in individual or group therapy (Gomes-Schwartz et al. 1984). A family approach is essential, but family therapy may be possible only much later in the family's development. When the parent's anxiety, more than the child's symptomatology, is most prominent, periodic consultations may be sufficient.

If child protective services are involved, they usually make the referral. If a parent or other adult has referred the child, a decision to report the abuse, based on state regulations, needs to be made.

Initial Goals of Crisis Intervention

- Find out what has happened (the "who, when, where, and how" of child protection reports), based on as many sources of information as are available.
- Begin the diagnostic assessment of the child; determine effects of the abuse.
- Make appropriate medical referral.
- Assess the acute safety of the child and family; make appropriate recommendations (e.g., incestuous father to leave the home), decisions (e.g., mother should file for a restraining order and needs help in doing it), and referrals (e.g., pediatric care, child protective services, police, district attorney).
- Assess the nonabusing parent's ability to protect.
- Assess the father's (or other alleged offender's) ability to cease his behavior and obtain help; assess the potential for immediate crisis reactions (e.g., suicide, revenge).
- Formulate initial findings and diagnostic impressions in a carefully worded report.
- Make (and implement) *initial* disposition plans.
- Help all family members deal with their reactions to the disclosure and its consequences.
- Assess need for long-term treatment.

Essential Tasks of Crisis Intervention

- *Interview the child alone.* This is essential for diagnostic purposes, to elicit the information necessary to plan for the child's safety and to begin the treatment process by supporting the child's strengths.
- *Interview the nonabusing parent.* Provide support and non-judgmental suggestions about how to help the abused child. Fos-

tering the highest level of functioning, despite the crisis of revelation, takes precedence over exploratory work at this point in time. Information regarding the parent's ability to protect the child from further harm should be gathered. Eliciting history of sexual victimization is important, but should be done carefully.

- *Interview the offender.* This essential component of the evaluation of an incestuous family provides information about the family dynamics and the child's safety. The object of the interview is not to force an admission of guilt, but to understand whom the family and the child have to deal with. The offender may react to the disclosure with serious psychopathology, including suicidal or homicidal impulses and actions. In a nonincestuous abuse situation, access to the offender may be limited but should always be sought.
- *Interview the siblings.* This may reveal other victims or may elicit reactions that can be detrimental to the victimized child (e.g., blaming the victim for the act and for the turmoil following the disclosure).
- *Provide a referral for a physical examination.* Referral for a physical examination, either to the family pediatrician or to a pediatric gynecologist familiar with and sensitive to the issues of sexually abused children, should be made. The physical examination may detect consequences of the abuse that require treatment or that may be important elements in case of legal action. The examiner should always respond to the child's and parent's spoken and unspoken fears (e.g., "Is the child physically marred for life?" "Will my child be promiscuous?" "Will my child become an offender?").
- *Cooperate with child protective and legal services.* This cooperation elicits their help and informs them of clinical needs and issues. Their work as investigators and case administrators is essential and leaves the clinician more freedom to maintain supportive and therapeutic roles.
- *Assess the child's safety.* This assessment is the primary consideration. Consideration needs to be given to the following:

    - The identity of the *offender*, the access he has to the child, his modus operandi (e.g., using violence or not), his acknowledgment or denial of the abuse.

- The age and the stage of development of the *child,* the child's strengths (e.g., a trusting relationship with mother, the therapist, or other adults; an ability to say no), weaknesses (e.g., mental retardation, any other impairment, ambivalence toward the nonabusing parent, need to side with the offender, provocative hypersexual behavior increasing the risk of revictimization).
- The response of the *mother,* whether she can side with the child without blame or punishment, whether she is appropriately angry with the offender, whether she can place the child's needs over her own attachment to the offender, and over her own needs.
- The response of *siblings,* their situation in the family (are they at risk?), their response toward the victim (e.g., blaming the victim and siding with the offender, thus increasing the mother's dilemma of choosing between them).

- *Recommendations.* Separation between the child and the alleged offender is always indicated. In cases of incest, the offender should leave the household, at least temporarily, thus acknowledging that he accepts the blame. Financial responsibilities, however, should continue to be met. Removing the victimized child from the home should be seen as the last resort in families that cannot protect the victim from further harm.

Evaluation Guidelines

- All the principles of good child assessment technique apply: finding the developmental level of the child, offering various modes of communication (e.g., play, talk, art), observing all communications (e.g., play, words, body), expressing empathy but *no* personal reaction to the material.
- A team approach works best for complex cases, with two (or more) clinicians evaluating the child, parents, and siblings.
- Know as much as possible before you see the child but keep an open mind. At the end of the evaluation you want to know:

- Who was the perpetrator (one or more)? Are there any other victims?
- Where did the abuse occur, under what circumstances, and where were other family members?
- When did the abuse occur (approximate start, frequency, last episode)?
- How did the perpetrator approach the child and enlist her cooperation or submission (e.g., threats, bribes, manipulation, violence). How did he enforce secrecy? What exactly did he do, make her do, and so on? Did anyone else know? Did the child ever try to tell?
- How was the abuse disclosed (accidental, purposeful, ambivalent)? What is the exact history and chronology of the disclosure process (e.g., who told whom, who believed, who did not, who enlisted help, who is now supportive or angry)?

- Take nothing for granted. Even when the abuse history is well established before you see the child, details need to be double-checked (e.g., who is "Pop"—a grandfatherly neighbor, grandfather, or someone's boyfriend who likes children? Is there more than one "Joe" in the child's life? Is the child describing more than one offender, more than one victim?).
- Make sure you and the child together define the words used. With the help of a doll or drawing, name the relevant anatomic parts. More difficult to define are the actions the child needs to describe. Do not impose a word, do not use "hurt" or "touch" indiscriminately (the sexual abuse may not have hurt, or may not be categorized as touching by the child).
- Listen for expressions of affect (in body, language, or play) that corroborate or confuse the emerging story and for idiosyncratic details that have made an impression on the child (e.g., what she saw through the window, or a particular smell).
- Try to ascertain the child's understanding of the abuse, and of the consequences of disclosure. Was she told why it was occurring (e.g., because she is bad or special, because her mother is bad or untouchable)? What did she think? Some children have constructed cause-and-effect theories to explain the unexplainable, which are

egocentric and guilt based. Even when the child does not feel ready to reveal her private theories, expressing interest can pave the way for later discussions.

- Make sure you do not impose your affective or countertransference responses. At the time of disclosure, the child may love the offender seemingly without ambivalence, or may correctly know that telling mother can only cause more harm. You may feel disbelief, disgust, horror, or a wish for revenge, but the victim needs the freedom to proceed at her own pace.
- Make sure to find the developmentally correct balance between infantilizing the child, thus disempowering her ("of course you did nothing bad, you were only 6 years old"—true, but the victim's concern implies she knows how complex her situation was) and provoking guilt with "why" questions ("Why didn't you say no?" "Why didn't you tell someone sooner?").
- Make sure you remember that the current consequences of the disclosure may sometimes feel worse to the child than her memory of the sexual abuse, and that she needs realistic help and support in her current life crisis.

Interviewing Guidelines

The passive, observing, and evaluating approach forms the initial baseline for assessing a sexually abused child. Getting acquainted, forming an alliance, getting a sense of the child's life, assessing areas of strength and weakness, and performing a mental status examination are all important features of the assessment; they may not lead, however, to any discussion of the sexual abuse. *Concrete and direct questioning about the alleged abuse is usually necessary.*

Some children are so eager to talk they get confused by an delay in addressing the topic. Most are somewhat to very reticent. The getting acquainted phase of the hour thus varies in length. Neutral topics need to be interwoven when the child seems too anxious or the talking leads nowhere. It is best to verbalize these shifts for the child (e.g., "this really seems hard right now; let's do something—or talk about something—else for a little while").

Introductions. Let the child know who you are, what your professional identity is, and what your role is expected to be. Many children have already been questioned, some in less than ideal settings (e.g., a police station, or sitting on their own bed where the abuse occurred). Do not give any false reassurances, either in general (e.g., "everything will be all right in no time") or to specific questions ("I'm sure your dad won't go to jail" or "I'm sure your mom will end up believing you").

Introducing the topic. "Do you know why your mom brought you here?", used in many child evaluations, can be used. "She told me to tell about Uncle Joe" is often the response of children ready to talk about the abuse. "She told me to tell you what my father does to me," in a divorce and custody battle situation, can lead to confusion about whose allegations are being investigated. A clinician who is not open-minded may either immediately conclude that the child has been coached or may fail to register the wording of the response. When a child responds with "I don't know" the discussion needs to address whether she thinks she has her parents' permission and support to talk about what has happened. If she does not, this issue needs to be addressed first as it may shed crucial light on the family dynamics and on the child's safety.

Talking about the abuse. Most children require direct questioning, going from the general ("I hear your family has had some difficult times lately") to the more particular ("what is it that happened to you to make your mother bring you here?"—but *not* "I hear you've been abused."). Facial reactions, body and hand movements, and use of play materials guide the direction and pace of questions as much as verbal responses.

Practically all sexual abuse evaluations require verbal communication. With a preverbal, barely verbal, or very scared child, it may be mostly the therapist who talks, while the child responds with body language (nodding or flinching or repeating the described act on a doll, or pointing to body parts).

Avoid leading questions, which provide the child with data. If you have to ask, "Was it your father?" you should then ask, "Or was it your brother, your uncle, your teacher . . . ?" and so on.

The balance between telling and showing varies from child to child, and from hour to hour. The showing can involve pointing to body parts on people, on drawings, or on any available doll or puppet.

Anatomically correct dolls are most useful for research purposes or in sexual abuse clinics in which large numbers of children are seen and evaluators have learned to interpret their various reactions (White 1991).

The length of time a child can stay with the disclosure material is quite variable. As the hour progresses, many children change the emphasis or seriousness of their story. Some may get overanxious, dissociate, act silly, regress, or become difficult to contain. Others may deny or minimize the abuse they described a few minutes or days earlier (the "yes, no, maybe so" syndrome) (MacFarlane and Krebs 1986). Some may add new important details when returning to the topic; others may confuse the evaluator with exaggerated, slightly implausible or clearly impossible answers (e.g., "he hit me so hard my skull broke and bled"); "we hid behind the couch when Mom came in and the curtain fell down"; "he tied me to a tree and then the Indians came"). Accounts and descriptions need to be understood in the context of the developmental stage of the child. The falling curtain, for example, may be a metaphor for how the sky fell down on the child's life, may be a condensation of several events, or may indicate confabulation.

Closure of the interview. Allowing time to end the sessions is particularly important in sexual abuse evaluations; the child may feel great anxiety about what she has just revealed and about the family she has to go back to. It is important to elicit the child's questions about the session and her concerns about the future. The discussion should be supportive and realistic. Confidentiality issues need to be addressed. If a child is afraid to go back home or if the evaluator is afraid to send a child back home, the child protective agency needs to be involved immediately. When placement of the child is considered, the protective agency is not only essential but may serve to reality test perceptions and detect possible countertransference interference.

Diagnoses

As stated in the description of the family, offenders, nonoffending parents, and victims present with a wide range of symptoms. Diagnoses commonly found are *posttraumatic stress disorder* in the child and *adjustment reactions* in the family members. In addition, it is imperative to investigate areas of strength as well as pathology of a more chronic nature. This may not be appropriate or possible in the immediate crisis, which may lower ego functioning considerably, but is crucial for long-term planning.

Victims

Blaming the victim is a universal defense. It serves to reduce the anxiety aroused and to contain the fear that "this could happen to me or my child." The psychiatric literature has sometimes participated by describing sexually abused children as seductive, precocious, and beautiful, implying they were responsible for seducing the adult (Bender and Blau 1937). The error lies in a confusion of cause and effect; some sexually abused children are indeed seductive with their therapists, as well as with anyone else, because they have been taught that this behavior pleases. Even precocious puberty may come to be seen as a physiologic consequence of sexual abuse (Putnam 1989).

More recent literature focuses on the wide range of presentations seen in sexually abused children (Finkelhor 1986). On average, they show more psychopathology than children in control groups but less than those in a psychiatric clinic population (Gomes-Schwartz et al. 1985). This confirms clinical observations that some sexually abused children show no signs of distress at revelation, whereas others show serious signs and symptoms. Self-esteem may be normal in younger children, particularly if the abuse was nonviolent and the response to the revelation was caring and supportive. They may not have yet perceived the pathologic nature of what has happened to them. It may be only later, sometimes as late as adolescence or adulthood, that they come to realize that they have been misled and abused by a trusted adult. The absence of symptoms in an abused child, shortly after revelation, thus needs to be carefully evaluated. Is there a "sleeper effect"? Can therapeutic intervention in the absence of current symptomatology prevent the later occurrence of serious psychopathology?

The victim-to-patient process. The victim-to-patient process refers to the course of events and experiences that lead some sexual abuse victims to become identified patients, either in childhood or later. In the Tufts-NEMC study (Gomes-Schwartz et al. 1984), increased symptomatology was seen when there was violence, when the abuser was a stepfather and the mother sided with him, when the nonabusing parent was punitive and rejecting, and when the child was removed from the home. Putnam's (1989) research indicated that biological changes occur (e.g., increased hormones, early puberty). Finkelhor and Browne (1985) focused on the importance of traumatic sexualization, betrayal, stigmatization, and powerlessness. Rieker and Carmen (1986) stressed the interplay between abuse events, family dynamics, and the victim's attempts to adjust to how others judge her during and after the abuse.

The disclosure process and its consequences, including our interventions, play a vital role in shaping the long-term outcome.

Mothers

In the older incest literature, mothers were seen as "pivotal" and as colluding with the abuser. Today there is growing awareness that there is a wide range of mothers in such situations (Gomes-Schwartz et al. 1990). Some know about the abuse but are just as intimidated as the child or respond with "better this than being alone." Others truly have no idea, are appalled at the revelation, and react appropriately to protect and support their child. Nonetheless, some form of denial is an almost universal finding in incestuous families.

The initial reaction of shock and disbelief makes many mothers appear to lack the capacity to empathize with, and support, their child. In cases of incest, she has to choose between her child and her partner. It cannot be stressed enough how difficult this choice can be. Situations in which a new partner, who represents a new chance, is found to be an abuser are often even *more* difficult than long-standing marital relationships that may already have been marred by chronic problems (Gomes-Schwartz et al. 1990).

The literature describes mothers of incest victims as having received poor mothering themselves and thus being unable to mother their children, often abdicating that role to one child (usually the oldest daughter). In the Tufts-NEMC study (Gomes-Schwartz et al. 1984), 34% of the mothers reported they had been physically abused and 41% sexually abused in their own childhood. These research findings speak to the complexity and the power of the intergenerational trend. What is not known yet is what differentiates those mothers who enter relationships with men who will abuse their children from those who choose partners who do not. No correlation was found between particular diagnoses and types of sexual abuse or types of reactions to the revelation. No significant difference was found between mothers of incest victims and mothers of children not victims of incest (Gomes-Schwartz et al. 1984).

With nonjudgmental therapeutic intervention, many mothers can assume the role of protector and act appropriately.

Offenders

The offender has the pivotal role. Research has focused mainly on those who are jailed. Although useful, this does not address the wide range of offenders seen in clinical practice where no single diagnostic profile or category identifies them. Groth (1979) made the differentiation between the fixated and the regressed offender. The *fixated offender* is a pedophile whose psychosexual development is arrested and whose preferred sexual partners are children. Although these men may be capable of relations with adults, this usually occurs as a means of reaching their partner's children. They are only rarely seen in clinical practice because their pedophilia is usually ego-syntonic.

The psychosexual development of *regressed offenders* does permit them to enjoy adult sexual relations, and they often present as invested and caring parents. In times of stress, however, they resort to the less demanding sexuality offered by a relationship with a child, often based on power and idealization. Because of their inability to react empathically to their victim as a child, they fail to see the distress they provoke and later state that they would have stopped if the child had said no. They thus feel little personal responsibility. Although many comply with therapeutic recommendations, the potential for relapse, given conducive circumstances, is always present.

Other categories of offenders include those who are *psychopathic*, whose main goal is satisfaction of their incessant need for gratification. These offenders, who may brutalize their whole family, are also often capable of presenting a trustworthy image to their environment. They react to the allegation with outrage, can challenge even the seasoned expert, and may well succeed in intimidating those who want to help the child. Their posture, threats, or punishments at home can lead the victim to retract allegations, thus further complicating the task of those attempting to protect the child. Prognosis for rehabilitation is always guarded, as with all psychopathic persons.

The rare *psychotic offender* or *mentally retarded offender* requires intervention to remediate the primary condition. The psychotic offender may be schizophrenic, manic, or depressed and may use the victim in ways particular to his delusional system (e.g., to "sacrifice" his daughter's virginity or to expiate some guilt). Prognosis after the treatment of the psychosis depends on character structure and family dynamics.

Offenders who are *alcoholic* or *substance abusing* often try to deny their responsibility by blaming their inebriated state. Some offenders get intoxicated after the abuse episode. Addiction to immediate gratification of pregenital needs may well be a common factor, but does not resolve the issue of personal responsibility.

Juvenile offenders have access to children as siblings, friends, or baby-sitters. Most of them are sexual abuse victims who have dealt with their trauma by identifying with the aggressor. Many adult abusers started abusing children as teenagers. Sibling incest takes many forms, from rape to relationships meeting some of both children's needs for security and affection in a barren or cruel home.

Rape of Children and Adolescents

Rape of children, like sexual abuse, is a criminal act more frequent than once thought.

Presentation

Rape victims are often brought to an emergency room by their parents, who are as upset as or more upset than their child. The psychological aspect of the trauma is often greater than the physical one. Although some offenders may hurt their victims for gratification of sadistic impulses, most violence occurs as means to gain the child's compliance and is usually less severe than in adult rape.

Childhood rape is usually disclosed by the child. In younger children, conflict about disclosure is related to their relationship to the offender; if there is none, there is less conflict. In older children, particularly adolescents, revelation of rape may be impeded by the same issues as seen in adult victims: self-recrimination, guilt, fear of being blamed or seen as "dirty," and fear of retaliation from the rapist.

Parental reactions vary from anxious disbelief, to denial, to panic.

Clinical Intervention

Medical, psychiatric, and legal interventions need to be coordinated. A *medical examination* of the child is essential and should be performed by a pediatrician comfortable with such examinations and willing to testify in court if necessary. As with adult victims, the gathering of corroborating data is an essential part of the medical examination. The medical record should be written as if ready for court.

A gynecologic examination should be performed in the context of a general medical examination and only after establishing a relationship with the child. Performing an internal examination on an uncooperative, panic-stricken child is a retraumatization that is never justifiable. If the examination cannot be delayed, it should be performed on a tranquilized or even anesthetized child. Hospitalization may be necessary.

A comprehensive physical examination includes the following:

- Medical history, including gynecologic history if appropriate
- History of the assault, recorded in a legible, precise, and nonprejudicial manner
- Recording of all observations on how the victim presents

- Physical examination, noting all signs of physical trauma, described in words as well as on a body chart
- Collection of medical-legal evidence (e.g., semen, blood, any foreign matter, loose hairs, material for DNA analyses)
- Pelvic examination and collection of laboratory specimens (e.g., for evidence of sexually transmitted disease)
- Medical therapy, if necessary, for physical injuries, pregnancy, or sexually transmitted disease

A rape kit, as used for adult victims, should be available. Follow-up is always necessary.

Psychiatric intervention should occur concurrently with the medical examination. Basic information and interviewing techniques are described in the paragraphs on sexually abused children.

Particular to rape victims is that they are being seen after an assault that has interrupted the flow of their usual life. The victim and the victim's family may have been functioning very well, adequately, or poorly before the rape. When seen in the emergency room, they are in a state of crisis and need to be responded to on that level. The parents' level of functioning may be seriously compromised, and they need pragmatic guidance as well as support.

There are no predetermined family patterns related to the rape of a child, but some children are more likely to be raped than others: those who have been sexually abused before, who dissociate under stress, who are lonely and needy, who have poorly developed social skills and cannot respond with adequate suspicion and self-protectiveness, and those who find themselves in violent surroundings (e.g., runaways and children in chaotic homes). These children may become victims of strangers, peers, or family members.

The victim and the family's tendency is to look for a cause, which easily leads to blaming the victim ("if only _______"). A child may be overtly blamed or punished for the rape when the parents cannot tolerate their helplessness or rage toward the offender. This requires intervention: no misbehavior or breaking of rules makes the child responsible for being raped. Intervention also decreases the potential for revictimization of the child.

Another relatively common finding is a reaction of overprotectiveness toward the child, sometimes with paranoid tendencies, which can be quite regressive and allow latent pathology to surface (e.g., school phobia). All parents have fears about the effects of the rape on the child and the whole family. Their anxiety has to be listened to without the child being present.

Legal Issues

The requirements vary from state to state. In Massachusetts, a report to child protective services has to be filed if the parents are not capable of responding adequately to their child and should be filed if services can thus be secured for the family. Criminal reporting and prosecution is separate from child protective service intervention. If the offender is a person the child will continue to see (e.g., if the offender lives in the neighborhood or goes to the same school), involving the police may be necessary to secure the child's safety.

Treatment Planning

Levels of functioning before the rape vary greatly, as do diagnoses. Some children exhibit a rape trauma syndrome similar to the one described in adults (Burgess and Holmstrom 1974; Sauzier 1984). Others may respond with behavior symptoms or with minimal symptoms. The level of parental anxiety strongly affects the child's reaction.

The first therapeutic intervention required is crisis intervention; individual meetings with the victim and individual couple meetings with the parents are necessary. Whether long-term therapy is necessary has to be decided in the course of crisis intervention.

Conclusion

The recent dramatic increase in reported sexual abuse challenges psychiatry with new issues. On a practical level, the need to cooperate with other agencies and in particular with the legal system conflicts with the traditionally more passive and isolated role of the psychotherapist. On a theoretical level, many questions arise. Is sexual abuse always linked to later psychopathology? Why do some victims identify with the aggressor, whereas others internalize a victim identity? What is the importance of trauma in human development? What are the costs and benefits of intervention?

Our increasing knowledge of the profound psychological and biological consequences, the intergenerational transmission, and the ability of one undetected offender to affect many children makes the task of intervening seem ever more daunting. Prevention and intervention remain great challenges for our society as much as for mental health professionals.

References

Adams-Tucker C: Proximate effects of sexual abuse in childhood: a report on 28 children. Am J Psychiatry 139:1252–1256, 1982

American Academy of Child and Adolescent Psychiatry: AACAP policy statement: guidelines for the clinical evaluation of child and adolescent sexual abuse. Washington, DC, American Academy of Child and Adolescent Psychiatry, 1990

Bender L, Blau A: The reaction of children to sexual relations with adults. Am J Orthopsychiatry 22:500–518, 1937

Bourne R, Newberger E: "Family autonomy" or "coercive intervention"? ambiguity and conflict in a proposed juvenile justice standard in child protection. Boston University Law Review 57:670–706, 1977

Brant RST, Tisza VB: The sexually misused child. Am J Orthopsychiatry 47:80–90, 1977

Bryer JB, Nelson BA, Miller JB, et al: Childhood sexual and physical abuse as factors in adult psychiatric illness. Am J Psychiatry 144:1426–1430, 1987

Burgess AW, Holmstrom LL: Rape trauma syndrome. Am J Psychiatry 131:981–986, 1974

Burgess AW, Nichols GA: Sexual Assault of Children and Adolescents. Lexington, MA, Lexington Books, 1978

Ferenczi S: Confusion of tongues between adults and the child (1933), in Final Contributions to the Problems and Methods of Psychoanalysis. Edited by Balint M. New York, Basic Books, 1955, pp 156–167

Finkelhor D: Sexually Victimized Children. New York, Free Press, 1979

Finkelhor D: Sourcebook on Child Sexual Abuse. Beverly Hills, CA, Sage, 1986

Finkelhor D, Browne A: The traumatic impact of child sexual abuse: a conceptualization. Am J Orthopsychiatry 55:530–541, 1985

Freud S: The etiology of hysteria (1896, 1924 footnote), in The Standard Edition of the Complete Psychological Works of Sigmund Freud, Vol 3. Translated and edited by Strachey J. London, Hogarth Press, 1962

Gomes-Schwartz B, Horowitz JM, Sauzier M: Sexually exploited children: service and research project. Washington, DC, Office of Juvenile Justice and Delinquency Prevention, 1984

Gomes-Schwartz B, Horowitz JM, Sauzier M: Severity of emotional distress among sexually abused preschool, school-aged and adolescent children. Hosp Community Psychiatry 36:503–508, 1985

Gomes-Schwartz B, Horowitz JM, Cardarelli AP: Child Sexual Abuse: The Initial Effects. Newbury Park, CA, Sage, 1990

Goodwin JM, Talwar N: Group psychotherapy for victims of incest. Psychiatr Clin North Am 12:279–293, 1989

Groth N: Men Who Rape: The Psychology of the Offender. New York, Plenum, 1979

Harper G, Irvin E: Alliance formation with parents: limit-setting and the effect of mandated reporting. Am J Orthopsychiatry 55:550–560, 1985

Herman J, Hirschman L: Father Daughter Incest. Cambridge, MA, Harvard University Press, 1981

Herman JL, Perry JC, van der Kolk BA: Childhood trauma in borderline personality disorders. Am J Psychiatry 146:490–495, 1989

Katan A: Children who were raped. Psychoanal Study Child 28:208–224, 1973

Kelley S: Stress responses of children to sexual abuse and ritualistic abuse in day care centers. Journal of Interpersonal Violence 4:502–513, 1989

Kinsey AC, Pomeroy WB, Martin CE, et al: Sexual Behavior in the Human Female. Philadelphia, PA, WB Saunders, 1953

Landis J: Experiences of 500 children with adult sexual deviants. Psychiatr Q 30 (suppl):91–109, 1956

Lewis M, Sarrel P: Some psychological aspects of seduction, incest and rape in childhood. J Am Acad Child Adolesc Psychiatry 8:606–619, 1969

MacFarlane K, Krebs S: Videotaping of interviews and court testimony, in Sexual Abuse of Young Children. Edited by MacFarlane K, Waterman J. New York, Guilford, 1986, pp 164–193

Massachusetts General Laws: Chapter 288 of the Acts of 1983, amending section 51B of Chapter 119

Peters JJ: Children who are the victims of sexual assault and the psychology of offenders. Am J Psychother 30:398–421, 1976

Pollak J, Levy S: Countertransference and failure to report child abuse and neglect. Child Abuse Negl 13:515–522, 1989

Putnam FW: Diagnosis and Treatment of Multiple Personality Disorder. New York, Guilford, 1989

Rieker PP, Carmen E: The victim-to-patient process: the disconfirmation and transformation of abuse. Am J Orthopsychiatry 56:360–370, 1986

Rimsza ME, Niggerman E: Medical evaluation of sexually abused children: a review of 311 cases. Pediatrics 69:8–14, 1982

Russell DEH: The Secret Trauma: Incest in the Lives of Girls and Women. New York, Basic Books, 1986

Sauzier M: Emergency care of rape victims, in Emergency Psychiatry. Edited by Bassuk E, Birk A. New York, Plenum, 1984, pp 271–283

Sauzier M: Disclosure of child sexual abuse: for better or for worse. Psychiatr Clin North Am 12:455–469, 1989

Sgroi S: Handbook of Clinical Intervention in Child Sexual Abuse. Lexington, MA, DC Heath, 1982

Summit R: The child sexual abuse accommodation syndrome. Child Abuse Negl 7:177–193, 1983

Summit R, Kryso J: Sexual abuse of children: a clinical spectrum. Am J Orthopsychiatry 48:237–251, 1978

Thoennes N, Tjaden PG: The extent, nature and validity of sexual abuse allegation in custody and visitation disputes. Child Abuse Negl 14:151–163, 1990

White S: Interviewing preschool children with sexually anatomically detailed dolls, in Play Diagnosis and Assessment. Edited by Schaefer C, Gitlan K, Sandgrun A. New York, Wiley, 1991, pp 317–330

Section III

Consultation and Special Clinical Problems

17

Consultations

Michael S. Jellinek, M.D.
Ourania Madias, M.D.

Child psychiatric consultation should integrate psychiatric diagnoses, child development, family dynamics, and understanding of systems—pediatric unit, court, or school—with the goal of enhancing a child's well-being. If successful psychiatric consultation frequently broadens to include training pediatric residents, schoolteachers, judges, and so on, as well as a "political" role as a child advocate, such advocacy can influence the policies and practices of courts, schools, and social service agencies as well as the level of funding provided by governmental agencies (Ahsanuddin and Adams 1982; Berlin 1980; Caplan 1963, 1970; Harper 1989; Herzog and Jellinek 1990; Jellinek 1990; Jellinek and Herzog 1991; Koocher 1974; Lewis 1980).

The consultant's role is complex as he or she encounters the issues involved in relating to large systems, groups, and hierarchies, all of whom, while asking in some way for expert guidance, may resist or actively discourage the consultant's activities and recommendations. Consultants are at the mercy of numerous forces beyond their control. In pediatric consultation there are reimbursement constraints and the attitudes of the pediatric or psychiatric chairpersons. In other areas of consultation, the shrinking budgets of agencies (i.e., courts and schools) often result in annual reevaluations of the need for consultation. Last, given the innumerable variables inherent in a case-by-case approach, consultants face a difficult task trying to conduct research that would validate their role.

It may be useful to enter the consultative setting with the expectation of being unloved, an outsider bringing more work for the consultee, a threatening and overpaid presence, and an expert who should not overemphasize his or her expertise (Jellinek 1985). Indeed, consultants, as in psychotherapeutic work, must attend to their powerful reactions, which include discouragement or resentment at not being valued and appreciated; reactions based on one's personal past; and grandiose perceptions of one's influence.

Nevertheless, whatever the setting, the consultant must begin with an empathic appreciation of the consultee's and patient's positions and perspectives. Only then can the consultant's expertise in clinical issues, development, group process, and systems issues be fully utilized.

The Process of Consultation

Although the specific nature of the consultative task will vary according to setting, as discussed later in this chapter, there are some common elements that are essential and in many respects parallel traditional therapeutic approaches. These include

- Contacting the consultant and clarifying specific questions.
- Focusing on key factors that contribute to the current problem.
- Differentiating long-term problems that need different approaches.
- Establishing empathic contact.
- Developing a psychiatric formulation and diagnosis.
- Speaking the "language" of the consultee (e.g., pediatricians pressed for time will not be able to use or tolerate a lengthy and anxiety-provoking psychodynamic explanation of patient and staff behavior. Such is the case even more with legislators).
- Becoming acquainted with the particular history and background

of the consultee's setting (e.g., program details, prior consultation, prior and current personnel).

- Gaining sanction from the system's leadership (e.g., school principal, chief of pediatric service, judge of the court).
- Establishing as clearly as possible from the outset "who wants what from whom." A consultant reads between the lines to avoid being used unwittingly to resolve or exacerbate internal systems' problems and thus destroy the potential usefulness of one's role to a child or, once asked, to a system.
- Recognizing the limitations of the consultation as early as possible. The achievement of modest, concrete goals often is more effective in establishing alliances and a positive consultative "niche" than the promise of more grandiose services.
- Retaining sufficient distance to avoid splitting in the consultative alliance. A rapport with only part of a system (e.g., the head nurse but not the attending on a pediatric service) often trades short-term comfort for long-term failure in the consultative task.

Specific Types of Consultation

Pediatric Consultation-Liaison

Consultation requests in pediatric settings often involve the following issues (Fritz 1990; Herzog and Jellinek 1990; Jellinek and Herzog 1991; Schowalter and Solnit 1966):

- Concerns about the child's reaction to illness and hospitalization (especially chronic disease, acute trauma)
- Suicidal behavior
- Dangerous or out-of-control behavior
- Depression-anxiety (often secondary to an illness, a specific treatment, or parental psychiatric disorders)
- Death and dying
- Problems specific to the preschool child (e.g., failure to thrive)
- Noncompliance with medical regimens
- Problems specific to the intensive care unit (e.g., delirium, massive trauma)

- Psychosomatic disorders
- Familial grief or behavior counterproductive to the patient's care (e.g., rigid denial that blocks critical procedures)
- Psychosis
- House-staff issues (Jellinek 1986; Schowalter 1970)

The two initial steps in addressing a pediatric consultation are to clarify with the pediatrician specific questions and to ensure that the pediatrician has informed the patient and family of the impending psychiatric consultation. (Sometimes the child psychiatric consultant's first educational task is to help the pediatric staff feel well grounded in suggesting to their patients and families that a psychiatric consultation is indicated.) These two initial steps are essential because the consultant must have the pediatrician's, child's, and family's endorsement both for proceeding to gather the necessary information and for the eventual implementation of any recommendations. The consultant's feedback to the physician and family must be direct, concise without psychiatric jargon, and prompt. The note in the chart must be legible, brief, and respectful of both the family's confidentiality and the pediatrician's practical goals.

The key points in consultation-liaison are as follows:

- Talk to the child's caretakers (nursery, house staff, attendings, social worker) and review the chart, including medical and laboratory findings.
- Establish a diagnostic impression.
- Be supportive. Support is communicated through tone, posture, questions, and choice of words, all of which indicate your understanding of the patient's and family's worries, fears, and hopes.
- Maintain realistic hope and adaptive denial (do not break adaptive defenses).
- Communicate clearly your interventions and objectives.
- Attend to possible team discord (e.g., dogmatic disagreements, scapegoating).
- Attend to parents' needs. Understand their likely feelings of guilt and anxiety as well as their wish to help.
- Empower parents and engage them as partners in their child's care

and well-being. Offer support and/or education. Respect coping styles that may be different.

In the best of circumstances, well-crafted consultations may lead to more frequent requests and, ultimately, a fuller liaison relationship with a ward, service, or subspecialty (Bernstein and Sussex 1984; Sherman 1982). Such connections can develop new clinical services (e.g., a Tourette clinic shared by child and adolescent psychiatry and neurology, support groups for nurses, enhanced child psychiatric teaching in the pediatric curriculum, additional funding of child psychiatric staff).

School Consultation

Because the school is the workplace of the child, and because increasingly available psychological services are being offered there (through PL 94-142 (1975), which mandates special services for children ages 3–21 with mental, emotional, or physical handicaps or local special educational programs), contact with the schools and school systems is an essential aspect of outpatient evaluation and therapy. Establishing contact with the teacher(s) and school of one's own patients is often necessary and always useful; such episodic contact can help develop an "outpatient milieu" (J. F. McDermott, personal communication, October 1991) that supports treatment.

In addition, a limited number of school districts have contracts with child psychiatrists for consultative purposes. Thoughtful efforts in establishing a contract, including proper sanction from the superintendent, defining whether the consultations will include direct psychiatric evaluations of children or work only through school staff, and ensuring adequate availability for difficult or emergent situations (Adler and Jellinek 1990; J. F. McDermott, personal communication, October 1991), will help ensure a mutually satisfactory consultation relationship.

It is especially important to understand the basis of the consultative arrangement within the school setting. If, for example, one is requested to evaluate individual children, are such evaluations to include family contacts? What safeguards exist to maintain confidentiality? To whom are you responsible? Is classroom observation acceptable to all faculty? How will you interface with existing staff psychologists or guidance counselors? Can you gain ready access to key members of the power structure (e.g., principal, superintendent)?

In asking and answering these questions, the consultant must keep in mind system, town, and district politics; funding issues and constraints; and the constant awareness that one is in an educational rather than medical service delivery system. Flexibility and patience can lead to increasing energies at the administrative levels of the school system where more constructive change can be implemented.

Currently school systems are under unusual stress (Jellinek 1990). Society at large has increased its expectations of schools so that the curriculum now may well include AIDS education, courses on human sexuality, and efforts to prevent substance abuse. In addition, special education laws now ask the schools to provide adequate or even optimum care of all children, even those with physical or psychiatric disorders. All of these demands are in the context of a declining school budget, a lower enrollment that results in the aging of the largely tenured faculty, and societal forces including a high divorce rate and a majority of two-career families. Although child psychiatrists are among the most skillful at integrating and balancing the child's emotional and medical status with the many forces confronting the school, declining budgets are forcing many districts to limit comprehensive planning and consultation.

Forensic Consultation

Child psychiatrists, in their clinical patient care as well as broader roles, are increasingly involved with courts, lawyers, and judges. Such involvement is sufficiently complex to require a chapter in its own right (see Chapter 18).

Adoption and Foster Care Consultation

The number of children involved in foster care and adoption is expanding. Many of these children are among the most seriously disturbed (see Chapter 20). Child psychiatrists can play a useful role in relation to adoption and foster care by consultation to agencies and institutions that serve such children and their families.

Agency Consultation

The agencies empowered to care for children and their families are increasingly numerous and complex. These include state and local welfare systems, child-care services (e.g., day care, group homes), residential settings, protective services, and advocacy structures. Several common problems appear to be present in these systems.

The roles of respective agencies are often redundant boundaries. Some services are duplicated; others are not available or permitted. For example, welfare, protective services, and mental health departments may all be responsible for intervention with and funding of services for troubled children. Who is "in charge" is less clear. Funds are often tied to specific services so that even regional managers do not have the freedom for innovative programs.

"Therapeutic" services are increasingly present within agencies where this was not previously true (e.g., group homes, emergency shelters). Although such changes are motivated primarily by fiscal concerns, they complicate the life of the child psychiatrist consultant. The consultant may have less to say about major decisions affecting children's lives. For example, a child's length of stay in a group home or residential treatment center is no longer the sole domain of the child psychiatrist. Many settings view their particular mandate as primary in a child's life; struggles between treatment programs, residencies, and state agencies for control can lead to extremely complicated situations. In the area of custody and foster care, the consultant can see such dilemmas in operation. In addition the courts are often slow and limited by availability of resources or ambiguity of what is best for the child.

Finally, the larger question of to what degree the agencies involved see themselves in loco parentis has begun to affect the consultative process and its problems. Agency interventions frequently cause different but similar difficulties than the initial clinical problem. (This situation can arise in incidents of alleged sexual abuse that immediately lead to family disruption, multiple losses, and related trauma).

Political Consultation

From the previous sections of this chapter it should be evident that the clinical arena is increasingly entwined in immediate and powerful political institutions and policies that *directly* affect questions of medical care and available services to children and families, reimbursement for these services, questions of professional competence and licensing, quality of care, viability of educational programs, and approval for necessary research studies.

Hence the child psychiatrist needs to appreciate the critical importance of his or her role as an advocate for children, families, and the professional agencies that serve them. Proactive involvement may be useful; passively ignoring such problems ensures further erosion of budgets and services essential for optimal levels of care for children who, of course, do not speak for themselves. These political consultants can perform a variety of tasks, including

- Knowing and maintaining contact with key legislators (local, state, and federal) sympathetic to children's issues and needs
- Testifying before legislative committees involved in decisions and policies affecting children
- Writing letters to legislators and their staff vis-à-vis pending legislation
- Educating legislators and their staff about the facts of many clinical situations; busy politicians make critical decisions on the basis of available knowledge (or supposition); brief fact sheets and personal contact can influence voting patterns and appropriations
- Remaining available to run for office in professional societies or public sector settings where expert knowledge can influence policy directions and budgets

Additional Considerations

The future of child psychiatric consultation is directly related to how well our society cares for children and families. Economic forces will determine whether there is reimbursement through the health care system or sufficient state and federal funding to provide expert consultation integrating developmental, psychiatric, familial, and cultural factors with a goal of developing comprehensive treatment recommendations. The child psychiatric consultant, partially because of economic pressures, will also have to decide who is being served and will face an ongoing challenge to maintain the child's and family's well-being as the central focus.

References

Adler RS, Jellinek MS: After teen suicide: issues for pediatricians who are asked to consult to schools. Pediatrics 86:982–987, 1990

Ahsanuddin KM, Adams JE: Setting up a pediatric consultation liaison service. Psychiatr Clin North Am 5:259–270, 1982

Berlin IN: Psychiatry and the school, in Comprehensive Textbook of Psychiatry, 3rd Edition, Vol 3. Edited by Kaplan H, Freedman A, Sadock B. Baltimore, MD, Williams & Wilkins, 1980, pp 2693–2706

Bernstein NR, Sussex J (eds): Handbook of Psychiatric Consultation With Children and Youth. New York, SP Medical & Scientific Books, 1984

Caplan G: Types of mental health consultation. Am J Orthopsychiatry 33:470–481, 1963

Caplan G: The Theory and Practice of Mental Health Consultation. New York, Basic Books, 1970

Fritz GK: Consultation liaison and child psychiatry and the evolution of pediatric psychiatry. Psychosomatics 1:85–90, 1990

Harper G: Focal inpatient treatment planning. J Am Acad Child Adolesc Psychiatry 28:31–37, 1989

Herzog DB, Jellinek MS: Psychiatric Aspects of General Hospital Pediatrics. Chicago, IL, Year Book Medical, 1990

Jellinek M: Consultation. Presentation to Child Psychiatry Board Review Course, Boston, MA, June 1985

Jellinek MS: Recognition and management of discord within house staff teams. JAMA 256:754–755, 1986

Jellinek MS: School consultation: evolving issues. J Am Acad Child Adolesc Psychiatry 29:311–314, 1990

Jellinek MJ, Herzog DB: Introduction to psychiatric consultation to children, in Handbook of General Hospital Psychiatry. Edited by Cassem N. St. Louis, MO, CV Mosby Yearbook, 1991

Koocher GP: Talking with children about death. Am J Orthopsychiatry 44:404–411, 1974

Lewis M: Residential treatment, in Comprehensive Textbook of Psychiatry, 3rd Edition, Vol 3. Edited by Kaplan H, Freedman A, Sadock B. Baltimore, MD, Williams & Wilkins, 1980, pp 2685–2692

PL 94-142: Education for All Handicapped Children Act, 1975

Schowalter JE: Death and the pediatric house officer. J Pediatr 76:706–710, 1970

Schowalter JE, Solnit AJ: Child psychiatry consultation in a general hospital emergency room. Journal of the American Academy of Child Psychiatry 5:534–551, 1966

Sherman M: Communicating: a practical guide for the liaison psychiatrist. Psychiatr Clin North Am 5:271–278, 1982

18

Forensic Child and Adolescent Psychiatry

Joseph J. Jankowski, M.D.
Stephen G. Porter, M.D.

During the past 15 years there has been an increased involvement of child and adolescent psychiatry with the judicial system (Densen-Gerber and Lothian 1985). The dependent status of children results in increased vulnerability to emotional and legal problems occurring in the family. It is often necessary but difficult to separate the child's legal rights from those of the parent. Only recently have the unique emotional and developmental issues of childhood been considered independently from parents' rights. This has resulted in an increased demand for child psychiatric clinicians to become the advocates for their patients within the judicial system.

Irrespective of the site of their work, child psychiatrists are expected by society and the courts to become more involved in legal matters concerning their patients. As a result, in this chapter we present aspects of forensic issues in the context of specific service delivery sites. In addition, we discuss more specialized forensic aspects of clinical care such as consultation to the courts and risk management.

Legal Issues Related to Service Delivery Sites

Emergency Room

Patients are usually brought to the emergency room by the patient, parent, agency, or medical care provider wishing to resolve a crisis and "normalize the situation." Since crisis issues often lead to controversies that need immediate attention, forensic issues are often encountered as follows:

Good samaritan rule. The patient without a clear legal status who comes to the emergency room for services can be evaluated and treated in his or her best interests for only one session. If the patient is at risk safety-wise, the patient must be taken to court to obtain approval for further services. If safe, the patient cannot be treated further without permission from the legal guardian and is discharged.

Legal guardian. The identity of the legal guardian must be determined so that either written or verbal consent to treatment can be obtained. Often children are brought for emergency services by schools, agencies, neighbors, and other health care providers without the parents (guardian) being informed. In those instances, the good samaritan rule applies unless the legal guardian can be located. (In this chapter, the term *parent* will be used, but may be understood to refer to a child's legal guardian as well.)

Right to refuse treatment. All patients and their parents have the right to refuse treatment (*In re Roe* 1981; *Rogers v. Okin* 1979). However, if the treatment is deemed necessary for the safety of the child, the right to refuse treatment can be challenged by filing either a commitment paper or a care and protection petition, both of which will need resolution by the court.

Emancipated minor. Children under age 18 are considered minors in most states. In some instances, children can be treated as a decision-making adult when they have a certain status (e.g., pregnancy, military service, living independently, parent of a child, married, widowed, or divorced) or when they have a dangerous public health illness. Such children can make decisions regarding medical and psychiatric care for themselves without input from their parent.

Civil commitment. If a child is deemed to be dangerous to self or others, the child can be committed by a licensed physician (in some states by psychologists and psychiatric nurses) to a secure facility for a time-limited period (e.g., 10 days), depending on state law (California Welfare and Institutions Code 1984; *Lessard v. Schmidt* 1972; Schwitzgebel 1981). During that time, the patient is evaluated at a secure facility to determine whether further commitment is necessary. During this process, a special commitment paper is completed by the clinician and sent with the patient to the commitment facility. This paper allows patients to be restrained and transported against their will. The evaluating clinician assumes responsibility for the patient to arrive at the receiving facility safely (e.g., use of ambulance, restraints).

Concern about parent's ability to provide for safety of child. The clinician must decide whether the parent is capable of determining what is in the best interests of the child. For example, it is necessary to assess whether the child will be safe if allowed to be discharged to the parent. Otherwise, the courts must be notified and action taken to ensure the child's safety. This can take the form of a restraining order on the parent or an emergency care and protection petition. In either case, the clinician will require the aid of an attorney and appear in court to provide testimony to support this decision.

Another consideration may be for the clinician or parent to request that the child be seen elsewhere (equivalent care) for a second opinion. If that option is selected, the other facility must be contacted, a copy of the initial evaluation will accompany the child, and transportation is provided by ambulance. Depending on the findings and decision of the parent and clinician, the child may either return to the first facility or remain at the second.

Restraints (physical or chemical). Restraints are used as needed to manage patients in the emergency room. Leather or cloth restraints (four-point) with a fifth point (sheet) around the chest and abdomen are used. Such restraints require the constant presence of a clinician observing and recording the patient's status regularly (e.g., every 15 minutes). Such patients are assigned a one-to-one sitter and not left alone. There must be adequate justification to restrain, and the reasons must be communicated in the hospital record.

Chemical restraints, such as benzodiazepines, can be useful. Neuroleptics are rarely used because of the *Rogers* decision (1982), which prohibits their use for more than one dose without obtaining consent from the patient or court for their further use (*Rogers v. Okin* 1979).

Seclusion. Minors cannot be legally secluded in locked rooms unattended according to most state laws. If a locked quiet room is used, there must be a clinician in attendance in the room at all times and its continued use justified regularly (e.g., every 15 minutes) in the record. Such rooms can be helpful to provide reassurance to out-of-control patients and relief from interpersonal demands and increased sensory overload. These rooms, however, can be abused or become institutionalized without rules or safeguards (Gutheil 1978).

Protective services. Children and adolescents who are victims of neglect and abuse (physically or sexually) often require protection from further abuse. In such cases, the patient can either be admitted to a pediatric inpatient service for 24 hours until a placement is made by the responsible state agency or court or an alternative placement occurs from the emergency room. Such patients can also be relocated to a responsible adult who can protect the child.

In these cases, the clinician is mandated by child protection laws to report the incident of abuse or neglect to the designated state agency. The emergency room clinician should refrain from extensive questioning about the abuse because the child will usually require referral to another clinician who will reexamine and treat the patient. To avoid further victimization, the emergency room clinician needs only to acknowledge and record that the abuse had taken place. This information should be well documented in the record.

Determination of suicide risk. During emergency room evaluations, the clinician is often faced with determining the risk of allowing the patient to be discharged. The clinician's findings and recommendations must be clearly documented in the record and a specific notation made concerning the element of risk and what the clinician's judgment is about that risk. If the risk is considerable, the patient should be hospitalized. However, if the risk is borderline and a decision is made to hospitalize, a written justification should be provided.

Substance abuse. Toxic screens of urine and blood are permissible to establish the clinical diagnosis that would dictate treatment or some other intervention. However, patients should be informed that these are being obtained and a notation made in the record to that effect. Patients who refuse such a test are refusing services. Either the patient must be discharged and referred elsewhere or, if the patient is not safe, the patient might require commitment.

In most cases, unless the patient is an emancipated minor or age 18, the parent has a right to be informed of the blood and urine test findings.

Weapons and gunshot wounds. The presence of weapons in the hands of minors must be reported to the security officers of the hospital. Recent gunshot wounds that have not been treated must be mandatorily reported to the police.

Rape. Victims of rape undergo a detailed physical examination with cultures of vaginal, urethral, anal, and oral orifices. In addition, blood studies for venereal disease are obtained, and an attempt is made to establish whether semen is present in the vaginal vault of the patient. During the interview of the patient, all details need to be carefully documented in the record since they will be used by the courts to obtain a conviction if an arrest and trial ensue. The information obtained is not confidential since it involves a crime that preempts the therapist privilege.

Physical searches. On occasion, it is necessary to search patients or their belongings because of the suspicion that they might be concealing a weapon to injure themselves or others. Patients who do not allow a search cannot be seen because they are not cooperating with the treatment or intervention and may be referred elsewhere. If the patient is considered suicidal, the patient's rights regarding a physical search can be overridden to maintain the patient's safety.

Pediatric Consultation-Liaison (C-L)

The pediatric hospital presents a setting where the likelihood of legal action being utilized in patient care is high. Patients referred in this setting often present complicated, crisis-oriented medical, psychiatric, or psychosocial problems that often have legal involvement. The C-L psychiatrist is frequently requested to co-manage such cases with the pediatric staff.

The types of legal issues encountered in this setting are as follows:

Informed consent. Parents initially bring their child to the pediatric hospital expecting intervention of a medical nature. However, while hospitalized, the child may manifest a behavioral or psychological problem that interferes in the child's medical care. When this happens, it is difficult initially for parents to accept a referral for a psychiatric consultation or evaluation. As a result, the referring pediatrician and C-L psychiatrist must sensitively inform the parent and child about the need for such a consultation, outlining what it entails and discussing issues of confidentiality and informed consent (Kaufmann 1983; Lidz et al. 1984).

The parent must give oral or written permission to the C-L psychiatrist to contact outside sources other than the primary medical caregiver during the evaluation or intervention. If oral permission is given, a note to that effect should be entered in the record. Additional consent must be obtained for psychological tests to be performed on the child during a C-L evaluation.

Lack of parental cooperation. If the parent does not cooperate with the C-L evaluation or intervention, the services must stop, and the psychiatrist should write a note in the record to that effect and inform the referring physician. If the child's life is at risk (e.g., Munchausen by proxy), a care and protection petition could be obtained or the patient transferred to another hospital for a second opinion (see concern about parent's ability to provide for safety of child in the emergency services section).

Confidentiality. Only case material relative to the immediate problem regarding the child should be shared with medical caregivers. Additional material of importance, but not immediately relevant, must be kept in the private records of the clinician. Medical records are open and not confidential.

Case material should not be discussed in the hallways, elevators, or common areas of the hospital. Patients have a personal right to privacy regarding their medical, personal, and psychosocial issues (Schmid et al. 1983). Conference rooms where such material is discussed with the parents or other staff should afford needed privacy.

Even though the C-L psychiatrist may see the patient only once or twice, the therapeutic privilege remains intact (*Robinson v. Commonwealth* 1987). The confidence of the patient-therapist privilege must be maintained unless the patient or court waives that privilege. Psychiatrists are, however, expected to reveal a privileged communication if a future dangerous act is intended. Another exception is in divulging information in order to place a patient in a medical or psychiatric facility for his or her own safety (Knapp and Vande Creek 1987).

Right to refuse treatment. Parents have a right to refuse treatment for a minor. If such a refusal does not place the child at risk to harm self or others, the parent is requested to sign a form entitled "Against Medical Advice" (AMA), and the child is discharged. If the child is placed at risk by a refusal of treatment, a restraining order is brought against the parent to maintain the child in the hospital and provide the necessary care. This is done by immediately petitioning the court for such an action. Such petitions are processed by 24-hour on-call judges who will make an emergency decision on the phone after speaking with the hospital attorney, the C-L psychiatrist, and the parents. Within 24 hours after that decision is made, all parties must appear in court for a formal hearing on the facts, unless it involves a weekend or holiday.

Munchausen by proxy. These cases present special problems of child's rights versus parent's rights and are difficult to manage clinically and legally (Waller 1983). In some states, surveillance aids such as hidden cameras are allowed; in other states they are not. Munchausen by proxy cases are frequently at some point in the spectrum of their evolution usually not clearly discernible. As a result, if the case is not obvious or cannot be substantiated medically, reports must be specifically written in the medical chart outlining the clinician's suspicions, which are not proven. Copies must be sent to the primary care provider, who will be expected to follow the patient after discharge.

Where the case has been medically substantiated, the parent is confronted with the findings. The child not allowed to leave the hospital, and an abuse or neglect petition is filed. Consideration is also given to whether a care and protection petition is needed. Such cases often require court involvement and placement of the child away from the offending parent, at least on a temporary basis.

The accused parent usually requires further psychiatric evaluation, which should be court ordered. The return of the child is usually predicated on the findings of that evaluation.

Transplantation of organs. Minors who are a potential donor match must consent themselves without coercion from parents. They and their parents must be independently evaluated by psychiatrists. The psychiatrist's reports are sent to the judge, who makes a substituted decision for the child after consulting with the child in closed chambers.

Psychological reasons for not permitting transplants include lack of treatment compliance, substance abuse, lack of family supports, and lack of a predictable living arrangement. These items are usually evaluated by the psychiatric clinician.

In some instances, the parent of the minor child who is being denied a transplant decides to seek recourse through the courts. In those instances, the court will request testimony from all parties and provide a substituted decision.

Written statements of findings and recommendations, either within the hospital record or personal documents of the child psychiatrist, will be subpoenaed by the court during these proceedings.

Acquired immunodeficiency syndrome (AIDS). Minor patients who are suspected of having AIDS are requested to have a diagnostic test either at the hospital or at an anonymous site, only after obtaining the person's written informal consent (Mass Law 70F 1986).

The information provided to the patient and/or the parent must include

- The voluntary nature of the test
- The purpose of the test
- An interpretation of the test and significance of test results, including variability
- Availability of counseling
- The recording of the test in the patient's medical record with a separate consent obtained for each release of information

If a minor child refuses to have the test, the child cannot be coerced by the parent or medical care provider. The patient's decision must be respected regardless of the patient's medical status or its personal and social ramifications. If the test is necessary to determine a lifesaving treatment, the case may be brought before the court for a substituted decision.

If the psychiatrist is notified about the test results, or if the psychiatrist knows the patient has AIDS, that knowledge must be maintained in strict confidence.

Recently, children with AIDS have been determined by the courts to be entitled to the rights of the handicapped as defined by statute. They, therefore, cannot be kept from attending school (Centers for Disease Control 1987; Kermani 1988).

Substituted judgment. This includes decisions made by the court in the best interests of the child. For example, decisions to withdraw life support, even in hopeless situations, cannot be made by parents or physicians. Such cases must be brought before the court; the judge, after collecting all of the evidence, will make a substituted judgment for the patient. Such judgments require examination of all records and testimony from all parties involved.

DNR (do not resuscitate) orders. Parents can provide this recommendation either verbally or in written form to the physicians caring for the child. This order indicates that the patient who is terminally ill and expected to die should not be exposed to extraordinary measures to prolong life. This order does not imply that all normal care, including feeding and medications, would cease. Only extraordinary care such as resuscitation is withheld.

Ethical decisions. Not infrequently, the child psychiatrist is asked to evaluate a child or adolescent who has a serious medical problem in whom it is not known whether further medical or surgical procedures are ethically warranted. Such decisions require an understanding of the illness, its treatment, compliance, family stability, coping ability of the child's parents, and the emotional and developmental status of the patient.

Such complex clinical decisions are frequently made jointly by several clinicians, including the psychiatrist, and reviewed by an ethics committee. Such a committee is composed of a variety of individuals (medical, legal, former patients, community representative, clergy, nursing, and hospital administration). After hearing and deliberating on the clinical and ethical aspects of the case, this committee helps the clinicians arrive at a decision that is ethically responsible to the patient and parent.

An ethics committee provides an opportunity for a humanistic decision to be made by peers and others who are not directly involved in the patient's care (Ethics Consultation Service 1987).

Medical foster care. Patients with serious medical illnesses often require inordinate daily medical care and follow-up that the parent cannot provide in a substantial, reliable, and sustained manner. As a result, an alternative caregiver must be sought. In such cases, the child psychiatrist is asked to help assess whether the biological parent is emotionally capable of providing this care for the child. If not, the parent can either voluntarily sign over the legal responsibility of the child to a responsible state agency or the case is taken to court as a care and protection petition.

If the care and protection petition is approved by the court, the child is placed in a medical foster home where he or she can receive needed care. The foster parents are carefully selected, usually have only one foster child, and are specially trained to provide medical care and emotional support for the child.

The parent is encouraged to remain in close contact with the child and to have liberal visitation. Such foster care can be short or long term, depending on the length of the child's medical illness and the emotional capacity of the parent to resume care of the child.

Accidents. Accident-prone patients are at high risk in terms of child, parent, or family instability and repeated emotional crises. As a result, the C-L child psychiatrist is often called to evaluate such cases. If the accident appears to be related to abuse or neglect, it must be decided whether the child can be returned to the care of the parent, and a mandatory report should be filed with the appropriate state agency. If the child cannot be returned home, a care and protection petition must be obtained from the court, and legal custody of the child must be assigned to the responsible state agency.

The impaired parent. An impaired parent is usually identified on a pediatric medical unit where the parent's behavior is interfering in the medical care of the parent's child. The C-L child psychiatrist is asked to evaluate such a problem; depending on the evaluation, the impaired parent may be referred for outpatient psychiatric treatment or taken to the adult psychiatric emergency service for a psychiatric evaluation and/or intervention. Visitations with the child are usually curtailed or supervised, with restricted phone calls to the unit. A restraining order is often needed to limit visitation and provide supervised visits until the parent receives a psychiatric evaluation.

Outpatient

Given the current litigious aspect of our society, it is not surprising that many child and adolescent psychiatrists who provide outpatient services (clinic or private office) are becoming more involved with legal issues. Below are the following forensic issues that are most commonly encountered by outpatient clinicians:

Legal guardian. It is necessary to establish who is the patient's legal guardian before outpatient services are provided since this person is the only one eligible to provide permission for treatment. Without approval from the legal guardian, the patient can be seen only once under the good samaritan rule (see the emergency room section).

The legal guardian can give either verbal or written permission for treatment. In some cases where there is no legal guardian and the patient is not an emancipated minor, the court must appoint a guardian.

Emancipated minors. Minors who, as mentioned previously, demonstrate personal recognizance and responsibility can be seen for treatment at their own request. In effect, they are making decisions for themselves and are treated legally as adults (see the emergency room section).

Permission to treat (informed consent). Permission to treat must be obtained from the parent for any minor child except one who is emancipated. The type of treatment, its length, family involvement, and side effects (medications) should be communicated to the parent (Noll 1976). Afterward, a notation needs to be placed in the record that the clinician has communicated the relevant information to the parent and that the parent has given approval to institute treatment (see the pediatric consultation-liaison section).

Trainees. Trainees must inform the patient and the parents of the patient's status and obtain permission as a trainee to provide services to the child and family. This communication should include a description of their own trainee status, the name of their immediate supervisor, and the length of their training period as it relates to this particular patient and family. The option of a meeting with the patient and parent with the supervisor to review the case must be presented. The trainee must also note in the record that this communication and approval to treat has taken place.

All recordings of trainees should ideally be read and countersigned by the supervisor. However, if the course of treatment is long term (e.g., greater than 6 months), a monthly summary note can be signed in lieu of more frequent countersigned notes by the supervisor.

Confidentiality. Clinicians are expected to observe the therapist privilege, namely that whatever is communicated by a patient is held in confidence. It is understood that this privilege begins with the very first appointment unless it is clear to the patient, preferably in writing, that whatever is communicated can be reported to, for example, the court if it is a court-ordered evaluation (*Robinson v. Commonwealth* 1987).

The therapist privilege must be maintained unless it is revoked by patient or court. Under unusual circumstances, such confidentiality can be broached. They are as follows: 1) if the patient is in danger to self or others, 2) if the therapist uncovers child abuse, 3) if the patient undergoes court-ordered psychiatric examination and is warned of the purpose of the examination, and 4) if a judge orders disclosure in a child custody proceeding. Privileged communications include actions, conversations, correspondence, and written notes or records of communications (Massachusetts General Law 1968).

Records. Since psychiatric data are sensitive and confidential, such data should not be entered in the general hospital record except for what is needed for billing (e.g., demographic, dates seen, and diagnosis). Instead, a separate psychiatric record should be kept where confidentiality can be provided reliably and access limited.

Progress notes should be written whenever there is patient contact, such as phone calls from the patient, a parent, outside agencies, and other sources; changes in medication; results of conferences; and supervisory recommendations.

Psychiatric medical records can be released only after obtaining informed consent or a specific court order. The exceptions to this include *Tarasoff* (*Tarasoff v. Regents of the University of California* 1974) issues (duty to warn or protect), hospitalization, and court order (Mass Law 70 1983).

Supervisors. The name of the case supervisor should be mentioned in the record. As previously reported, supervisors must countersign the notes of their trainees and, if a case is particularly difficult to diagnose or manage, are expected to make their own notations in the record to clarify the issues and supervisory input.

Supervisors, at their own discretion, can interview the patient and the parent to obtain information in making their own decisions. Supervision of case management should be provided by staff who have clinical staff appointments and can assume clinical responsibility for the care of the patient. Supervisors without clinical appointments, but only teaching appointments, cannot be legally held responsible for the clinical care of the patient. As viewed by the court, their role is that of teacher, not clinical staff or supervisor.

24-hour coverage. Patients receiving outpatient care are expected to receive 24-hour clinical coverage by a responsible clinician. This is in keeping with the patient's right to receive aftercare (*Dixon v. Weinberger* 1975; *Halderman v. Pennhurst State School and Hospital* 1981). According to most state statutes, clinical services cannot be provided only from 9:00 A.M. to 5:00 P.M. without an arrangement for backup during off-hours. Patients and parents need to be formally told where and how they can access backup coverage during off-hours. This is preferably done in writing.

Consultation with other caregivers. Clinical data can be provided only to other medical or psychiatric care providers with the approval of the parent or emancipated minor. Such permission should be noted in the patient record as being verbally given or as a formal permission form, a copy of which is included in the psychiatric record.

Whenever possible, it is beneficial to include the parent or emancipated minor in a meeting of providers. This reduces the concerns about confidentiality violations and allows an open forum to discuss clinical issues optimally.

Medications. Informed consent must be obtained from the parent or emancipated minor to use psychiatric medications. In this process the benefits and side effects of the medication must be communicated. Afterward, a dated notation must be made in the record that the informed consent was obtained, mentioning specifically what was told to the parent.

A medication flow sheet consisting of necessary prior medical tests and psychiatric evaluations, the name of the medication, date prescribed, dosage, schedule of administration, and number of refills must be available. Medication side effects and dosage changes are also maintained on this flow sheet, which should be kept in the patient's record.

Some medications are approved by the Food and Drug Administration (FDA) for certain age levels. However, in some areas of the country, medications are given to children younger than at FDA-approved age levels for specific clinical entities. If there is a question about this, determine from other clinicians in your area what the standard of practice is before giving such medications. A regional professional society can be helpful in directing you to the proper resource person concerning this issue. The courts generally abide by the accepted clinical standards practiced in the medical and psychiatric community of the prescribing physician.

Mandated reporter. All mental health clinicians are mandated to report all cases of suspected or actual sexual or physical abuse and neglect to the designated state agency. In some cases, the reporting of these events can be postponed if the patient and parent are cooperative in the treatment plan and there is reasonable certainty that the child is not being further abused.

In some cases, it is helpful to present the case to a multidisciplinary committee of mental health and medical care providers for discussion. Such groups function as a clearinghouse for reporting and sharing decision making about reporting abuse cases and carry substantial weight in the courtroom. These committees or groups often exist in general hospitals where the potential incidence of abuse and neglect reports is high and where many other providers (e.g., nurses, nonpsychiatric physicians, aides) are present.

The mandated reporter is protected by law from being sued by the person being reported. The report is not an allegation or indictment; it is merely a report of the suspiciousness or concern that abuse or neglect might be occurring. An actual indictment must await the results of the evaluation of the problem by the responsible state agency.

Inpatient

Inpatient child and adolescent psychiatry programs serve very disturbed youngsters in a self-contained, emotionally intense setting for a relatively short period (e.g., 3–4 weeks). Such a clinical program, by its very nature, is at high risk to encounter forensic issues, which are listed as follows:

Psychiatric hospitalization of minors. Parents have the authority to make decisions about their minor children regarding medical and psychiatric treatment, including hospitalization. Minor children who resist are considered incompetent to decide for themselves what is in their best interests. The U.S. Supreme Court (*Parham v. JR*) in 1979 upheld these parental rights as long as they were supported by a neutral fact finder or decision maker (e.g., physician). The court accepts the parents' good intentions toward their children and assumes that physicians would admit only children who are in need and not at the whim of a parent who is seeking admission of a child who is disruptive at home and school.

In some states, judicial hearings are still held if an adolescent resists hospitalization, and legal counsel is provided for the patient. This occurs despite the *Parham* ruling because of the perceived loss of liberty and stigmatization incurred by psychiatric hospitalization (Patterson 1982).

Patient safety. Inpatient child and adolescent units often utilize locked entrance doors or one-to-one sitters to maintain patients on the unit in a safe manner. Troubled children and adolescents, as psychiatric inpatients, are not expected to be under control of their impulses at all times. Therefore, the inpatient unit must have the capacity to lock its doors when needed to prevent elopement and to contain high-risk patients.

One-to-one sitters (24 hours). Whenever possible, a staff-secure environment should ideally be provided rather than restraints or locked doors. Individuals employed to provide a staff-secure environment (one-to-one sitters) should have training and supervision to perform their task and be prepared to ask other staff for help whenever necessary. The inpatient unit is clinically responsible for defining their roles and boundaries on the unit and for providing internal supports within the unit to help them function optimally.

Restraints. Physical and chemical restraints are utilized on inpatient units as in the emergency room. If a patient is placed in physical restraints, the patient should have a one-to-one staff person or sitter with them at all times and a flow sheet kept with notations at 15-minute intervals describing the patient's condition and status. As the patient regains control, the restraints are reduced and discontinued as rapidly as possible. The record must document the need to institute restraints and their continued use, if needed (see the emergency room section).

Chemical restraints are optimally provided by benzodiazepines rather than neuroleptics because of tardive dyskinesia and the *Rogers* decision (*Rogers v. Okin* 1979). The *Rogers* decision does not allow neuroleptics to be given to a patient without the patient or parent's informed consent. Chemical restraints should be tapered and discontinued as soon as possible (see the emergency room section).

Seclusion. By statute in many states, it is not legal to seclude children in locked rooms by themselves. This has led to the use of open-door seclusion or quiet room (Joshi et al. 1988). Such rooms can be helpful to reduce stimuli, to allow psychological reintegration, and to defuse emotional lability. However, as with restraints, such rooms must have clinical staff available at all times and such seclusion should be used only for as short a time as necessary (e.g., 15-minute intervals) (see the emergency room section).

AMA (sign out against medical advice). On occasion, patients or parents determine for themselves that the treatment being provided is either not adequate or not what they expected and want to leave the hospital. These are generally ill advised and represent a patient population where the children have likely been physically abused and where violence exists in the home (Green et al. 1986). If the patient is clinically ready to leave, the patient is discharged. If it is felt that the patient is not clinically ready to leave, the parent must sign the patient out against medical advice (AMA). If the patient is unsafe to leave, the patient must be either committed or transferred to another facility. If the patient is to be kept in the same facility, this action must be court ordered. Generally this results in either obtaining a restraining order on the parent or the filing of a care and protection petition (see right to refuse treatment—pediatric consultation-liaison section.)

Elopement. In the event a patient elopes from the unit, the parent, community police, and hospital security services must be informed. If the patient is found, the patient is returned for a psychiatric reevaluation regarding future potential for elopement risk and consideration for placement in a more secure facility to avoid future elopements and maintenance of safety.

Strong efforts must be made by inpatient psychiatric staff to avoid elopement, including placing those at risk with one-to-one sitters or in locked facilities. A daily note must be placed in the record documenting the elopement risk of a patient with such potential.

Use of neuroleptics/*Rogers* decision. The *Rogers* decision of 1983 outlines the guidelines for the use of neuroleptics (*Rogers v. Okin* 1979). Since psychiatric inpatients receive these medications more often than patients in other settings, this issue is presented here.

Permission must always be obtained from the parent to use such medication. If the parent refuses and the patient cannot be treated and managed on the unit without the medication, arrangements must proceed for transfer to a unit that will provide treatment and management without using neuroleptics.

If the patient's guardian is a state agency, a substituted decision is provided by the court. Such requests to the court for the use of neuroleptic medication must be specific. When requesting such permission, it is necessary to have in mind the expected dosage ranges of all medications expected to be used and to consider all contingencies at that hearing so the clinician does not have to return repeatedly to court for minor adjustments in the dosage schedule.

***Tarasoff* decision.** Clinicians are expected by society and the courts to warn and protect those persons being threatened verbally by the clinician's patients. If a patient is making threats to injure or kill a person, the person to whom the threats are directed must be warned and protected, even if it requires commitment of the patient.

Usually the patient needs to be retained until the threat subsides.

Such patients, if already on an inpatient psychiatric unit, must be managed with increased vigilance regarding elopement. Passes to leave the unit should be canceled until the threat is modified or ends. If necessary, the patient can be committed to a locked inpatient unit if considered dangerous. In such decisions, the therapist privilege is waived.

Consultation to Courts

Delinquency

Since the turn of the century, legal reformers and child advocates have helped create a separate judicial system for children, the mission of which was to rehabilitate rather than to punish or deter (Healy and Bronner 1926). Efforts were made to consider the developmental needs of children in legal dispositions. The duty of the state to provide for the welfare of those without another protector emanates from the English common law doctrine of *parens patriae.* This doctrine fostered a special relationship between the juvenile court and its wards. This paternal concern was, unfortunately, a double-edged sword. Interventions to rehabilitate led to less formal judicial proceedings, which took on an "extra-legal" air. As a result, juvenile courts paid increasingly little attention to due process safeguards that protect adults in criminal court.

Trials, often informal affairs aimed at finding placements or interventions, varied with the respective training, compassion, and commitment of judges, probation officers, and other court personnel. The system was ripe for abuse, with children being separated from their families and confined to institutions for extended periods without proper legal representation or right of appeal. The quality of care provided was variable and could not be differentiated from punishment. In *Kent v. United States* (1966) and *In re Gault* (1967), the U.S. Supreme Court reversed these informal traditions, mandating that juveniles were entitled to due process protection in all legal proceedings. Combined with 1975 legislation (PL 94-142), the Education for the Handicapped Law, in which Congress required states seeking federal funding to desist from placing children who had committed status offenses in locked correctional facilities along with adjudicated delinquents, these rulings have dramatically altered the juvenile courts.

Criminal behavior in children is pathognomonic of the presence of psychosocial and/or organic pathology. It may indicate a failure of the family or community to provide authority and nurturance by protecting the child from abuse, neglect, and poverty (Glueck and Glueck 1950; Patterson 1982). Or it may indicate the failure of the child to adapt to a complex world, as in a child suffering with a neurological deficit manifested by low intelligence, attention deficit, or a learning delay (Lewis et al. 1987). The juvenile courts must rely on trained clinicians to provide a proper diagnosis of a defendant's problems, including comprehensive evaluations of individual, family, and school functioning, as well as appropriate treatment planning and ongoing consultation to the court.

There are several common forensic issues related to delinquent youth:

Court-ordered evaluations. Child psychiatrists are frequently asked to evaluate children who have committed crimes. Such a request may come as an emergency or as part of an extended diagnostic evaluation. A child psychiatrist might be involved at the very beginning of the proceedings at the request of a juvenile probation officer to render an opinion on that child's "amenability to treatment." Another common point of consultation is at the end of a court case when recommendations are needed for disposition planning.

All evaluations conducted for the courts should be comprehensive and include a history from family members and agencies, interviews with the child and family including a history of past antisocial behavior, events surrounding the alleged crime, and arrangements for any needed medical evaluations and psychological testing. If a psychiatric emergency exists, the consultant should arrange with the court and family for a hospitalization in an appropriate facility. Otherwise, the evaluation should be completed in a timely manner, and proper reports and findings should be made available to the court.

Competency and criminal responsibility. As part of the initial screening, it is important for the child psychiatrist to consider the issues of competency to stand trial and criminal responsibility. Traditionally, English common law considered children under age 7 to be incompetent to stand trial and to lack *mens rea,* criminal intent. Before age 14, English common law presumed children to be *doli incapax,* incapable of entertaining criminal intent. Thus, prior to *In re Gault* (1967), legal tradition and the rehabilitative focus of the juvenile court rendered issues of competency and criminal responsibility virtually irrelevant. With the advent of due process guarantees, especially involving serious crime, these issues emerge.

Age is not itself an indication of understanding; developmental issues as well must be considered for each child. For older children, it is necessary to consider whether they 1) have the capacity to understand the charges made against them; 2) understand the workings of the court, including the functions of various court personnel; 3) can cooperate with an attorney in the preparation and conduct of their defense; and 4) understand the potential outcomes of their trial.

Additionally, with respect to criminal responsibility, the clinician must consider whether a particular child is suffering from a mental illness or neurological defect and whether those problems prevent the child from appreciating the wrongfulness of his or her actions or conforming behavior to the law.

Substance abuse. The abuse of alcohol and drugs is widespread among latency-age children and adolescents, especially in impoverished urban environs, and is an intimate companion of crime. Detoxification of the child or adolescent is often necessary before one can render an informed diagnostic opinion about basic psychological problems. Some states allow for the civil commitment of children who are addicted. However, secure detoxification facilities are often scarce.

Gangs and cults. Criminal behavior in juveniles is often linked to participation in peer groups such as gangs or groups of mixed age with a charismatic or manipulative leadership. Various cults may require criminal or violent behavior as an initiation rite of passage. Membership in such groups should be questioned during all evaluations.

Parents have the right to request hospitalization for their child who is involved with a cult (*Parham v. JR* 1979). However, whether the child psychiatrist complies depends on the clinical needs of the child. Experience with such cases reveals that the parents receive more benefit from the hospitalization than the child. The child psychiatrist must answer the question, "Is being a cult member justification for psychiatric hospitalization?" A controversial topic, this can be answered affirmatively if there are covarying psychiatric problems and negatively if not (Berland et al. 1990; Bohn and Gutman 1987).

Transfer hearings. Due to the seriousness of certain crimes and the perception that adjudicated juveniles receive minimal punishment before they are set free, there has been recurrent controversy concerning procedures that allow the criminal justice system to transfer jurisdiction of a juvenile into the adult court (Benedek 1985). The basic guidelines for such a change are contained in the 1966 United States Supreme Court case of *Kent v. United States.* In that decision, a juvenile is entitled to a special transfer hearing, during which five areas must be considered by the court: 1) obtaining a careful psychiatric history, including the child's past criminal record; 2) weighing the seriousness of the alleged crime; 3) assessing the child's amenability to treatment; 4) determining the appropriateness of available juvenile court programs for the child; and 5) deciding whether the public welfare would be best served by trying the juvenile as an adult.

These hearings require expert evaluation and testimony regarding the child's rehabilitative potential. There are no specific guidelines for these opinions, and a finding that permits transfer to the adult court is often accompanied by a serious punishment. These evaluations pose an uncomfortable dilemma for the clinician. The child psychiatrist must be certain that he or she is not providing results simply to please the prosecution or solely out of sympathy for the involved juvenile. As in the controversy that surrounds testimony in insanity defense cases, forming an opinion about a child's potential for rehabilitation or for dangerousness can easily be construed as a finding of fact rather than as an expert opinion (Stone 1984). In this manner, the psychiatrist could be viewed as meddling with justice by allowing a child accused of a serious crime potentially to go free. These evaluations should be undertaken with caution, restraint, and thoroughness (Barnum 1987).

Juvenile homicide. No other crime stirs up as much passion and confusion as murder. No other crime leads to such intense pressure on the state to conduct a transfer hearing to be able to prosecute a child in adult criminal court. The best studies to date of juveniles accused of murder consistently conclude that there are no simple ways to characterize this population of juvenile offenders. Each must be examined for his or her own peculiarities and themes, including parental abuse and abnormal neuropsychiatric findings (Corder et al. 1976; Cornell et al. 1987; Lewis et al. 1979). Homicide may occur within or external to a child's family, or as part of another crime such as theft, rape, or drug use. It is important to avoid oversimplifications of motive and character, which might deviate a clinician from utilizing important clinical information (Stearns 1957).

Status offenses. Because of their "minor status," children are expected to be obedient and respectful of adult authority. Acts of truancy, defiance of parental authority and limit setting, and running away demonstrate a disregard of societal norms. These are acts that would not be considered criminal if done by adults. The juvenile court's effort to intervene in these matters represents an effort to shore up parental authority and help return a child to some degree of control for the family. Just as adult offenses such as drunkenness have been decriminalized, so too have status offenses been removed from the criminal proceedings of the juvenile courts in most jurisdictions. These problems are more generally remanded to proper state agencies.

Contested Custody

Through the early 19th century a father ruled over his property inclusive of wife and children with absolute authority and entitlement. It was a rare occasion for a court to find against the father even when his cruelty led to his family's dissolution. Change began most notably in 1817 when the poet, Shelley, was denied custody of his children due to his atheistic beliefs. Gradually the mother's claim to the children began to be entertained more seriously and was given its first legislative impetus with the passage of the Talfourd's Act in 1839. Through this law the courts were authorized to award custody of a child to the mother during that child's early years up through age 7. This standard would later come to be known as the "tender years" doctrine. The law specified that the child, once turned 7, would return to the father's care.

Legally the mother's importance to her children slowly evolved, and in the latter half of the 19th century the laws were rewritten to extend the period of childhood that children spent with their mothers first to age 16 and then to age 21 years. In the 1920s, the absolute rights of the father were challenged and lost. With remarkable speed mothers became the preferred parent to raise children. The rapidity of this change is linked to such factors as urbanization, industrialization, and psychology's focus on the importance of the mother in child rearing. By the 1960s, approximately 90% of all contested custody cases were awarded to the mother unless overwhelming evidence demonstrated her unfitness.

Attention eventually shifted to assessing the needs and rights of particular children, and the focus became "the best interests of the child." This new perspective elevated the rights of the child over the rights of parents. In 1964 the courts initiated the practice of appointing a guardian ad litem (GAL) to evaluate cases of contested custody (Hansen 1964). Through such efforts there emerged a greater awareness of children's needs and of maternal fallibility. As a result, over the last three decades, the importance of an ongoing relationship with the father and his role in parenting has been reclarified (Derdeyn 1976). The current position is that mothers and fathers are now equal in importance to the child's welfare, as shown in a 1971 Missouri court case, *Garrett v. Garrett,* when custody was awarded to a father in the absence of maternal unfitness. The decision (p. 742) stated that "the rule giving the mother preferential right to custody is considerably softened by the realization that 'All things never are exactly equal' (*Garber v. Tyree,* Mo App, 400 SW 2nd 193, 199) and is predicated upon the acts of motherhood—not the fact of motherhood." The court went on to comment that the "tender years" doctrine of children needing to be maintained in the custody of their mother is outmoded. It stated that

> This precept, gutted into most every opinion on the subject, is not based upon any superior right of the mother, for our statute provides that in al proceedings in which shall be involved the right to custody and control of minor children, neither parent as such shall have any right paramount to that of the other parent, but in each case the court shall decide only as the best interests of the child itself may seem to require.

Current standards do not assume that either parent is the preferred custodian. All efforts are made to determine which custody and visitation arrangement is in the best interests of the child (Goldstein et al. 1973). The ambiguities spawned by this doctrine have led the courts to seek professional guidance from experts such as child psychiatrists, who may be appointed as GAL, or as a special investigator for the court (Ash and Guyer 1984). In this capacity they are expected to conduct a comprehensive evaluation of the children and parents of a divorcing family, prepare a report for the court with a specific set of recommendations, and provide testimony as needed.

Custody is divided into two parts: legal and physical. Legal custody refers to a parent's right to participate in all of the important decisions of the children's lives such as schooling, medical treatment, and religious orientation. In many states it is now assumed that both parents will assume joint legal custody unless there is a compelling reason to the contrary. Physical custody indicates with whom the child physically lives during the majority of time. A specific visitation plan is developed with the noncustodial parent. Typically, custody is given primarily to one parent (custodial parent) with regular visitation scheduled for the other. Recently joint physical custody where the children spend an equal amount of time at each parent's residence has become a popular option for courts, parents, and children. In some states, the courts presume that initial custody arrangements be jointly shared. If that is not effective, the parents can return to court for further hearings (*Dodd v. Dodd* 1978; New Hampshire Revised Statutes Annotated 1983).

There are two entry points in the custody process that are determined by the nature of the divorcing parents' relationship. The first entry point occurs when couples are able to speak to one another and share a common concern for their children that is well differentiated from their own needs. They often are able to seek help from a child psychiatrist before they embark on a legal struggle. In these instances the child psychiatrist may act as an expert consultant advising the parents about the potential consequences of their divorce, especially in regard to the children's developmental stages and issues. These can be satisfying cases where everyone emerges from the consultation better able to compromise and plan effectively.

The second entry point occurs when a child psychiatrist becomes involved in a divorce case at the request of the court or at the request of the parents' respective lawyers. Such a request usually comes after all routine efforts by lawyers and the courts have failed to bring resolution to an acrimonious divorce proceeding. These cases frequently include serious issues such as a parent suffering from a major psychiatric illness or when allegations of abuse and neglect are a prominent feature. In these cases the court may appoint the psychiatrist as a GAL or as a special investigator to the court. In lieu of that, the parents, through their lawyers, may privately agree to abide by the findings and recommendations of a child psychiatrist concerning custody and visitation of their children. In such cases any decision reached will be accepted with serious reservation and often interference from the parents. The importance of hurting the other often takes precedence over any consideration for the welfare of the children. Unfortunately, the fight over custody simply brings the children into the cross fire of the parents.

The recommended format for a child custody evaluation is as follows:

- The evaluation should not begin until there is a written agreement specifying 1) the task of the psychiatrist, 2) who will pay for the evaluation, 3) the limits of confidentiality, and 4) to whom the final report will be made available. It is best to proceed with a specific appointment by the court and be certain that all reports become the property of the court.

- The evaluation should consist of a review of all relevant medical, psychiatric, court, and school reports. The parties should provide all relevant written material in their possession. It is helpful to have each parent write a history of the family highlighting the issues of concern to them from their perspective.
- The psychiatrist must conduct interviews of the parents, children, and all relevant individuals such as significant relatives, family friends, teachers, clergy, clinicians, and counselors. Each parent's relationship with their children and parental fitness must be assessed. Parental fitness includes the ability to provide for the physical and emotional needs of one's child.
- The report will include 1) a narrative of family life and the specific circumstances associated with the dissolution of the family, 2) a summary of findings, and 3) recommendations including a specific plan for custody and visitation (several options along with their pros and cons can be presented for the court's consideration.) The child psychiatrist must be prepared to defend this report through expert testimony if requested by the court.

Termination of Parental Rights

In the aftermath of severe abuse and neglect it is often necessary to begin proceedings that will permanently separate children from their parents. As a society, we tend to believe that either all problems can be fixed or all deserve a try at fixing. It is our first impulse to help heal even the most desperate of families. By the time a child psychiatrist becomes involved, there is always a long and complex history. The efforts of multiple social agencies often result in repeated attempts at therapeutic interventions on the individual or family level as well as placement in foster care. It is the failure of these efforts to mend the matrix of the child's biological family that leads to the initiation of legal proceedings to terminate parental rights formally. The decision to pursue such a course of action often rests with a child provider agency, whose attorney organizes the case and presents it to court.

The severance of parental rights requires a formal trial at which the parents and the involved children are entitled to counsel. The child psychiatrist is most often an expert witness who is asked to evaluate the entire family and prepare a report for the court.

It is imperative that the child psychiatrist conduct a thorough evaluation that renders a determination of current as well as past parental fitness. The U.S. Supreme Court in *Santosky v. Kramer* (1982) viewed termination of parental rights as a process by which government interferes with the privacy of family life and renders an irreversible decision. Whereas custody and visitation decisions are based on a "preponderance of the evidence," which requires a simple majority of the evidence, the standard of proof for terminating parental rights must be "by clear and convincing evidence," requiring that the evidence be 98% in favor of the decision being made. Additionally, the Supreme Court required that proof of parental unfitness be current and continuing at the time of the hearing.

Similar in format to a custody evaluation, a termination of parental rights case includes a careful review of family history, agency involvement, school and therapeutic interventions, interviews with all relevant parties, and home or school visits. The child psychiatrist must not rely on old data for a determination of parental functioning. The evaluation must provide an assessment of current parental fitness based on data from recent interviews and observations, as well as recent historical data of the involved child providers and agencies. The final report should contain reference to how the parents responded to efforts to help them reunite with their child and why it is unlikely that any further efforts in this regard would succeed. Without these data, an expert's report and testimony may be deemed insufficient by the court for such a serious determination.

The child psychiatrist may also be asked to 1) evaluate the appropriateness of a preadoptive family, 2) mediate issues between all of the involved parties, 3) help parents to recognize their limitations, and 4) elevate the interests of their children over the parents' own needs. Compromise and out-of-court settlements are always possibilities, even in the most desperate of situations.

Forensic Evaluation Guidelines

An evaluation conducted expressly for a legal purpose differs from traditional clinical evaluations in a number of important ways as follows:

- Forensic evaluations are most often involuntary court-ordered investigations. It is essential to establish the boundaries of the investigation with the court, the involved family, and the participating attorneys. The child psychiatrist must work out a unique contract for each case that specifies payment, confidentiality, the availability of information, and access of the final report.
- A comprehensive forensic evaluation may require 3–6 months for completion. Often it is necessary to observe a family over time to distill truth from the allegations and innuendo. It also is helpful for the child psychiatrist functioning as a GAL to work with the court in allowing a gradual evolution in the format of a family's visitation plan. Such clinical orchestration may allow a family to settle into a reasonably cooperative venture while fostering trust and mutual respect. This often necessitates taking a family systems approach to the understanding of family pathology (Jacob 1986).
- Direct observation of parents and children at home is an essential part of a forensic evaluation. The ability to see how a house is organized and maintained provides valuable insights into a child's existence. School visits or visits to other major sites in a child's life may also provide valuable information. In this way, the child psychiatrist assumes an expanded role as clinician correlating environmental life-space observations with office-bound clinical findings.
- Forensic evaluations cannot be used as emergency interventions. The treatment of substance abuse, psychosis, or suicide must be done in a neutral clinical setting before a forensic evaluation can proceed.
- The court-appointed evaluator should avoid becoming the therapist of the family being evaluated. Although there are many points at which a forensic evaluator may offer therapeutically informed suggestions, one cannot perform a legal evaluation while offering treatment. Conversely, therapists should not accept assignment by the court to do a forensic evaluation of a family for whom they have provided treatment.
- Whenever possible, a court appointment allows the child psychiatrist to assume a nonadversarial role. It is always best in these family cases not to become a "hired-gun" for one side against the other. A child-centered focus can be best maintained when one is working

for the court and for the best interests of the involved children. If one is contacted by an attorney for one party, it is important to direct counsel to join with the opposing attorney to have the court appoint a child psychiatrist evaluator to the case.

- Any case that involves a potential conflict of interest for the child psychiatrist should be avoided. Business or personal relationships with any of the involved parties will militate against involvement.
- Cases that provoke intense countertransference reactions in the evaluator should be referred to another clinician. A child psychiatrist cannot perform a balanced nonjudgmental evaluation if repelled by, frightened by, or attracted to any of the persons being evaluated.
- Reports and testimony must be rendered in clear, nontechnical language. Jargon and abstract concepts are to be avoided. Clear narratives of a family's life and difficulties are necessary for the court to understand the rationale for the child psychiatrist's findings and recommendations.
- Recommendations should be clearly delineated and relate to the body of the narrative and findings.
- The evaluator should be prepared to defend any and all statements during cross-examination. Statements should be objective and include a synthesis of the material, avoiding subjectivity.
- The basis of the evaluation must be maintained on the best interests of the child.

Risk Management

Prior to 1971, risk management received only little attention. However, during the early 1970s and early 1980s three important Supreme Court decisions were handed down regarding the right to treatment. The first ruling, *Wyatt v. Stickney* (1971) provided for "individualized treatment plans, humane physical and psychological environments, qualified staff in sufficient numbers and established environmental standards" for patients involuntarily committed. The second case, *O'Conner v. Donaldson* (1975), noted that patients being involuntarily committed were eligible to have their constitutional rights be properly protected. The third case, *Youngberg v. Romero* (1982), noted that involuntarily committed patients had a constitutional right to treatment in the least restrictive manner as a "fundamental liberty interest." As a result of these rulings, the era of holding institutions, governments, and eventually individual practitioners legally responsible for the care they provided was initiated.

There are several special malpractice issues with which child psychiatrists are most involved.

Abandonment of Patients

- The patient is not getting better, and something different needs to be done. This usually requires referral to another clinician for consultation. Terminating treatment can be misinterpreted as abandonment.
- The patient or family develops a grievance with the clinician. Instead of terminating the relationship, a referral should be made to another clinician.
- The patient or family refuses to accept your recommendations for treatment (e.g., psychopharmacology, inpatient psychiatric care). If, in your judgment, you cannot treat this patient properly without such modalities being used, refer the patient to another therapist who utilizes other modalities (e.g., behavior techniques, individual or family psychotherapy).
- Patients who miss appointments should not be terminated without having letters sent to them stating the dates and time of their next appointment. If they do not show up for that appointment after written notice, a final letter should be sent telling them that they could contact you if they have further difficulties or you could refer them to another clinician.
- Patients require having their phone calls returned within a reasonable period (e.g., 24–48 hours). If they are not, this can be construed as abandonment or lack of follow-up, especially if the patient is at risk for suicide or psychological decompensation or needs more medication.

Informed Consent

This usually occurs as a problem when the patient or parents have not been properly informed or warned about the possibilities of adverse reactions to medications. As with other medical providers who must abide by informed consent laws, the child psychiatrist must also outline all potential side effects of the medications being prescribed and write in the record afterward what exactly was told to the patient and/or parent. The benefits, risks, and alternatives to the procedures being recommended need to be communicated in such a fashion that the patient and parents understand them and can make their own decision (Kaufmann 1983). This topic was discussed in the pediatric consultation-liaison section but it can apply as well to all sites where services are provided.

Report Writing and Progress Notes

All written material should stand the test of public scrutiny. Most, if not all, written clinical material can be subpoenaed by the court. Also, patients have a right to see their own records, and parents have a right to see the records of their minor child.

Reports should be written objectively, avoiding subjective remarks, with statements being substantiated by direct quotes from the patient. They should be written with the intent that you will need to defend your statements in court.

Reports involving the child should contain only issues related to that child and the problem at hand. Other issues related to the parent or siblings, but not involving the child directly, should be maintained independently in the parent's folder. This is especially true when evaluating younger children, where the tendency is to add parent and sibling material in the identified child-patient record.

Relationship With Patient and Parents

Relationships can be misconstrued by patients and parents who are vulnerable when seeing a therapist. Undue familiarity has become a common allegation of patients and parents. Visiting the homes of patients without it being scheduled as a professional visit, sharing vacations, physical contact, and excessive gift giving have led to common allegations. Society and the courts expect reasonable boundaries to be maintained in the professional relationship, especially with psychotherapists. On the other hand, a good professional working relationship with patient and parents often helps to avoid adverse legal action.

Verbal Versus Written Communication

In the parlance of the legal profession, "if it is not written down, it did not take place." Verbal communications are used each day by all clinicians, and we expect them to continue in our profession. However, a written note substantiating a verbal communication with a patient is vital and necessary. When a patient or parent calls on the phone, it is helpful to note and date the summary of what was discussed and communicated. Patients who do not come for several appointments should have letters sent giving them another opportunity for a session so that abandonment does not become an allegation.

If you explain the potential side effects of medications to a patient or parent, the explanation should be written in the patient's record as you presented it.

If a case is taken to court, the written documents become your major defense. Verbal statements, although helpful and clarifying, do not match the importance of the written word.

Attorneys

If you are involved in a risk-management issue, you should contact your attorney as quickly as possible. In fact, that attorney should be appraised of potential problems as they occur. Often the attorney's guidance is helpful in avoiding further difficulty.

Generally, you will be told not to contact the patient or parent to discuss the case. Instead, all material regarding the case should be forwarded to your attorney for review. After your attorney receives your material, the attorney will arrange to meet with you to discuss potential strategies for reply and possible action. Your attorney may be an independent, hospital, or risk-management attorney, depending on the site and circumstances of the case.

Your attorney is your legal representative with the court and will act in your best interests. Other attorneys who contact you regarding material about the case should be directed to your attorney.

Keeping the Patient Safe

All actions that maintain the safety of the patient are viewed positively by society and the courts. Deviance from this standard will result in problems. Issues such as parents refusing to allow their suicidal children to be psychiatrically hospitalized will pose a major risk-management problem if the child is allowed to go home and commits suicide shortly after. It is expected of the clinician that he or she take legal steps to advocate for the child's safety. This may require contacting an attorney and taking the case to court for a substituted decision. Rarely will the courts decide against the clinician who is taking steps to protect the patient. This is an especially common occurrence in the emergency room where the parents of teenagers do not think their child is suicidal, either because the child is convincing them that they did not intend their act or the parent cannot narcissistically accept the recommendation.

Managed Care Issues

Managed care providers employ clinical reviewers to decide on the appropriateness of care for patients. These reviewers have usually not seen these patients and make judgments on incomplete evidence. Also, unfortunately, such decisions (e.g., whether to hospitalize a child) are at times influenced by financial considerations.

If a patient requires a specific treatment (e.g., inpatient care) and the managed care reviewer is not in agreement, the case can be taken initially to an internal appeal arranged by the managed care provider. If after the appeal the clinician remains concerned about the safety or best interests of the child, the case can be taken to court and the judge asked to make a substituted judgment.

Society and the courts will hold the clinician, not the managed care provider, responsible for the safety, care, and well-being of the patient. In their eyes, the managed care provider is a health care administrator whereas the clinician is the professional care provider. Rarely will the courts overrule the wishes of the clinician in favor of the managed care provider.

Sexual Exploitation

In the field of child and adolescent psychiatry, sexual exploitation of patients can include parents as well since they are often intimately involved with the process. Clinicians who sexually exploit patients are subject to civil and criminal actions as well as professional licensure revocation proceedings. In such cases, the plaintiff will have the difficulty of overcoming the burden of proof by a "preponderance of the evidence" (>50% chance) that exploitation actually took place. If medication is used either to induce compliance or reduce resistance, then it becomes a criminal act and the burden of proof is "beyond a reasonable doubt" (90%–95% certainty).

In the case of a minor patient, the issue of consent or coercion is irrelevant since by law minors and certain identified adults are incompetent and considered unable to give consent.

Summary

As can be seen from this chapter, child psychiatrists have many opportunities and requirements for becoming involved in forensic issues on a daily basis as part of their everyday work, regardless of service-delivery site. As part of this work, child psychiatrists are being called on 1) to have a working knowledge of forensic issues; 2) to evaluate children, parents, and families forensically; 3) to help make decisions about custody, placement, commitment, organ transplants, care and protection, and approval for medications; and 4) to maintain the safety of patients and society.

The child psychiatrist is also called on to evaluate the child in a number of different contexts (e.g., courts, pediatric inpatient services, child and adolescent psychiatry outpatient and inpatient services, emergency rooms, and private offices). The need for forensic work to be provided by child psychiatrists is growing rapidly and will become greater over time. In this chapter, we attempted to familiarize child psychiatrists with current areas of necessary involvement with forensic issues in their daily practice.

References

Ash P, Guyer MD: Court implementation of mental health professionals' recommendations in contested child custody and visitation cases. Bull Am Acad Psychiatry Law 12:137–148, 1984

Barnum R: Clinical evaluation of juvenile delinquents facing transfer to adult court. J Am Acad Child Adolesc Psychiatry 26:922–927, 1987

Benedek E: Waiver of juveniles to adult court, in Emerging Issues in Child Psychiatry and the Law. Edited by Schetky DH, Benedek EP. New York, Brunner/Mazel, 1985, pp 180–190

Berland DI, Spinazzola VL, Brayer E, et al: Ethical, legal and psychodynamic considerations in intervention of a possible cult member. J Am Acad Child Adolesc Psychiatry 29:975–981, 1990

Bohn T, Gutman JS: The civil liberties of religious minorities, in Cults and New Religious Movements. Edited by Galanter M. Washington, DC, American Psychiatric Association, 1987

California Welfare and Institutions Code, Sec 5000-5401, 1984 (Suppl 1993)

Centers for Disease Control, Public Health Service: Guideline for counseling and antibody testing to prevent HIV infection and AIDS. MMWR 36:509–513, 1987

Corder BF, Ball BC, Haizlip TM, et al: Adolescent parricide: a comparison with other adolescent murder. Am J Psychiatry 133:957–961, 1976

Cornell DG, Benedek EP, Benedek BA: Juvenile homicide: prior adjustment and a proposed typology. Am J Orthopsychiatry 57:383–393, 1987

Densen-Gerber J, Lothian J: Emergency issues at the interface of law and medicine concerning children of the 1980s, in Emerging Issues in Child Psychiatry and the Law. Edited by Schetky DH, Benedek EP. New York, Brunner/Mazel, 1985, pp 332–345

Derdeyn AP: Child custody contests in historical perspective. Am J Psychiatry 133:1369–1376, 1976

Dixon v Weinberger, 405 F Supp 974 (D DC 1975)

Dodd v Dodd, Family Law Review, 4:2302–2304 (1978)

Ethics Consultation Service: Administrative Memorandum No 3-87-4. Boston, MA, New England Medical Center Hospitals, 1987

Garrett v Garrett, 464 SW 2d 240 Miss (1971)
Glueck S, Glueck E: Unraveling Juvenile Delinquency. New York, Commonwealth Fund, 1950
Goldstein J, Freud A, Solnit AJ: Beyond the Best Interests of the Child. New York, Free Press, 1973
Green WH, Padron-Gayol M, Whiteman KN, et al: Child psychiatric discharges against medical advice. Journal of the American Academy of Child Psychiatry 25:260–265, 1986
Gutheil T: Observations on the theoretical bases for seclusion for the psychiatric inpatient. Am J Psychiatry 135:325–328, 1978
Halderman v Pennhurst State School and Hospital, 673 F 2d, 652, quoting in re Schmidt, 429 A 2d 635-363 (Pa Sup Ct 1981)
Hansen RW: Guardian ad litem in divorce and custody cases: protection of the child's interests. Journal of Family Law 4:182–184, 1964
Healy W, Bronner AF: Delinquents and Criminals. New York, Macmillan, 1926
In re Gault (387 VS 1) (1967)
In re Roe III, 421 NE 2d 40 (Mass Sup Jud Ct 1981)
Jacob JW: Divorce and child custody resolution: conflicting legal and psychological paradigms. Am J Psychiatry 143:192–197, 1986
Joshi PT, Capozzoli RN, Coyle JT: Use of a quiet room on an inpatient unit. J Am Acad Child Adolesc Psychiatry 27:642–644, 1988
Kaufmann CL: Informed consent and patient decision making: two decades of research. Soc Sci Med 17:1657–1664, 1983
Kent v United States, 383 US 541, 556 (1966)
Kermani EJ: Handicapped children and the law: children afflicted with AIDS. J Am Acad Child Adolesc Psychiatry 27:152–154, 1988
Knapp S, Vande Creek L: Privileged Communications in the Mental Health Professions. New York, Van Nostrand Reinhold, 1987
Lessard v Schmidt 349 F Supp 1078 (ED Wis 1972)
Lewis DO, Sharrok SS, Pincus JH, et al: Violent juvenile delinquents: psychiatric, neurological, psychological and abuse factors. Journal of the American Academy of Child Psychiatry 18:307–319, 1979
Lewis DO, Pincus JH, Lovely R, et al: Biopsychosocial characteristics of matched samples of delinquents and non-delinquents. J Am Acad Child Adolesc Psychiatry 26:744–752, 1987
Lidz CW, Meisel A, Zerubavel E, et al: Informed Consent: A Study of Decision-Making in Psychiatry. New York, Guilford, 1984
Mass Law (General Laws, c 111, Sect 70), 1983 (Supp 1993)
Mass Law (MEL c 111 Sect 70F), 1986
Massachusetts General Law (GL c 233 S20B), 1968
New Hampshire Revised Statutes Annotated, Section 458:17, 1983

Noll JO: The psychotherapist and informed consent. Am J Psychiatry 133:1451–1453, 1976

O'Conner v Donaldson, 422 VS 563 (1975)

Parham v JR (442 VS 584), 1979

Patterson GR: Coercive Family Processes. Eugene, OR, Castalia, 1982

PL 94-142: Education for All Handicapped Children Act, 1975

Robinson v Commonwealth 399 Mass (133-136) (1987)

Rogers v Okin 478 F Supp 1342 (D Mass 1979), mod 634 F 2nd 650 (1 Cir 1980), vacated and remanded sub nom Mills v Rogers—US-102 S Ct 2442 (1982)

Santosky v Kramer, 455 US 745,769–770 (1982)

Schmid D, Appelbaum PS, Roth LH, et al: Confidentiality in psychiatry: a study of the patient's view. Hosp Community Psychiatry 34:353–355, 1983

Schwitzgebel RK: Survey of state commitment statutes, in Civil Commitment and Social Policy: An Evaluation of the Massachusetts Mental Health Reform Act of 1970. Edited by McGarry AL, Schwitzgebel RK, Lipsett PO, et al. Rockville, MD, National Institute of Mental Health, 1981, pp 47–57

Stearns AW: Murder by adolescents with obscure motivation. Am J Psychiatry 114:303–305, 1957

Stone A: Psychiatry and violence, in Law, Psychiatry and Morality. Edited by Stone A. Washington, DC, American Psychiatric Press, 1984

Tarasoff v Regents of the University of California, 118 Cal Rptr 129, 529 P2d 553 (1974)

Waller D: Obstacles to the treatment of Munchausen by proxy syndrome. Journal of the American Academy of Child Psychiatry 22:80–85, 1983

Wyatt v Stickney, 325 F Supp 781 (MD Ala 1971)

Youngberg v Romero, US-102 S Ct 2452 (1982)

Additional Readings

Ash P, Guyer M: The functions of a psychiatric evaluation in contested child custody and visitation cases. Journal of the American Academy of Child Psychiatry 25:554–561, 1986

Barnum R: Integrating multiple perspectives in forensic child psychiatry consultation. Journal of the American Academy of Child Psychiatry 25:718–723, 1986

Beck JC: Confidentiality Versus the Duty to Protect: Foreseeable Harm in the Practice of Psychiatry. Washington, DC, American Psychiatric Press, 1990

Benedek EP, Schetky DH: Custody and visitation problems and perspectives. Psychiatr Clin North Am 8:857–873, 1985

Berlin FS, Malin HM, Dean S: Effects of statutes requiring psychiatrists to report suspected sexual abuse of children. Am J Psychiatry 148:449–453, 1991

Cotton NS: The developmental-clinical rationale for the use of seclusion in the psychiatric treatment of children. Am J Orthopsychiatry 59:442–450, 1989

Davis SM, Schwartz MD: Children's Rights and the Law. Lexington, MA, Lexington Books, 1987

Gari DS: Guidelines for children and adolescents, in The Psychiatric Uses of Seclusion and Restraint. Edited by Tardiff K. Washington, DC, American Psychiatric Press, 1984, pp 69–85

Guyer MJ: Child psychiatry and legal liability: implications of recent case law. J Am Acad Child Adolesc Psychiatry 29:958–962, 1990

Guyer MJ, Harrison SI, Rieveschl JL: Development rights to privacy and independent decision-making. Journal of the American Academy of Child Psychiatry 21:298–302, 1982

Herman SP: Special issues in child custody evaluations. J Am Acad Child Adolesc Psychiatry 29:969–974, 1990

Millstein KH, Cotton NS: Predictors of the use of seclusion on an inpatient child psychiatric unit. J Am Acad Child Adolesc Psychiatry 29:256–264, 1990

Schetky DH, Benedek EP: Emerging Issues in Child Psychiatry and the Law. New York, Brunner/Mazel, 1985

Schetky DH, Benedek EP (eds): Clinical Handbook of Child Psychiatry and the Law. Baltimore, MD, Williams & Wilkins, 1991

Schetky DH, Cavanaugh JL: Psychiatric malpractice. Journal of the American Academy of Child Psychiatry 21:521–526, 1982

Schetky DH, Guyer MJ: Civil litigation and the child psychiatrist. J Am Acad Child Adolesc Psychiatry 29:963–968, 1990

Schetky DH, Angell R, Morrison CV, et al: Parents who fail—a study of 51 cases of termination of parental rights. Journal of the American Academy of Child Psychiatry 18:366–383, 1979

Schoettle UC: Termination of parental rights—ethical issues and role conflicts. Journal of the American Academy of Child Psychiatry 23:629–632, 1984

19

Alcohol and Substance Abuse

George W. Bailey, M.D.

Despite encouraging declines in youthful use of illicit psychoactive substances (Johnston 1990), the issue remains one of major concern and high priority. This is particularly true for underage use and abuse of tobacco and alcohol products. Concern is no longer limited to adolescents, but extends to preadolescent youth also. Clinicians dealing with children, adolescents, and families should be keenly aware of the diagnostic, therapeutic, and preventive aspects of this major public health problem.

The purpose of this chapter is to provide physicians with a framework for assessing a substance abuse problem and determining the appropriate type and setting for treatment. Evaluating youngsters for substance use and abuse should not be seen as esoteric or mystical. The format presented here uses the basic medical diagnostic model familiar to all physicians.

History and Physical

Identifying Information

Youths who use substances represent a highly heterogeneous group with a broad spectrum of degree and types of use and abuse. The spectrum begins with curiosity and progresses through experimentation, casual use, regular use, heavy use, and, for some, the development of chemical dependency. Significant morbidity and mortality may occur at any point along this broad spectrum.

Any individual youth may experience the use of psychoactive substances in a variety of ways and with a highly individualized outcome. The current state of the art precludes our ability to predict definitively what will happen to any particular youth. We can, however, enhance our ability to do so by considering the following factors.

Who Is at Risk?

Most late-prepubertal and adolescent youth are statistically at risk for at least trying alcohol, tobacco, and other substances of abuse (Johnston et al. 1990). Some youth, however, are more at risk for developing significant problems than others, including those who 1) are children of substance-abusing parents, 2) are aggressive and antisocial, 3) are school dropouts, 4) are pregnant, 5) are abused or neglected, 6) are physically handicapped, 7) are socioeconomically disadvantaged, 8) have learning and language disorders, and 9) have mental health problems, especially if suicidal and depressed (Kumpfer 1987).

What Are They Using?

Although often classified as legal drugs, it is important to note that use of alcohol and tobacco by underage youth is illegal. These two drug classes represent substances most frequently used and abused by youth, and together carry more potential morbidity and mortality than all the others combined. Alcohol products include beer, wine, and hard liquor. Tobacco includes smokable (cigarettes, cigars, and pipe tobacco) and smokeless (chewing tobacco and snuff) varieties. Other legal psychoactive substances include prescription medications (including steroids), nonprescription medications (e.g., "over-the-counter"), and inhalants.

Illegal substances of abuse include cannabinoids (marijuana, hashish, tetrahydrocannabinol [THC]); cocaine and "crack"; hallucinogens (lysergic acid diethylamide [LSD], phencyclidine [PCP], mescaline, psilocybin); and heroin, opioids, and synthetic analogs (often inappropriately referred to as "designer drugs").

Chief Complaint

Children and adolescents with substance-related problems may present with medical, psychological, social, or school-related problems or a combination. Few will identify substance use or abuse as a major concern, although parents may bring them for evaluation because of their own concern.

History of Present Illness

Typical histories for substance-abusing youth include significant and persistent changes in mood, behavior, dress, peer group, interpersonal relationships, school attendance, school performance and behavior, leisure activities, attitudes, and goals. There may also be problems with depression, suicidal issues, anxiety, disordered eating patterns, disturbances of impulse control and conduct, and disturbances of self-esteem and identity. Some have legal difficulties such as driving while intoxicated (DWI) or under the influence (DUI), drunk in public, shoplifting, breaking and entering, and disorderly conduct.

Frequently, symptoms of substance use and abuse are masked and distorted by other issues and become known only on careful evaluation and after prolonged delay between onset of use and detection (Williams et al. 1989).

It is important for clinicians to note that all youthful substance users and abusers do not exhibit these typical patterns. Some can use casually or even regularly for significant periods of time, especially on weekends, and may manage to avoid both serious consequences and detection. Continued use, however, generally leads to negative consequences in their lives.

Medical History

With some exceptions, children and adolescents who use and abuse alcohol and other drugs typically escape major medical complications.

When present, typical findings include weight loss, chronic fatigue, chronic cough, and recurrent upper respiratory symptoms. History of repeated accidents and injuries may also signal psychoactive substance use.

Psychiatric History

Of note, both the medical history and the psychiatric history in substance-using and substance-abusing children and adolescents may be clean. For many, however, common findings may include disorders such as attention-deficit/hyperactivity disorder, learning and language disturbances, conduct disorder, oppositional defiant disorder, affective disturbances (depression, bipolar), anxiety disorders, and posttraumatic stress disorder (especially if abused or if the child of a substance-abusing parent). A history of suicidal ideations and attempts is often noted in those more seriously affected.

Family History

Careful review of these youngsters' family history is helpful. It is not uncommon to find various manifestations of cardiovascular-respiratory disorders (e.g., hypertension, emphysema), gastrointestinal disorders (e.g., irritable bowel syndrome, ulcer disease), stress-related disorders (e.g., migraines, low-back pain), and alcohol- or drug-related illness (e.g., pancreatitis, hepatitis) in a carefully taken family *medical* history.

Common family *psychiatric* histories may include alcohol and other drug use, affective disorders, anxiety disturbances, eating disorders, physical abuse and neglect, sexual abuse, violence and other antisocial behaviors, impulse-control disturbances, and family discord such as separation and divorce.

Developmental and Social History

There are important indices to assess carefully in a substance-using child or adolescent. Development of impulse control and reality resting; ability to delay gratification; ability to identify, express, and tolerate unpleasant affective states appropriately; acceptance of rules, limit setting, and respect for the rights of others; and ability to form and sustain appropriate interpersonal relationships are all important milestones that help determine the course that any particular child's or adolescent's substance use may take. This information is particularly important when deciding treatment options.

The course for any child or adolescent is multiply determined by an interplay of factors involving genetic predisposition, response to familial stressors, response to social and environmental stressors, psychological vulnerabilities, and personality traits (Newcomb et al. 1986).

The powerful influence of parental and peer role models cannot be denied. Situations, environments, and relationships that accept, condone, and promote substance use and abuse, and those that do not, need to be carefully assessed.

Physical, Neurological, and Mental Status Examinations

As noted above, it is uncommon to find significant physical findings in substance-using children and adolescents, especially in early stages and in controlled use. Despite this, it is crucial that any evaluation include a physical and neurological examination and a formal mental status examination. Depending on the type, degree, amount, frequency, and timing of drug use, there may be transient or persistent neurological or mental status findings. These tend to be drug specific.

Making the Diagnosis

In addition to a carefully taken history, several assessment instruments are available to assist clinicians with diagnosing substance abuse (see Farrell and Strang 1991 for an excellent review). Such assessment instruments include screening instruments, semistructured and structured diagnostic interviews, and self-report scales.

DSM-IV (American Psychiatric Association 1994) is of limited value in diagnosing substance abuse in youth because it fails to distinguish between preadolescent, adolescent, and adult substance abuse

(Bailey 1989) and lacks valid and reliable age-appropriate diagnostic criteria (Bukstein et al. 1989).

Laboratory Examination

Routine laboratory examinations generally reveal little, if any, definitive information for diagnosing substance use and abuse. However, certain tests may be indicated in some substance users. These include pregnancy tests, tests for sexually transmitted diseases, and evaluation for human immunodeficiency virus (HIV) in sexually active youth.

Toxicological testing is an important adjunct for detecting substance use and abuse. The American Academy of Child and Adolescent Psychiatry (1990b) prepared a policy statement to guide clinicians in the appropriate utilization of drug testing.

Clinical indicators for using toxicology screens include the following: all adolescents with psychiatric symptoms; high-risk adolescents (e.g., children of substance-abusing parents, runaways, delinquents); adolescents with changes in mental status or performance; adolescents exhibiting acute behavior changes; adolescents with recurrent respiratory ailments, recurrent accidents, or unexplained somatic symptoms; and for monitoring abstinence (Gold and Dakis 1986).

The use of breath analysis and blood for alcohol content remains the mainstay for alcohol testing. Both qualitative and quantitative tests are useful for detecting other substances in clinical practice (for a review, see Council on Scientific Affairs 1987).

Qualitative tests are less expensive, easier to perform, and highly sensitive at drug concentrations equal to or greater than the cutoff level determined by the laboratory performing the test. Blood, urine, and saliva are typically used for these types of tests. Such tests, however, lack appropriate specificity to be used without quantitative confirmation.

Typical examples of commonly used *qualitative* or *screening tests* include color or spot tests, thin-layer chromatography, and immunoassays. Color or spot tests are inexpensive, quick, and easy to perform. They are, however, highly sensitive to contamination by other drugs and their metabolites, and the drugs must be present in sufficient quantity for detection.

Thin-layer chromatography is the most commonly used screening test because it detects a broad spectrum of commonly used drugs. Technical difficulties such as extracting and concentrating the specimen to avoid contamination by other compounds, preparing printable reports of the various colors, more than one drug sharing the same chromatographic stain, and lack of specificity due to the broad spectrum of drugs screened limit its usefulness for anything other than a presumptive screening technique.

Two types of immunoassays are commonly used. Radioimmunoassay (RIA) utilizes techniques in which specimens labeled and unlabeled with radioisotopes compete for antibody binding sites. This type of testing requires special training, experience, and equipment; can screen for only one drug at a time; and is prone to false-negative results when adulterated by other drugs.

Enzyme-multiplied immunoassay technique (EMIT) has the advantage of being quick, semiquantitative, and capable of screening for several drugs at a time. The drawbacks include expensive reagents and cross-reactivity with other medications. More recent use of fluorescent polarization techniques provides a greater range of immunoassay testing capabilities.

Of grave concern is the recent introduction of sprays and urine tests available to the lay public. Such tests are prone to cross-reactivity and false positives, lack the benefit of confirmation, and stretch the limits of confidentiality and invasion of privacy. Clinicians should advise parents to refrain from these measures.

Qualitative screening tests that are positive should be followed with appropriate confirmation by a *quantitative* test. These typically utilize gas chromatography, gas chromatography/mass spectrometry, or high-performance liquid chromatography. Each is highly specific and sensitive, yet expensive, time-consuming, and requiring training and experience to do properly.

A negative test indicates only that drugs were not detected; it does not eliminate the possibility of substance use. A positive test, on the other hand, merely indicates that drugs were detected and provides no indication of when, where, how, and under what circumstances the drug was used. Also, a positive test does not necessarily mean that drugs are causing the immediate symptoms or that the youth is under the influence at the time of the test (Stewart 1982).

A confirmed positive drug screen is only one step in an otherwise critical process. Appropriate utilization of these clinical data must be integrated into a comprehensive clinical assessment and cogent presentation to the child and the child's family (Bailey 1989).

Child and adolescent psychiatrists and other clinicians have two primary responsibilities in the area of drug testing (Bailey 1989). First, it is important to know the various types of qualitative and quantitative tests available and the advantages and disadvantages of each. Second, they must know how to order, understand, and interpret these tests for patients, for their families, and for consultees.

Treatment

Clinicians should remain mindful that all children and adolescents who use and abuse alcohol and other drugs may not necessarily require specific substance abuse treatment. Because of the considerable heterogeneity and variation in youthful substance use, thoughtful and comprehensive assessment of the nature, extent, and circumstances of use must be done. Some may not need treatment at that time, yet bear careful monitoring. Others may be in the early stages of use and may warrant attention to other more primary issues such as coexisting biological, emotional, or social disturbances. Some will definitely require treatment. The important bottom line is that substance use and abuse should not be deemed as benign normative behavior, but should be carefully and comprehensively assessed, and treatment decisions should be highly individualized.

There are many treatment philosophies and modalities for treatment of substance abuse in youth. Most tend to share general features including abstinence from substances of abuse, group therapy with other substance abusers, adjunctive use of self-help groups, and the philosophy that the problem is "arrested" rather than cured (Hoffman et al. 1987). Most treatment programs use 12-step principles based on the Alcoholics Anonymous (AA) model (Ehrlich 1987).

Finding the most appropriate treatment for a specific child or adolescent is often a difficult task, limited in large part by available options. The optimal arrangement would provide a broad continuum of treatment services with different levels of care. Each child or adolescent would enter at the most appropriate level of care based on a careful, comprehensive individualized diagnostic assessment. Within such a system, there is the option of transition from higher to lower levels of care and vice versa as clinically indicated (American Society of Addiction Medicine 1991).

The "continuum of care" (American Academy of Child and Adolescent Psychiatry 1991a) involves many options, including 1) acute inpatient, residential treatment; 2) partial hospitalization or day treatment; 3) intensive outpatient treatment; 4) traditional outpatient treatment; and 5) self-help groups. Clinicians are familiar with most aspects of this continuum of care, although some aspects have changed in recent years and warrant review.

Inpatient

The number of pure chemical-dependency inpatient treatment units for adolescents is decreasing, and more units designed for the assessment and treatment of *dual diagnosis* (comorbidity of psychiatric illness and substance abuse) are available.

Deciding to hospitalize a child or adolescent for any reason (including substance abuse) should be a thoughtful and carefully assessed determination. The American Academy of Child and Adolescent Psychiatry (1990a) outlined specific guidelines to help clinicians determine this need; posed important questions to ask regarding inpatient substance abuse treatment (1991b); and delineated the integral role of the child and adolescent psychiatrist in such treatment (1987).

Partial Hospitalization or Day Treatment

Although the concept of partial hospitalization began approximately 60 years ago (Parker and Knoll 1990), the use of this treatment modality for children and adolescents has been more recent. The terms *partial hospitalization, day hospital,* and *day treatment* are often used interchangeably. Each offers structured, comprehensive, multidisciplinary care in a more flexible, less expensive, and less restrictive environment than inpatient treatment while continuing to deliver an intensive level of therapeutic programming.

Partial hospitalization or day-treatment programs are designed to assist children and adolescents not needing the intensive level of intervention found in an inpatient unit, yet needing a highly structured, well-supervised milieu with academic, behavioral, and therapeutic interventions available. Candidates may be youth being discharged from an inpatient unit in need of a "step-down" program, those who are being given a trial of outpatient treatment prior to the more restrictive environment of inpatient treatment, and those in need of more intensive intervention than can be attained in traditional outpatient treatment.

Considerations for partial hospitalization or day treatment involve both patient and familial factors. Patients must have an emotional or behavioral disturbance significant enough to require intensive treatment, yet not requiring inpatient treatment; must be willing to strive for abstinence from all forms of psychoactive substance use (including nicotine in some programs); must be motivated and willing to attend all aspects of the programming; must be capable of interacting verbally; must be able to tolerate and benefit from group therapy; must be able to work toward realistic therapeutic goals; and must possess sufficient impulse control toward self and others to participate safely. Familial factors include motivation and willingness to participate in the treatment and ability to maintain adequate and appropriate structure and security at home.

Partial hospitalization or day treatment provides structure and supervision for periods ranging from 6 to 12 hours each day. Patients return to their homes or other places of residence at the end of the day and on weekends.

Therapeutic programming includes comprehensive biopsychosocial assessment techniques and treatment modalities similar to inpatient units. Typical programs use various types of individual, group, and family therapies (including multifamily education and therapy); substance abuse education and treatment; milieu therapy; expressive therapies (e.g., art, music, psychodrama, recreational); pharmacotherapy; academic instruction; and vocational rehabilitation.

Intensive Outpatient Treatment

Intensive outpatient treatment is also a structured, typically time-limited course of treatment that supplements traditional outpatient treatment and generally occurs in conjunction with individual psychotherapy and/or pharmacotherapy conducted in a clinician's office. It occurs after school or on weekends for periods between 2 and 4 hours a session and may occur one or more times each week. Modalities include group therapy in the form of substance abuse education; confrontation and process groups; and aftercare, recovery, and relapse prevention groups. Twelve-step or self-help groups such as AA, Narcotics Anonymous (NA), codependency groups, Alateen, Alanon, and Children of Alcoholics (COA) are generally incorporated into the programming. Individual family and multifamily education and group therapy are often included in intensive outpatient treatment.

Outcome

Outcome is extremely variable and highly individualized. Some youth will experiment and stop; others will continue to use casually without significant consequences; some will use regularly and experience varying degrees of difficulty; and some will become chemically dependent or addicted (Bailey 1991).

There are limited data that define, measure, and longitudinally track treatment outcome, especially in regard to partial hospitalization and intensive outpatient treatment for substance abuse in youth. This is an important area for future research.

Reimbursement Issues

The course that reimbursement issues for child and adolescent psychiatric and substance abuse disorders will take is uncertain. Current trends have dramatically shifted toward sharply limited reimbursement for inpatient services while not necessarily providing for outpatient coverage. Some third-party payers are covering partial hospitalization, day treatment, and intensive outpatient treatment; others are not. Child and adolescent psychiatrists and other clinicians must become keenly aware of and knowledgeable about treatment options in their communities to assist patients and their families to attain appropriate and adequate care.

References

American Academy of Child and Adolescent Psychiatry: Position statement on substance abuse, part 2: the role of the child and adolescent psychiatrist. Washington, DC, American Academy of Child and Adolescent Psychiatry, 1987

American Academy of Child and Adolescent Psychiatry: Eleven questions to ask before psychiatric hospital treatment of children and adolescents (Facts for Families No 32). Washington, DC, American Academy of Child and Adolescent Psychiatry, 1990a

American Academy of Child and Adolescent Psychiatry: Position statement on drug and alcohol screening. Washington, DC, American Academy of Child and Adolescent Psychiatry, 1990b

American Academy of Child and Adolescent Psychiatry: The continuum of care (Facts for Families No 42). Washington, DC, American Academy of Child and Adolescent Psychiatry, 1991a

American Academy of Child and Adolescent Psychiatry: Making decisions about substance abuse treatment (Facts for Families No 41). Washington, DC, American Academy of Child and Adolescent Psychiatry, 1991b

American Psychiatric Association: Diagnostic and Statistical Manual of Mental Disorders, 4th Edition. Washington, DC, American Psychiatric Association, 1994

American Society of Addiction Medicine and National Association of Addiction Treatment Providers: Patient Placement Criteria. Washington, DC, American Association of Addiction Medicine, 1991

Bailey GW: Current perspectives on substance abuse in youth. J Am Acad Child Adolesc Psychiatry 28:151–162, 1989

Bailey GW: Substance use and abuse, in Textbook of Child and Adolescent Psychiatry. Edited by Wiener JM. Washington, DC, American Psychiatric Press, 1991, pp 439–451

Bukstein OG, Brent DA, Kaminer Y: Comorbidity of substance abuse and other psychiatric disorders in adolescents. Am J Psychiatry 146:1131–1141, 1989

Council on Scientific Affairs: Scientific issues in drug testing. JAMA 257:3110–3114, 1987

Ehrlich P: 12 step principles and adolescent chemical dependency treatment. J Psychoactive Drugs 19:311–317, 1987

Farrell M, Strang J: Substance use and misuse in childhood and adolescence. J Child Psychol Psychiatry 32:109–128, 1991

Gold MS, Dakis GA: Role of the laboratory in the evaluation of suspected drug abuse. J Clin Psychiatry 47:17–23, 1986

Hoffman NG, Sonis WA, Halikas JA: Issues in the evaluation of chemical dependency treatment programs for adolescents. Pediatr Clin North Am 34:449–459, 1987

Johnston LD, Bachman JG, O'Malley PM: High school senior survey: monitoring the future. Rockville, MD, National Institute on Drug Abuse, 1990

Kumpfer KL: Prevention of drug abuse: a critical review of risk factors and prevention strategies, in Prevention of Mental Disorders, Alcohol and Other Drug Use in Children and Adolescents (OSAP Prevention Monogr No 2 [DHHS Publ No ADM-89-1646]). Washington, DC, US Department of Health and Human Services, 1989, pp 309–372

Newcomb MD, Maddahian E, Bentler PM: Risk factors for drug use among adolescents. Am J Public Health 76:525–531, 1986

Parker S, Knoll JL: Partial hospitalization: an update. Am J Psychiatry 147:156–160, 1990

Stewart DC: The use of the clinical laboratory in the diagnosis and treatment of substance abuse. Pediatr Ann 11:669–682, 1982

Williams RA, Feibelman ND, Moulder C: Events precipitating hospital treatment of adolescent drug abusers. J Am Acad Child Adolesc Psychiatry 28:70–73, 1989

20

Adoption and Foster Care

Steven L. Nickman, M.D.
Marie Armentano, M.D.

Adoption of children and their placement in foster care are complex aspects of the care of children when their biological families of origin cannot or will not care for them. With an increase in older age and handicapped adoptions, as well as foster care settings for troubled children and youth, the "at-risk" population of such children comes increasingly to the attention of child and adolescent psychiatrists. Familiarity with these populations of young people is essential in the practice of contemporary child and adolescent psychiatry.

Adoption

Approximately 1.5% of children in the United States are adopted by parents to whom they are unrelated by blood; another 1.5% are adopted by a stepparent or blood relatives. Studies suggest that the child psychiatrist will encounter adopted children (primarily those unrelated to their adopters) out of proportion to prevalence in the population (Brinich 1980; Schechter et al. 1964).

Until the early 1970s, most children placed for adoption were white infants. Societal changes have profoundly affected the pattern of adoption in America. Increased availability of contraception and abortion and lessened stigma for unmarried mothers who keep their babies have caused a "baby famine" and led to the emergence of hitherto unfamiliar forms of adoption. The definition of an "adoptable child" has undergone a radical broadening in response to pressure from would-be adopters and with the support of social work professionals who have pioneered new kinds of placement (Dikette 1984). These include

- Transracial adoptions
- Transnational adoptions
- "Special-needs adoptions" of developmentally disabled and physically or emotionally handicapped children, many of whom are toddlers or older
- "Legal risk adoptions" of children in the foster care system, whose legal freedom to be adopted has not yet been established
- "Open" and "identified" adoptions
- Increasingly frequent formal adoption of black children by black families

Other changes include state subsidy of placement in recognition of certain children's unusual needs, and a greater acceptance of "nonmainstream" adoptive parents. Single persons, couples past childbearing age, and gay individuals or couples are increasingly regarded as potential adopters.

Most adoptive parents cannot procreate. They have suffered a complex loss involving body image and identity as members of a genealogical chain (Blum 1983). Nonmainstream adopters may have sustained similar or other losses. Society exerts pressure on couples to have children and encourages adoption when procreation is impossible, yet there is a subtle undercurrent of prejudice against adoptive families and adopted children (Kirk 1964). The adoptive process is affected by these stresses (Blum 1983; Kirk 1964; Schechter 1970).

Factors Affecting Personality Development in Adoptees

Prenatal care and inherited constitution. Most important is the possibility of poor nutrition or substance abuse during pregnancy, affecting biological substrates for cognition. (Heritability of intelligence and of psychiatric disorder is generally accepted by placement workers, but rarely precludes adoption because many workers and parents believe strongly in environmental influences.)

Early infant-caretaker interactions. Some children have had "good enough" experiences in infancy, with biological mothers or during brief fostering and after placement in adoptive homes. The greater the number of disruptions a child undergoes, the more likely it is that later personality formation will be affected. The later the adoptive placement, the more difficult the "take." Acting out in child and adolescent adoptees may be related to Winnicott's (1958) theory relating the "antisocial tendency" to early discontinuities in experience.

Adopter-adoptee relationships. Procreators "have" a child; adopters "get" one. The "gotten" child may be experienced as alien. Parents may have little support to cope with such feelings (Schechter 1970). Likewise, when an infant or toddler shows a grieving reaction for what is lost, this may be misinterpreted as rejection of the new parent. Adoptive ties may need help to get off to a good start.

"Telling," status losses, and fantasy formation. This factor is described later in this chapter.

Adolescence and entry into adult life. Many young adoptees speculate about birth-parents and whether to seek them out. They may experience themselves as incomplete without such knowledge. In response to pressure from adoptees, many birth-parents, and some adoptive parents, bills have been introduced into state legislatures to make original birth certificates available to adoptees at age 18. Four states now have such laws; five have partial "mutual consent" laws.

Opposition to reform is vigorous and appears to come largely from adoptive parents. Adoption professionals are divided, but increasingly recognize the legitimacy of pressures for change (Dikette 1984; Feigelman and Silverman 1986; Howe 1983; Sorosky et al. 1979).

Clinical Interventions With Adopted Children

Child psychiatrists may be approached at various stages of an adoptive placement. Requests include

- Intervention around the adoptive process
- Assessments shortly after a child is placed in a home
- Requests for advice or psychotherapeutic help in established adoptive families

The first type of request has resemblances to the divorce custody evaluations with which child psychiatrists are familiar; the last is similar to traditional office or clinic practice.

Intervention Around the Adoptive Process

This may involve a request by a court, a social service agency, prospective adoptive parents, or an attorney to assess a child, a birth-mother, or the quality of the bond between a child and foster parents who hope to adopt. The child psychiatrist brings expertise to bear on emotionally charged areas in which hard scientific evidence is still scant. A written report or court testimony may be requested.

The child psychiatrist need not assume more responsibility than his or her experience warrants. If the psychiatrist has substantial knowledge of child placement, placement-related recommendations can be incorporated into the report with greater confidence than would be the case with a less experienced psychiatrist. The latter, however, can still help by reporting clinical observations and providing diagnostic assessments. Ultimately the responsibility for placements belongs to the placing agency and the court.

Requests may be for assessments of individual children or sibling groups, or (more commonly) they may involve evaluation of child-adult interactions or of parental capability in the context of a "bonding study" or a court case involving the rights of a biological parent (Goldstein et al. 1979; Rutter 1981; Schoettle 1984; Steinhauer 1983).

Clinical assessment of children. Questions raised include the suitability of a child for adoption, as opposed to long-term foster care or group placement; less frequently, the appropriateness of placement in a specific family is considered. These questions are not usually posed "up front." Agencies do not assume that psychiatrists are expert in placement issues, and those questions may emerge in discussion when a child is referred for evaluation. The clinician needs to know the child's full background. When practical, the prospective adoptive parents should be met, and the clinician should request access to the agency's home study because assessment of a child may be more useful in conjunction with knowledge of potential caretakers.

The question for a psychiatrist, when considering "adoptability," is whether the child has sufficient emotional health to make use of a family as opposed to life in a foster or group home, which makes fewer demands for object-relatedness. This question is usually asked about children from 4 years old through adolescence, who have had substantial life experience and possibly neglect or abuse. Increasingly such borderline cases are tried in adoptive homes when the alternative is that the child will grow up essentially "objectless" in a series of foster placements or a group home.

Clinical procedure includes

- Careful reading of the record, assessing developmental influences on the child
- Full clinical evaluation, with special reference to the child's depth and style of relating
- Referral for pediatric, psychological, and neurological evaluations when warranted
- Observation of interactions between the child and the present caretakers
- Full documentation of the clinician's observations, conclusions, and recommendations

- Verbal contact with the referring placement worker, preferably in person

Bonding studies and "rights of natural parent" situations. A situation that arises with increasing frequency is the so-called legal risk adoption in which a child who is not yet legally free for adoption is placed with a family that hopes to adopt that child, expecting that the court will abrogate the natural parents' right to the child based on past events. A child psychiatrist may be asked to assess the emotional bond between the child and the prospective adopters and to establish whether it would be harmful to the child to be removed from present surroundings. This need arises when the birth-parent has shown a degree of interest that makes it impossible for the judge to terminate parental rights without hearing the cases on its merits.

Another request may be to assess a birth-parent with respect to ability to be a caretaking or visiting parent to the child.

These situations constitute a new and complex challenge to law, custom, and the mental health professions. "Permanency planning," as now promoted by child welfare agencies, encourages early placement of children in adoptive homes or early return to natural parents. Such treatment plans respond to important clinical findings (Goldstein et al. 1979; Rutter 1981), but they also aid the public treasury because children in foster care are supported by public funds whereas adoptions are not usually subsidized.

The important difference between this type of court contest and divorce custody litigation is that in the latter case the best interest of the child is virtually the only legal standard now in use; in contrast, although best interest is followed increasingly, many judges still use fitness of the natural parent as the more important standard (Derdeyn et al. 1982). Biological ties may be deemed so important that unless a parent is unfit, the child's present attachments are given little weight. In the presence of different standards, one clinician is often not asked to evaluate all parties (as is the custom with divorce custody evaluations) because best interest may be addressed when dealing with the child and present caretakers, and fitness addressed when reporting to the court about birth-parents. Different experts may be asked to fill the two roles; clinicians who insist on retaining "impartial expert" status and assessing the relative merits of two sets of parents may be excluded.

Countertransference may interfere if the clinician has personal experience with adopting or with losing a child or has other personal feelings about such situations, or if there has been a de facto abandonment of the child by the natural parent, which seems partly an agency failure, due to inadequate attempts to rehabilitate the parent-child connection. The clinician's heart may go out to the natural parent as victim, and the clinician may be less inclined to appreciate deficiencies. The clinician may, instead, identify with the child's attachment to the prospective adopters.

With older children who retain emotional ties to parents who cannot care for them, the controversial alternative of "open adoption" is used in some situations. Many would formerly have been kept in long-term foster care. Open adoption implies that the child will have contact with the original parent while living in a stable adoptive home.

Adoptive parents entering such arrangements must be able to feel secure in their roles. Some, because of their personal notion of parenthood, cannot raise a child under these conditions. Psychiatrists may be asked to make recommendations in such dilemmas. From the standpoint of the child's welfare, the psychiatrist may be the only advocate of continued relationship with an emotionally impaired parent. A significant arguing point in favor of open adoption is that complete loss of a prior caretaker may be unfair to the child and may even make it harder for the child to commit to a new home.

Paramount in the consideration of return to parental custody, or continued relationships with birth-parents, are the following questions:

- Has the child shown evidence of regression or distress around the time of visits with biological parents?
- What interactions have been noted by observers during supervised visits?
- Would continued contact with a birth-parent be unacceptable to a preadoptive family with whom the child has a psychological right to stay?

Clinical procedure includes all the steps mentioned in the previous section. Additional procedures include the assessment of interaction and the assessment of parental capability (Steinhauer 1983).

Assessment of interaction. This can be applied to child-with-prospective-adoptive parents, as well as to child-with-birth-parents. The goal is to observe and describe what the child *does* and *seems to be feeling* in the presence of one or more adults, and vice versa, keeping in mind what would be expected developmentally considering the child's age and any existing neurological or intellectual impairment. The adult should be invited to talk first with the psychiatrist. An invitation is issued to make use of the playroom and materials with the child in whatever way seems most natural. Assurance should be given of the clinician's awareness that this is a stressful situation. (This is indeed a stressful interview, but parents have to cope with stress.) At times interaction with biological or prospective adoptive siblings is important to observe as well.

Relevant observations include: How often does the child approach the adult? How does the adult respond? Is there physical contact? Initiated by whom? How often? For how long? Is the adult alert to a young child's rapprochement behaviors, such as seeking eye contact, "checking back" for emotional refueling, and so on? Do the adult's facial expressions betray pleasure in the child? Do nonverbal cues match the emotional implications of words? Is the adult passive, controlling, or involved in comfortable mutuality while interacting with the child? Is the child's response to the examiner, a stranger, substantially different from the way the child behaves with the caretaker, or is there evidence of indiscriminate attachment? (A detailed description of procedures in assessing young children and their parents' interactions with them is found in Chapter 21.)

The clinician should be somewhat passive during the interview, but may need to facilitate interaction. The degree to which this is necessary should be noted.

A useful maneuver when assessing attachment in babies and younger children is to ask the adult to leave the room unobtrusively while the child plays. One then watches the child's behavior, including facial expression, whether attempts are made to find the adult, and how soon and persistently such attempts are made. Equally important is the child's behavior after the parent or parent-substitute is found. Does the child grin, with a decrease in bodily tension? Does the child seem indifferent? Does the adult seem confident, overly worried, or uninvolved during this procedure?

Assessment of parental capability. These evaluations may or may not progress to an interaction assessment as described above. Initially one interviews the adult, usually a biological parent from whom the child has been removed because of neglect or abuse. The format should be semistructured; several interviews may be necessary. Questions to be addressed include:

- Mental status, with particular reference to present level of functioning, intellectual and emotional. (Referral for psychological testing may be indicated if cognitive functioning is in question; projective testing may be called for if a thought disorder or serious character pathology is suspected but not obvious.)
- Attitude toward the child during pregnancy, neonatal period, and subsequently; expectations and hopes for the child's future.
- Community supports, including family, friends, social contacts, and religious contacts.
- Reality testing, including understanding of how the present situation came about; degree of insight versus projection of fault onto others.
- Understanding and knowledge of children's needs and development; specific knowledge of the child: What is at issue is the parent's ability to empathize with the child (e.g., to understand that important bonds may have been formed with foster parents). How narcissistic or self-serving is the parent's attitude? Is the child seen primarily as a separate person, an extension of self, someone who can help the parent in time of trouble, or a piece of property the parent has a right to control? Was the child's removal experienced primarily as a narcissistic blow or as the loss of a loved child? The ability to respond to specific factual questions about the child (e.g., what the child wants to become in adult life, or what activities the child presently enjoys) is often telling.

Assessment of other members of the adult's household (particularly new spouses or live-in friends). If the parent is found potentially capable, the next stage is observation of parent-child interaction. If visits have been ongoing, arranging this should not pose a problem. But if the child is in a preadoptive home and visits with the natural parent have been cut off or allowed to lapse, the psychiatrist, along with the court and social service agency, must struggle with the question of whether to reopen the relationship.

Reports should be free of jargon and include illustrations and descriptions to support one's conclusions. Judgmental language should be avoided. The clinician should be clear from the start as to who has a right to get copies of the report.

Requests to Assess a Child Soon After Placement

Often the covert message is: "Our whole family is having trouble since this child came to live with us. We aren't sure we can stick it out, but would feel terrible guilt if we decided not to keep him. Please help us figure out how to make things better, or how to bow out gracefully." Often the overt request is to assess a child's disturbance, with a view to possible psychotherapy. "Listening with the third ear" comes in handy at such times.

These situations need to be recognized for what they are—stages in a child's life when he or she exists, even if no longer in a legal limbo, then still in an emotional one. (The adoption may already have been finalized). Parents may have been encouraged to "tough it out" by agency personnel, family, or friends, or may feel compelled to follow through on an initial commitment despite misgivings. Such considerations are especially relevant now because of the increase in "new wave" adoptions involving older and traumatized children.

Child psychiatric intervention at this stage of a placement will generally require some or all of the following:

- Obtain consent to talk to the placing agency.
- Catalyze creative working together of agency and family so they can together address whether the placement should continue.
- Remain available to see the child for extended evaluation, being

open to hear parents' and workers' concerns.
- When necessary, help parents disengage from an initial commitment.
- In the event of disruption, maintain availability to all parties; offer to see the child again, and provide therapy or management as a valuable bridge.
- Remain alert to countertransference difficulties (e.g., over-identification with the child or the adoptive parents).

Requests for Help by Established Adoptive Families

Parents and children may deny the relevance of adoption to presenting complaints because of personal discomfort with the topic and because of society's lack of recognition of adoption as a stressor. Yet a disproportionate number of adopted children and adolescents experience difficulty. It seems wise to assume, until one is convinced otherwise, that adoption is an important issue. One wonders during the assessment of parents and child: How deeply should the psychiatrist inquire about adoption as a source of chronically injured self-esteem, in the face of initial denial?

Much attention has been paid to the identity problems of the adopted child, but little to those of the adoptive parent. Both have sustained losses. The therapist's role involves primary, secondary, and tertiary interventions.

Primary Intervention

The first aspect of primary intervention is conveying current knowledge to parents and pediatric colleagues concerning vulnerabilities of adoptive families, "age of telling," curiosity about birth-parents, the wish to search, and related issues.

With respect to age of disclosure about adoption, matters are no longer as clear as they seemed 25 years ago. The question of disclosure does not even arise with many children who are placed during the oedipal years and later, and who retain memories of their families of origin. (With those children, however, it is increasingly recognized that an appropriate kind of dialogue needs to take place between the adoptive parents and the child concerning the period before they lived together as a family. In such families, finding this kind of communication is analogous to disclosure of adoption, with ensuing dialogue, in infant adoptions.)

In the past 40 years, children placed as infants or toddlers have traditionally been told of their adoption prior to age 4. The common question—"Did I grow in your belly?"—has appeared to many to require a truthful answer. Questions have been raised about this procedure, however, and cases are cited in which disclosure when the child was between ages 3 and 6 interfered with resolution of the oedipal dilemma or with developing self-esteem. The debate is still active (MacIntyre and Donovan 1990), and it is clear that many mental health professionals have appreciated how traumatic it can be to learn of an adoptive status.

The debate in the professional literature has generally addressed the issue as though it were a question of chronology. We maintain, however, that the adoptive parents' confidence in their ability to support their child through a painful disclosure is the salient aspect of the problem. It can be taken for granted that most young children will be troubled by the initial disclosure, and troubled subsequently throughout their development as they reflect on the sadness inherent in relinquishment or a lost connection. Sadness can be dealt with openly, however, whereas prolonged secrecy can have subtle and far-reaching effects, both during the period while secrecy is maintained and after it has been broken. To disrupt a child's sense of personal history at, for example, age 8 or 9, when the child has already constructed a picture of personal origins, is likely to introduce an idea of hidden truths about the self that is just as risky for the child's self-regard as the more traditional early initiation of disclosure.

It is true that telling, once initiated, is irreversible. Yet it should be borne in mind that disclosure and dialogue about adoption constitute a long process of give-and-take within the family, with many opportunities for discussion, reassurance, and correction of false impressions. Thus parents should not enter into it out of a sense of urgency prompted by the child's cognitive stage ("He might ask about tummies any day now!") or by the parents' need to unburden themselves to the child. Instead, the parents need to master their own feelings.

They need to be confident that imparting a piece of unwelcome news will not destroy their child, themselves, or the child-parent relationship.

Clinicians should advise parents that a policy of watchful waiting is advisable when a child begins asking questions. Often the earliest "tummy" questions are intended by the child to obtain reassurance that he or she truly belongs to the parents, and they to him or her; thus to take a 3- or 4-year-old's first tummy question as requiring disclosure about adoption may be a fallacy of misplaced concreteness. A concrete answer at this point may be experienced by the child as an empathic failure on the parent's part. If the child continues to ask questions related to reproduction and personal origin, parents may then reasonably conclude that the child has been satisfied on the first point—that of family membership—and is now truly interested in learning the facts concerning his or her biological origin.

Thus the best age for disclosure cannot be legislated. In a given case, it is defined by two simultaneous parameters: the developmental stage and maturity of the child and the ability of the parents at a give time to carry out the task with sensitivity and remain in touch with the child emotionally. If the parents are psychologically prepared, then probably moderately early disclosure (e.g., between ages 48 and 60 months, in some cases earlier) is appropriate. It is always to be hoped that these discussions will arise from the child's spontaneously expressed curiosity (Pannor and Baran 1984). (For some cognitively impaired children, these recommendations would have to be modified.) But if a 4-year-old's parents are not sure they can disclose the adoption with a degree of comfort and confidence or if there is depression or family turmoil, they are better advised to get some help for themselves and wait a while, rather than embark with their child on a journey at a time when the weather is stormy and the omens unpropitious.

Concerns about original parents need to be dealt with. Such questions are legitimate and deserve to be answered with factual material. But it must be recognized that they also often represent the adopted child's or adolescent's way of expressing normal impulses to individuate or to rebel. The response, "I'll help you search," may be given in anger and may arise from the parent's own insecurities. In such circumstances it is equivalent to the hostile retort to a child who threatens to run away: "I'll help you pack your bags." But it may be experienced as profoundly reassuring if a parent can say, "When you're 18, if you still wish, I'll try to help you find out who and where they are."

Identifying adoption-related elements in developmental crises of childhood. Nodal points may occur at which parents and children can be helped to become more comfortable with their feelings about adoption. Mild disturbance can be influenced in the direction of spontaneous resolution, rather than becoming entrenched as long-standing problems of adjustment (Brinich 1990; Brodzinsky 1987, 1990).

Problems with "open adoptions." Open adoptions are one of two kinds: those in which a child in foster care is placed in an adoptive home with the understanding that there will be some kind of ongoing contact between the birth-parent(s) and the child or the adoptive parents, and those that are initially set up by the relinquishing parents and the adoptive parents together, usually including formal or legal agreements (Nickman 1986; Pannor and Baran 1984). Not much has appeared in the literature concerning outcomes with the second type, since it is quite new. The first type is often problematic. A birth-parent may be mentally ill or characterologically disturbed and may make the occasional visits an uncomfortable experience for the child. Or the court that finalized the adoption may have put in place such frequent visits that the adoption agreement looks more like a divorce custody and visitation document. Finally, some birth-parents who have contact with a child in an adoptive home are in competition with the adoptive parents and convey to the child in various ways that they have not given "emotional permission" for the child to be a member of the adoptive family. These situations frequently need the help of a child psychiatrist to sort out what is in the child's interest and to work sensitively with the adults involved, if necessary, providing a report or testimony if the case is actively before the court.

Early identification of attachment problems. This is a supremely important task. Alert pediatricians and child psychiatrists can do great service in this regard. Even in early placed children, cycles of mutual understanding and rejection that lead eventually to serious conflict can be set up. In extreme cases, children placed in early infancy may be extruded by the family during adolescence.

Parents adopting older children are usually more prepared for problems with parent-child "fit" and may deal with them better. But infants may sense a discontinuity in their caretaking even before the conventionally recognized age for object constancy and may respond by sleep, eating, or mood disturbances. Parents may be vulnerable and feel rejected. The clinician can explain that the child is mourning what has been lost, and that the parents are the best ones to help the child through it. Ongoing psychiatric advice may be required.

Secondary Intervention

When an adopted child becomes symptomatic to the extent that regular therapy is needed, feelings about adoptive status are high on the list of possible etiologic factors (Brinich 1980, 1990; Brodzinsky 1987, 1990; Nickman 1985; Schechter et al. 1964; Sorosky et al. 1979). Many adopted children, particularly those in midlatency, demonstrate vulnerable self-esteem in relation to their knowledge of not having been kept by their birth-parents, experiencing themselves as cast-off or worthless. They may be moody, underachieve in school, or become aggressive. Psychiatric intervention can take as its goal the sensitive fostering of a grieving process so that the child can be freed-up to go on with the tasks of development. Responses need to be timed to a child's intermittent ability to bear painful affect. What is being grieved, in the case of early adopted children, is the fact that the child was not born into a family that wanted and could care for the child (Nickman 1985). With later-adopted children, object loss and various confusional states related to changes of caretaker also are involved. Some children feel stigmatized among peers because of adopted status, particularly if their appearance is different from that of their parents or the local peer group. (It still occurs frequently, however, that even in the absence of such a difference, children who know a member of their group's adoptive status will taunt the child, saying things like "Your mother didn't want you.")

Parents who deal poorly with unpleasant feelings will need help in tolerating the sadness their child may express. "Isn't our love enough? Why does he have to keep thinking about those people he doesn't even know?" They might be encouraged to reflect on misfortunes they have experienced—particularly infertility, if present—to help them empathize with their child's pain (Blum 1983; Kirk 1964).

The child can be encouraged to share fantasies of the original parents. Many adoptees fantasize extensively, and at times these fantasies crystallize into negative or shifting figures that maintain a hold on the growing child's imagination and influence in the direction of a "negative identity," with subsequent alienation and acting out in adolescence. Family dialogue about adoption that is neither perfunctory nor excessive should be encouraged, and by means of which the child can find a way to connect inner fantasies with real surroundings.

When adoptees have difficulty in childhood or adolescence it is often in the form of problems with aggression and impulse control. Many are considered hyperactive and given medication. This is sometimes appropriate, but a more psychodynamic approach may be in order.

Extended psychotherapy is often needed, and the parents need access to the child's therapist perhaps more than do nonadoptive parents because of their own vulnerability to feelings of guilt and decreased self-esteem. In other situations, a case-management approach is useful.

Clinicians should be alert to parents who stonewall the topics of adoption and infertility, because children in such families often feel foreclosed from an important part of their personal histories. Often much help is needed in these families.

Tertiary Intervention

Some adolescent adoptees suffer long-standing neurotic or characterological impairment, in whose genesis the fact of their adoption, or the life circumstances surrounding it, play an important part (Brinich 1980; Nickman 1985; Schechter et al. 1964; Sorosky et al. 1979).

Adolescent developmental issues involving separation and individuation are particularly hard for some adoptees and their parents to negotiate, and at times families present in states of profound crisis (Berman and Bufferd 1986). The child psychiatrist must help the family decide whether outpatient psychotherapy has been given an adequate try in the past, and should now be vigorously pursued, or whether the adolescent and the family need some distance from each other. When feasible, boarding school or some alternative living situation (such as having the teenager live with relatives for a time) is a sanity-saving measure—particularly when the adolescent provokes the parents continually and a battle has been set up in which there are no winners. Under such circumstances, the boy or girl will often do better if given a chance for self-definition in a new peer group and with adults whose approach is warm but relatively impersonal, rather than with parents whose love and concern he or she is not able to make use of at this stage.

Two sensitive and related issues with older child placement are 1) the frequent inadequacy of postplacement services by the placing agency, contributing to chronic difficulty, and 2) the lack of sensitivity on the part of inpatient and outpatient therapists, social service agencies, and courts to the complex nature of these placements, resulting in discouragement of further attempts to save the family. These individuals may fail to see existing bonds between adolescents and adoptive parents and may identify with one while labeling the other as unempathic or bad, and thus may contribute to a disruption that was not inevitable.

Occasionally the degree of mutual hostility is impossible to break through, or the parents are implacably rejecting toward a son or daughter who appears to the clinician to be a manageable teenager. When this occurs and the expedients mentioned above are not available, the psychiatrist may eventually have to "preside" over the breakup of a family. If extrusion of the adolescent seems inevitable, the clinician does best not to fight the emotional realities, but rather should try to help each member of the group understand how things came to be so difficult in the family, to facilitate grieving, and to remain available to parents, adolescents, and siblings in whatever way seems feasible. When teenagers must go into foster care or group care, it is important for the therapist to initiate contact with the child's new caretakers; often the teenager will be greatly reassured by this continued manifestation of interest. It is better if continued clinical contact is possible; often such contact represents the most stable continuity in an adolescent's life over a turbulent time.

Conclusion

Although the emotional development of adoptees within their families (especially adoptees with traumatic histories) is often troubled to some extent, the majority do well in the long run. Child psychiatrists can assume an attitude of watchful hopefulness with adoptees and their families, helping them to face difficult issues while maintaining a justified belief that long-standing ties are likely to survive present crises.

Foster Care

Half a million American children are in foster homes (Geiser 1973). Such care may be required transiently or for longer periods, at parents' request, or involuntarily when parents are unable to care for or control a child. Some are eventually placed in group-care facilities.

Removal may occur at so young an age that the child retains no memories. Older children suffer from separations, even when parents are neglectful or abusive. Both groups are traumatized by impersonal treatment, lack of continuity of foster homes and social workers, and lack of connection with families of origin.

Children hope for a reconstituted family, although aware of parental failings. The role reversals forced on many such children lead to conflict between ego progression and the role-reversed regressions involved in looking out for an impaired parent.

Foster homes have the task of providing emotional support, structure, and caring commitment, while not becoming so invested that they make subsequent planning (e.g., for placement back with natural parents, or in an adoptive home) difficult. The foster parents' attitude toward the natural parents should be helpful rather than competitive, and they should not downgrade them to the child. Ideally they should receive substantial initial training and ongoing supervision as paraprofessionals.

Most are conscientious and well-motivated people selected by social agencies. At times scarce funding and heavy caseloads, however, compromise the quality of agency work. Some foster homes are neglectful, abusive, or overcrowded. Professionals involved with individual children can help agencies in their monitoring function.

Permanency planning refers to existing social policy that encourages early decisions in child placement. Too often in the past, foster children were left in limbo without clear goals on the part of those in charge. Children deserve a permanent home; increasingly this principle displaces that of parental rights. Guidelines include

- Children should not remain in homes that cannot meet their needs.
- Foster children deserve timely decisions regarding their parents' potential to care for them again.
- If such potential is judged lacking, other plans should be made and put into effect.

Some children do better in long-term foster placements than in adoptive homes, for various reasons. Under certain conditions, foster parents may become adoptive parents for a child in their care. Services to natural parents, including counseling and visitation with the child, are important; in their absence, not only does the child suffer, but subsequent attempts to terminate parental rights become difficult even when appropriate.

Disturbances of foster children arise from early deprivation, subsequent disruption, or both. Many foster children have transient adjustment reactions when placed, including regression in sphincter control, withdrawal, aggression, and problems with sleep and appetite. Underlying psychological causes include

- Grief at separation from parents and guilt toward them
- Anxiety and confusion about what will happen in their lives and when
- Anger at authorities for disrupting their lives, at foster parents for exerting authority, and at parents for abuse or neglect
- Lowered self-esteem and depression due to feeling abandoned by parents (whatever the circumstances of removal)

Interventions include

- *Routine monitoring.* A child psychiatrist who sees a foster child should consider:
    - Does this placement seem to be working for the child? Is there evidence of good care? Are there signs of neglect or physical or sexual abuse?
    - Is the child likely to return to the family of origin? Are there criteria for deciding if and when the child should be returned? Are parents being offered appropriate services and visitation?
    - Has the child been evaluated adequately from the pediatric, dental, neurological, cognitive, and emotional standpoints, as may be indicated (Schor 1982)?
    - In the absence of indicators for reunion, are appropriate steps being taken to try to free the child for adoption or to make alternate arrangements such as specialized or long-term foster care or group care?

- *Evaluations* with respect to the child's overall treatment plan. Assessment may be required of an emotional and cognitive status in relation to possible placements (e.g., back with parents, in a specialized foster home, or in group care).
- *Psychotherapy* for reactive or long-standing problems. Continued placement in a foster home may be threatened and the therapist seen as one who may help save it. Therapy is often an essential lifeline for a foster child. Even at a time of turmoil, when therapy cannot accomplish structural changes in personality, it can serve as an important stabilizing force.

Children in group homes have much in common with foster children. Many have been in both kinds of settings. These children have an importance disproportionate to their numbers because they represent the most deprived and volatile segment of the child population. Group-care facilities often have access to child psychiatric consultation, but only the best of them provide regular psychotherapy for the children in their care.

Conclusion

Children living in substitute care form a continuum. At one end are group homes; at the other, adoption with the formation of permanent bonds. The themes of abandonment, loss, and diminished self-esteem pertain to all such children to some degree.

References

Berman LC, Bufferd RK: Family treatment to address loss in adoptive families. Social Casework 67:3–11, 1986

Blum H: Adoptive parents: generative conflict and generational continuity. Psychoanal Study Child 38:141–163, 1983

Brinich P: Some potential effects of adoption on self and object representations. Psychoanal Study Child 35:107–133, 1980

Brinich P: Adoption from the inside out: a psychoanalytic perspective, in The Psychology of Adoption. Edited by Brodzinsky D, Schechter MD. Oxford, Oxford University Press, 1990

Brodzinsky D: Adjustment to adoption: a psychosocial perspective. Clinical Psychology Review 7:25–47, 1987

Brodzinsky D: A stress and coping model of adoption adjustment, In The Psychology of Adoption. Edited by Brodzinsky D, Schechter MD. Oxford, Oxford University Press, 1990, pp 3–24

Derdeyn AP, Levy AM, Looney JG, et al: Child Custody Consultation: Report on the Task Force on Clinical Assessment in Child Custody. Washington, DC, American Psychiatric Association, 1982

Dikette R: Value issues in present-day adoption. Child Welfare 53:223–243, 1984

Feigelman W, Silverman AR: Adoptive parents, adoptees and the sealed record controversy. Social Casework 67:219–226, 1986

Geiser RL: The Illusion of Caring: Children in Foster Care. Boston, MA, Beacon Press, 1973

Goldstein J, Freud A, Solnit AJ: Beyond the Best Interests of the Child. New York, Free Press, 1979

Howe RW: Adoption practice, issues and laws 1958–1983. Family Law Quarterly 17:173–197, 1983

Kirk HD: Shared Fate: A Theory of Adoption and Mental Health. New York, Free Press, 1964

MacIntyre J, Donovan D: Debate forum: resolved: children should (should not) be told of their adoption before they ask. J Am Acad Child Adolesc Psychiatry 19:828–833, 1990

Nickman SL: Losses in adoption. Psychoanal Study Child 40:365–398, 1985

Nickman SL: Open adoptions—for whom? a clinician's view. Boston Bar Journal 30:32–35, 1986

Pannor R, Baran A: Open adoption as standard practice. Child Welfare 63:245–249, 1984

Rutter M: Maternal Deprivation Reassessed, 2nd Edition. New York, Penguin, 1981

Schechter MD: About adoptive parents, in Parenthood: Its Psychology and Psychopathology. Edited by Anthony EJ, Benedek T. Boston, MA, Little, Brown, 1970

Schechter MD, Carlson PV, Simmons JQ, et al: Emotional problems in the adopted. Arch Gen Psychiatry 10:100–118, 1964

Schoettle UC: Termination of parental rights—ethical issues and role conflicts. Journal of the American Academy of Child Psychiatry 23:629–632, 1984

Schor EL: The foster care system and health status of foster children. Pediatrics 69:521–528, 1982

Sorosky AD, Baran A, Pannor R: The Adoption Triangle. Garden City, NY, Anchor Books, 1979

Steinhauer PD: Assessing for parenting capacity. Am J Orthopsychiatry 53:468–481, 1983

Winnicott DW: The antisocial tendency, in DW Winnicott: Collected Papers. New York, Basic Books, 1958, pp 306–315

21

Infant and Toddler Psychiatry

Margaret P. Gean, M.D.

Child psychiatrists have been intrigued with infants and toddlers for most of the 20th century. Such noted clinicians and researchers as Winnicott, Spitz, Bowlby, Anna Freud, Mahler, and Klein have contributed to present-day enthusiasm and investigation. It is essential that the child psychiatrist be aware that extensive information exists delineating the unique and complex capacities of this age group. It is no longer sufficient to evaluate a very young child solely by speaking with the parent and observing the child from afar. Signs and symptoms of autism, mental retardation, failure to thrive, abuse, anxiety disorders, developmental deviations, and reactive disorders may be identified and treated. Children with vulnerabilities to major mental illness may need to be monitored and have early treatment. Additionally, difficulties in parenting styles warrant attention as early as possible to prevent dysfunctional parent-child relationships and primary psychiatric illness in the child (Anthony and Koupernik 1973; Bayley 1969; Call 1974; Call et al. 1985a, 1985b; Greenspan 1981; Noshpitz 1979; Osofsky 1979; Sherman 1982).

Evaluation

To formulate a diagnosis and treatment plan, several appointments are usually needed, whether the child is seen as an outpatient or while hospitalized (Gaensbauer and Harmon 1981; Minde and Minde 1986). An initial interview with the parents alone is optimal; talking candidly in the presence of all but the youngest infant may be disturbing to the child. Furthermore, it is difficult for a parent to focus on the child psychiatrist's detailed questions while simultaneously attending to the child's needs. Occasionally parents feel such anxiety and urgency to have the child seen that they may refuse to come without the child. In these circumstances, the order of appointments may have to be modified, and the history can be gathered later. If parents must bring the child or young siblings to the appointments scheduled for the parents, on-site baby-sitting arrangements (a grandparent or baby-sitter) should be made. This will ensure that the parents may be talked with privately without leaving the children unsupervised or stressed by the separation from adults with whom they are familiar.

The chief complaint; expectations of the evaluation; details of the pregnancy, labor, and delivery; and the medical history of the child should be covered. Maximum data about the chief complaint are helpful in formulating an approach to the problem and help to clarify the style and degree of parental involvement with the child. Such information as when, how long, after what, how frequently, and family and marital circumstances should be inquired about if not spontaneously provided. A description of the personality of the child and the parents' theory as to the etiology of the problem should be elicited. Ages at which developmental landmarks were achieved (e.g., smiling, sitting, self-feeding, first words, separation anxiety, walking, toileting), history of parent-child separations, and precipitants of affective responses such as anger and sadness are essential data. One should also gather information concerning the child's daily schedule of meals, naps, sleep patterns, toileting, and play activities. More information about the expectable ages for these landmarks and descriptions of social, emotional, and attachment development is provided elsewhere (Ainsworth 1978; Bayley 1969; Greenspan 1981; Noshpitz 1979; Osofsky 1979). Inquiries into the parents' own life are warranted as current family stress, moves, pregnancy, job changes, and history of trauma (e.g., loss of parent, abuse, depressed parent, illness, separation) in the parents' own younger years may elucidate why a parent is having difficulty parenting during a particular developmental phase.

A second appointment should be scheduled at an optimal time for the child (i.e., not nap times, mealtimes, or, in general, late in the day). Observations of the child begin in the waiting room and should include the child's response to any unfamiliar people present and the introduction to the child psychiatrist. The parents' interactions with the child should be noted, including the manner in which the child is held, whether eye contact is made, whether the parents engage the child in socially reciprocal interchanges, and how they attend to the child's response to the strange environment. Feeding and diapering may be observed during the evaluation process, and permission should be given to the parent to do these tasks as necessary.

An assessment of an infant or toddler requires that the child psychiatrist develop a standard format of "interviewing." As language and elaborative fantasy play are limited, a broad array of interactions must be elicited. An opportunity to evaluate the child's social skills, emotional development, cognitive level, language progression, motor skills, physical development, and temperament as well as the status of the parent-child attachment are necessary. The circumstances that will allow for systematic assessment of these capacities are the following:

- History from parents and other caregivers
- Observation of parent-child interaction in structured and unstructured play
- Observation of child in independent, structured, and unstructured play
- Observation of child's interaction with the evaluator in structured and unstructured tasks
- Developmental assessment (e.g., Bayley Scales of Infant Development [Bayley 1969])
- Observation of child's response to a brief separation and reunion with the parent
- Review of medical records including birth records, day-care reports, and developmental and psychiatry evaluations

Given the needs of young children for a sense of security in stressful circumstances, the infant-toddler evaluation is carried out with a parent (primary attachment figure) present. Observations of the child without the parent present are incomplete and may distort or make an accurate diagnosis impossible. Even with the parent present, a decrease in vocalizing is common for young children under stress and should not be misinterpreted as mutism or language delay. Free play at the end of a session will often facilitate vocalizing if it has not previously been demonstrated.

In addition to test items, other toys that cover the full zero to 3-year age range should be available:

- Small rattle (safe for mouthing)
- Ball (stuffed or soft to prevent injury or breakage when thrown)
- Pull toy
- Blocks (8–10 will suffice)
- Toy telephone or other item with motion and noise
- Doll or stuffed animal

Such toys will help the parent and child feel comfortable as well as facilitate unstructured play observations. In general, asking the parent to help the child adjust to the unfamiliar setting will initiate a parent-child interaction.

Depending on the age, temperament, and presenting problems of the child, the child psychiatrist can create a structured interaction with the child using a developmental test to assess cognitive, language, motor, and behavior skills. During phases of stranger anxiety or when there is discomfort on the part of the parents, the child's hesitancy to engage can usually be alleviated by having the child observe (hear) a comfortable verbal interchange between the parent and the child psychiatrist. Positioning the child in the parent's lap so that the child sees the parent's face also helps reduce discomfort. If a child cannot be comforted adequately for the evaluation, the child psychiatrist should inquire about an alternative time for an appointment. The parents' speculations as to why the child is inconsolable can help in planning the next session. Occasionally, the problem occurs because the child's primary caregiver may be someone other than the person who accompanied the child to the evaluation. This may occur with adolescent parents, with foster parents, and in cases of unsettled custody. A grandmother, teenage or adult child of a foster parent, father, or live-in baby-sitter may be the absent primary attachment figure. Having all caretakers come for the evaluation will usually clarify the child's hierarchy of attachments and allow for completion of the evaluation.

The choice of a standardized test to measure cognitive and motor development should vary depending on the needs and interests of the child psychiatrist. If a screening assessment is needed or if the physician infrequently evaluates infants and toddlers, the Denver Developmental Screening Test (Minde and Minde 1986) may be used. If in-depth diagnostic and treatment planning is called for and the child psychiatrist anticipates seeing many young children, the Bayley Scales of Infant Development would be preferable and are widely used for both clinical and research purposes. The Bayley scales have been standardized across various economic, ethnic, geographic, and sex groupings in the United States and have subsequently been used internationally. Experience through testing a number of children of various ages is essential in developing one's skill and familiarity with this tool. If neither standard tool is available, a structured approach to interacting with young children during part of the interview will allow the clinician to develop his or her own comparative view of young children's development. Winnicott (1975) outlined a method and the rationale for this approach.

After completion of the structured and unstructured observations and interactions, a direct observation of a separation and reunion between the child and the primary caregiver is warranted. As reported by Ainsworth (1978) in a detailed description of the procedure and research, the response of the child on separation from the parent and more clearly on reunion provides information about the security of the child's attachment to the parent. From a practical standpoint, placing the separation and reunion at the end of the appointment prevents interference with other aspects of the evaluation. The stress from the separation can be significant and may prevent the child from returning to a comfortable state for further evaluation.

To initiate this task, the parent is asked to leave the office for a brief period and to wait close by. If more than one caregiver is present, a separation-reunion event should be carried out with each adult-child combination. This will allow the child psychiatrist to compare the child's differential reaction to each adult separately. The child psychiatrist should observe the parents' method of departure from the child and the child's response. Children with both age-appropriate and heightened separation anxiety may show immediate distress. Other securely attached children may have a delayed reaction or only look to the door, point, or approach the place where the parent had been sitting. Older and unattached children may appear not to have noticed the parents' departure and continue to play. This is also observed if the person leaving the room is not the primary attachment figure. Several minutes should elapse prior to the reunion to observe the child's response of delayed distress and self-soothing techniques. The child psychiatrist should observe the child's immediate response to the return of the parent and should note three major distinguishing patterns of reunion:

- The child who shows no reaction to the parent
- The child who makes brief contact (e.g., tactile, visual, vocal) and returns to play or test items
- The child who actively avoids the parent, is angry at the parent, or clings to the parent and does not reengage in play

The first of these patterns is likely to reflect a child with a lack of attachment to the person who left the room. The second pattern can be expected from children with secure attachments to the parent. The third group of reactions is associated with ambivalent and insecure attachments. It should be noted that some children will demonstrate attachment behavior (e.g., approaching, physical contact, clinging) toward strangers, including the child psychiatrist. Indiscriminate attachment behavior is frequently seen in children who have attachment disorders or who have experienced abuse or neglect.

Before the evaluation is completed, the child's birth records and pediatric evaluation as well as any prior medical, psychiatric, and social service records must be reviewed. Essential information may be inadvertently overlooked or not known to a parent during the history taking. Distortion of information about stressful situations such as labor and delivery, emergency room visits, or prior psychiatric evaluations may be misleading if acquired only from the parents' memory. Permission to obtain these records should be requested in writing at the first appointment and ideally reviewed prior to seeing the child. In custodial or foster care circumstances, care must be taken to have the releases for this information signed by the authorized legal custodian. This is often someone other than the primary caregiver. An additional source of information comes from observations of a child in his or her day care. If the presenting problem is occurring at day care, on-site observation and discussion with the staff may expand areas of information significantly.

As with the first appointment of the evaluation, arrangements should be made to speak with the parents about the findings of the assessment without the child present. In formulating the conclusions of the evaluation, it is important to describe the unique strengths and weaknesses of the child. Covering social, emotional, motor, physical, cognitive, language, and attachment issues will give parents and other clinicians a comprehensive picture. Young children in this age range are complex and rapidly changing in their manifestations of normal development. Describing the findings in terms of the developmental age of the child (e.g., chronologic age of 15 months, social development age of 9 months) gives the parents a way to conceptualize the information. This also helps parents adjust their expectations of the child more effectively than the use of diagnostic labels and test scores (e.g., "mental retardation"). The child psychiatrist must also note whether the development is progressing in an expectable pattern for the chronologic age or whether the pattern is deviant and not appropriate at any age (e.g., social impairments of a depressed or autistic child, motor tics, language-processing problems, or articulation problems). Some possible combinations that would describe a child's development are

- Being ahead or delayed by a specific number of months, or progressing in the range consistent with the child's chronologic age
- Being deviant in some areas but not delayed

- A combination of deviance in one area, delay in another, and age appropriate in others

It should be noted that when reporting the results of evaluations for children born prematurely, correction for gestational age may be needed.

Diagnosis

Throughout the evaluation the child psychiatrist is constantly developing hypotheses and attempting to understand the meaning and origin of the presenting problem and the data from his or her interviews. The complexity of most situations warrants uninterrupted time, without the family present, for the child psychiatrist to review and integrate all of the data, score the test materials, and formulate a diagnosis and treatment plan.

At the present time, there is no widely accepted nosology for use in the diagnosis of infants and toddlers. DSM-IV (American Psychiatric Association 1994) has a section of childhood categories. Useful descriptions of particular symptoms and approaches to formulating diagnoses can be found elsewhere (Anthony and Koupernik 1973; Call et al. 1985a; Noshpitz 1979).

There is little correlation between a symptom and its etiology in infants and toddlers. For example, a child with an attachment disorder may present with symptoms suggestive of organic illness or developmental delays instead of problems in the parent-child relationship. Children with prematurity may appear to have symptoms of an attachment disorder due to the gaze aversion and passivity often seen following a premature birth (Brazelton and Als 1981). Likewise, common presenting complaints such as sleep disturbances, feeding disturbances, temper tantrums, and toileting problems have an extensive differential diagnosis—from organic origins to emotional conflict.

Careful observations in all areas of development and an ability to consider combinations of temperament, interactional, intrapsychic, environmental, and physiologic contributors to a problem make it feasible to describe the nature of the difficulties and to develop a treatment plan. DSM-IV Axis I has a significant number of categories available that do apply to very young children (e.g., anxiety, attachment, oppositional, or communication disorders, feeding disorders of infancy or early childhood). Axis II of DSM-IV includes Mental Retardation. A notation can be used to describe whether this diagnosis is suspected to be of an organic etiology (e.g., fetal alcohol syndrome, chromosomal abnormality, perinatal compromise) or due to environmental difficulties such as lack of appropriate stimulation.

Additional DSM-IV categories not listed under childhood disorders may be adjusted for age if the clinical circumstances are appropriate. Posttraumatic stress disorder may be diagnosed in children with trauma such as facial dog bites, physical or sexual abuse, and other extraordinary events that have exceeded the child's age-limited capacity to master intense emotional stress. In cases of suspected physical and sexual abuse, a physical examination is essential to rule out fractures, infections, and soft tissue injury. A negative physical examination does not, however, rule out the possibility of abuse. Behavioral information and psychiatric evaluation can aid in planning interventions to ensure the child's safety.

Affective disorders should be considered in young children whose presentations approximate DSM-IV descriptive criteria (adjusted for age), especially if a family history of mental illness is present. Because a combination of genetic and environmental factors may contribute to symptom formation in schizophrenia, the findings of developmental deviations in infants of parents with schizophrenia make it appropriate to provide early clinical interventions. These deviations, however, are not predictive of schizophrenia but seem to place children at risk for a variety of childhood disturbances.

Infants and toddlers may have adjustment disorders in response to external stresses. These can occur as the result of life stresses that exceed the age-adjusted emotional and cognitive capacities of young children. Additionally, the lack of empathic responses by a parent to the arrival of a sibling, a move, parental stress, or illness may result in symptoms. DSM-IV Axis IV includes a number of notations that are useful in describing family circumstances.

Treatment

Interventions for the vast array of symptoms in infants and toddlers must be based on the etiology of the signs and symptoms as well as the availability of resources and the parents' motivation for help.

- Direct interventions to child
    - Individual psychotherapy
    - Individual or group cognitive and sensorimotor stimulation
    - Day care
    - Hospitalization
    - Placement in foster care

- Indirect interventions via parent
    - Individual or group parent guidance and education
    - Psychiatric treatment of parent
    - Case management and protective services

- Dyadic parent-child intervention
    - Family treatment
    - Day-care program with parent participation
    - Parent-child observations, role modeling, video feedback, and developmental assessments
    - Outreach to child's home as site of treatment

Treatment ranges from individual counseling of the parents to direct individual work with the infant or toddler. Varying combinations of these approaches are usually undertaken with young children. Both regular and therapeutic day-care centers that include parental involvement may be able to incorporate particular suggestions into the program. Specific problem-focused therapies can be designed for children with cognitive delays, visual and hearing impairments, and medical problems requiring special treatments. These usually entail multidisciplinary and multiagency collaboration. Children who are at risk due to emotional, physical, and environmental compromises may require periodic evaluations to adjust the treatment plan as development and progress occur. Programs that offer outreach and case management to assist parents in utilizing other services such as pediatric care, day care, and social services may be warranted in addition to psychiatric therapies.

Psychopharmacologic treatment for young children is infrequent but may be an adjunct while other interventions are undertaken (e.g., antihistamines for sedation). Common psychotropic medications used for older children and adults are not approved for use in the first 3 years of life.

In conclusion, evaluation, diagnosis, and treatment of children from birth to age 3 years provide an opportunity to assist families with specific problems and may contribute to prevention of future difficulties. The child psychiatrist has a opportunity to draw on the breadth of his or her medical training and has the challenge of accomplishing a unique piece of detective work. Interventions call on individual therapy, family therapy, and consultation-liaison skills.

References

Ainsworth MD: Patterns of Attachment: A Psychological Study of the Strange Situation. Hillsdale, NJ, Lawrence Erlbaum, 1978

American Psychiatric Association: Diagnostic and Statistical Manual of Mental Disorders, 4th Edition. Washington, DC, American Psychiatric Association, 1994

Anthony EJ, Koupernik C: The Child in His Family, Vol 3. New York, Wiley, 1973

Bayley N: Bayley Scales of Infant Development. New York, Psychological Corporation, 1969

Brazelton B, Als H: A new model of assessing behavioral organization in pre-term and full-term infants. Journal of the American Academy of Child Psychiatry 20:239–263, 1981

Call JD: Helping infants cope with change. Early Child Development and Care 3:229–247, 1974

Call JD, Galenson E, Tyson R (eds): Frontiers of Infant Psychiatry, Vol 1. New York, Basic Books, 1985a

Call JD, Galenson E, Tyson R (eds): Frontiers of Infant Psychiatry, Vol 2. New York, Basic Books, 1985b

Gaensbauer TJ, Harmon RJ: Clinical assessment in infancy utilizing structured playroom situations. Journal of the American Academy of Child Psychiatry 20:264–280, 1981

Greenspan S: Psychopathology and Adaptation in Infancy and Early Childhood. New York, International Universities Press, 1981

Minde K, Minde R: Infant Psychiatry. Developmental Clinical Psychology and Psychiatry Series, Vol 4. Beverly Hills, CA, Sage, 1986

Noshpitz JD (ed): Basic Handbook of Child Psychiatry. New York, Basic Books, 1979

Osofsky JD (ed): The Handbook of Infant Development. New York, Wiley, 1979

Sherman M: The neonatal intensive care unit. Psychiatr Clin North Am 5:433–443, 1982

Winnicott DW: The Observation of Infants in a Set Situation, Through Paediatrics to Psycho-Analysis. New York, Basic Books, 1975

22

Mental Retardation and Genetics

James C. Harris, M.D.

Human genetics has been defined as the "science of variation and heredity in human beings" (Thompson et al. 1991, p. 432). It addresses genetic variation of medical and behavioral significance. There are an estimated 50,000–100,000 human genes, and approximately 5%–10% of these have been identified. In a genetic disease there are variations in the chemical makeup of genes, the units of heredity, which result in the production of abnormal proteins (e.g., enzymes, structural proteins, signal receptors, and intercellular signals).

The application of genetic study is becoming increasingly important in psychiatry, where advances in psychiatric diagnosis in children and adults, improved research methodology, and new developments in medical genetics techniques are now being utilized. The increased prevalence of mental disorders in the parents of children who are seen in psychiatric clinics has been recognized for many years. Since these families have serious individual and interpersonal difficulties, considerable attention has been focused on how psychiatric disturbance in

---

This chapter is adapted, in part, from Harris JC: *Developmental Neuropsychiatry: Mind, Brain, and Development*. New York, Oxford University Press (in press).

their children has been environmentally determined. In the past, this psychosocial risk for psychiatric disorder for children has been the primary emphasis. Recently a new focus has been placed on the importance of genetic factors in child psychiatric disorders. This change has come about because of improvements in genetic research strategies (standardized diagnosis, improved sampling of cases, appropriate selection of controls) and advances in molecular biology that allow more specific localizations and identification of genes. These advances are helping to specify the relationship of genetics and environment as new approaches emphasize an understanding of both shared and nonshared environments. An important aspect of the new genetic research is a better understanding of how to define psychiatric disorders and how to establish boundaries between the various disorders.

The interest in genetics has also resulted in an increased emphasis on the family history and consideration of both genetic and social transmission. This is apparent for children whose parents have major mental disorders as well as in mental retardation where there is considerable knowledge about genetic transmission. The application of genetic approaches is particularly important where there is the co-occurrence of a mental disorder and a mental retardation syndrome. When child psychiatrists treat children with serious mental disorders and mental retardation, a knowledge of genetics is of considerable importance.

In this chapter, I provide a background in genetics as it relates to mental retardation syndromes and psychiatric disorders. I include a rationale for genetic study and a basic definition of patterns of inheritance, review traditional and new molecular genetic approaches, and provide information on genetic factors in psychiatric disorders in children.

Importance of Genetics in Psychiatry and Mental Retardation

Identification of Treatable Conditions

Phenylketonuria (PKU) serves as a model in the prevention of a genetic metabolic disorder. Untreated PKU leads to severe mental retardation. An associated diagnosis that has been reported with untreated PKU is autistic disorder; attention-deficit/hyperactivity disorder has been described in children with treated PKU.

Genetic Counseling and Potential Prevention of a Genetic Disorder

Prevention is based on early recognition of the presence of a genetic disorder and on an acknowledgement of sensitivity to risk environments. Reduced exposure to risk environments may affect expression of the disorder. For example, there may be a genetic sensitivity in some individuals to alcoholism so that exposure to alcohol leads to expression of the disorder. Screening for genetic disorder in utero may lead to early recognition and provides the parent with a choice concerning continuation of the pregnancy. Prenatal diagnosis of Down's syndrome may lead to the start of adaptation to the disorder by parents, consideration of adoption plans, or termination of pregnancy.

Tsuang et al. (1990) suggested seven stages for psychiatric genetic counseling. The person counseled may be the identified patient, a relative, an adolescent, or sometimes a younger sibling. The first step is to clarify the accuracy of the diagnosis. The second step is the establishment of a formulation of the family psychiatric history, which may involve interviews with several family members. The next step is the establishment of risks, either empirical risks or exact risks. Empirical risks are based on psychiatric genetic research but are drawn from epidemiologic studies of morbidity. There is considerable variability between studies, but the range of research findings can be presented. Exact genetic risks can be predicted for several mental retardation syndromes, but not for the major psychiatric disorders (for depression, see Tsuang and Faraone 1990).

Definition of the Limits of Diagnostic Groups

For mood disorders, schizophrenia, and developmental neuropsychiatric disorders such as autism, the presence of heterogeneity and comorbidity requires careful designation of the phenotype. Since there may be a spectrum of presentations of a disorder, defining what is inherited is of importance. This is an issue of particular importance for the early recognition of major mental disorders in children. With a careful family history, diagnosis may be accomplished through a higher index of suspicion in conjunction with the use of standardized methods of assessment.

Recognition of Differential Effects of Shared and Nonshared Environments

Genetic approaches may help to define the impact of shared and nonshared family, school, and community environments. For example, if individual children in the same family are vulnerable to disorder, why does one child develop the disorder and a sibling does not? The term *shared environment* refers to the exposure of all children in a family to shared experiences, such as parental discord, that may increase the risk of disorder. However, these children may have other nonshared life experiences that are protective. For example, one child may have different experiences in social support from family members, increased peer support, and different school experiences. Consideration must be give to which aspects of the nonshared environments are protective and which ones increase risk. This may be important in understanding why one family member is affected and another is not.

Understanding of the Course of a Disorder

By careful study of children at risk, a better understanding may be gained of how genetic factors influence development. For example, temperament may shape life experiences by leading to the choice of certain environments that may place an individual at greater risk for developing a disorder. Furthermore, careful longitudinal study of cases recognized in childhood may lead to the recognition of subtypes of mental disorders.

Better Understanding of Potential Advantages for Heterozygotes

In a number of genetic conditions where the affected person rarely reproduces or does not reproduce at all, study of family members may demonstrate the selective advantage for the heterozygote.

Classification of Genetic Disorders

All clinical conditions are the result of combined activity of gene and environment, but genetic effects may be variable, small or large. There are three main types of genetic disorders:

Single-Gene Disorders (Abnormal Gene and Gene Product)

Single-gene disorders are caused by mutant genes. The mutation may be on one of a pair of chromosomes, matched with a normal one, or on both of the chromosomes of a pair. The result is an error in genetic information. Family studies show abnormal pedigrees. These conditions are rare, although their occurrence may be as frequent as 1 in 500 births. Of the 4,000 single-gene phenotypes, 3,000 are genetic disorders. In many of these conditions the gene is isolated and cloned; that is, segments have been purified so that large amounts of the purified segment can be produced for study.

Single-gene traits are often referred to as Mendelian because these traits segregate within families and, on average, are found in specific and fixed proportions when offspring of parents who have the trait are studied. Many single-gene diseases have been shown to have abnormalities at the protein or DNA level. The patterns of single-gene transmission depend on the location of the chromosomal focus, either autosomal or X-linked, and whether the phenotype is dominant or recessive. Dominant inheritance is expressed when carried by one chromosome of a pair, and recessive inheritance is expressed when both of a pair of chromosomes carry the variant gene. Classically the following Mendelian patterns of the inheritance have been demonstrated for single genes. There are four patterns of single-gene disorders: autosomal and X-linked, dominant or recessive.

Autosomal recessive. Autosomal recessive phenotypes account for approximately one-third of Mendelian phenotypes. Recessive disorders are only homozygous. An autosomal recessive phenotype has a recurrence risk of 1 in 4 for each sibling of the proband. Parents may be consanguineous; for most types, males and females are equally affected. When seen in more than one member of a kindred, an autosomal recessive phenotype is found only in the sibling of the proband and not in the proband's parents, children, or other relatives.

Autosomal dominant. Of 4,500 known Mendelian phenotypes, more than half are autosomal dominant traits. The phenotype appears in every generation, with each person having an affected parent. (Exceptions are fresh mutations and nonpenetrance.) Children of affected parents have a 50% chance of inheriting the phenotype. Phenotypically normal individuals do not transmit. Males and females are equally likely to transmit to male or female offspring. Males can produce unaffected daughters, and male transmission can occur.

X-linked recessive. The incidence for X-linked recessive disorder is much greater in males than females. The gene is transmitted from an affected male through all of his daughters. The daughters' sons have a 50% chance of inheriting the disorder. It is not transmitted from father to son, but is transmitted to all daughters. The gene may be transmitted via a series of females who are carriers. Ordinarily, heterozygous females are not affected, but some may show the condition with varying degrees of severity.

X-linked dominant. In this form of inheritance, in affected males with nonaffected mates, all the daughters and none of the sons are affected. Each child of an affected family member has a 50% chance of having the disorder. Both sexes are affected. However, because of the severity of the condition, they do not reproduce. Male and female children of carriers have a 50% chance of having the phenotype as in the autosomal dominance. In very rare phenotypes, females are affected about twice as often as males, but often have a milder form of the disorder.

Chromosomal Disorders (No Abnormal Gene or Gene Product)

Chromosome abnormalities have been shown in more than 60 identifiable syndromes, represent 0.7% of live births, and account for half of spontaneous first-trimester abortions (Thompson et al. 1991). The major disorders of chromosomes are three autosomal trisomies (13, 18, 21) and the four types of sex chromosomal aneuploidy: 1) Turner's syndrome (ordinarily 45, X); 2) Klinefelter's syndrome (47, XXY); 3) 47, XYY; and 4) 47, XXX. There is no error in genetic information but there is an excess or deficiency of genes in the whole chromosome or chromosomal segment. The chromosomal basis of a growing number of significant disorders has been demonstrated. These disorders occur in 7 of 1,000 births and are responsible for about 50% of the abortions (Thompson et al. 1991). In a condition like Down's syndrome, there is no abnormal gene.

Multifactorial Disorders (No Single Error in Genetic Information)

The largest number of genetic phenotypes are those that run in families but have neither a single gene nor a chromosomal basis. Multifactorial inheritance is defined as an inheritance of genetic factors and nongenetic factors, each of which is thought to have a small effect. The role of the environment may be relatively large. In the multifactorial model, the disorder is familial but no distinctive pattern of inheritance is demonstrated in a family. However, the recurrence risk is higher when more than one family member is affected; this is in contrast to single-gene disorders, where the risk is unchanged from one child to the next. The risk is much lower for second-degree relatives than for first-degree relatives; this is in contrast to the autosomal dominant condition, where it drops by half, and to the autosomal recessive condition, where it is siblings who are at risk. These conditions do not show a characteristic pedigree of single genetic traits. An example is cleft palate. Other possible examples are depression and schizophrenia.

Nonclassical Patterns of Inheritance

Although uncommon, recent genetic study has resulted in the description of non-Mendelian patterns of inheritance, for example:

- *Genomic imprinting:* differential expression of chromosomal material, depending on whether the material is inherited from the male or female parent
- *Uniparental disomy:* the presence of two chromosomes of a pair inherited from one parent with no representation of that chromosome from the other parent
- *Mosaicism:* the presence of two or more cell lines having the same origin in the same single zygote but genetically different due to postzygotic mutation or nondisjunction
- *Mitochondrial inheritance:* inheritance of a disorder that is encoded in the mitochondrial genome

Of particular interest is the occurrence of mosaicism and genomic imprinting.

Penetrance and Expressivity

Penetrance refers to the probability that a gene will have any phenotypic expression. It refers to those who are actively affected. The term is used primarily for dominant traits in heterozygous carriers. It denotes the all-or-none expression of genotypes. If less than 100% of carriers show the disorder, penetrance is reduced. If 60% of the carriers express it, it is 60% penetrant.

Expressivity indicates the degree or extent of expression of a genetic defect. This defect may be variously expressed from a mild to severe degree. In variable expression, the trait is always expressed but the extent of expression varies.

Methodology for Genetic Studies

Because of problems in separating genetic and environmental factors, twin and adoption studies (in addition to family studies) are necessary. The twin and adoption studies allow calculation of the strength of genetic differences (i.e., characteristics or predispositions). These studies help define the disorder, but neither provides evidence of the mode of genetic transmission.

Twin Studies

The comparison of monozygotic (MZ) with dizygotic (DZ) twin pairs is recognized as one of the best-established genetic procedures. It is based on the fact that MZ twins share all their genes in common, whereas DZ twins (on average) share half of their genes. Within-pair correlations allow an estimate of the role of genetic factors in individual variation expressed as a disorder, as a manifest trait, or as a behavioral characteristic. Twin research designs are strengthened when pairs who are discordant for the trait are studied, when the offspring of twins concordant or discordant for the trait are studied, and when twins separated in infancy and brought up in different environments are investigated.

Adoption Studies

Investigation of adopted children is an important genetic strategy since it allows for comparison of biological parents with adoptive parents. Furthermore, comparison of rates of disorder in biological and adoptive relatives is feasible. There are a variety of research designs: the assessment of the adoptee, cross-fostering designs, adopted sibling designs, and parent-offspring adoption designs. An issue that must be considered is the effects of the types of adoptive home (e.g., selective placement), since not all homes are the same. Analysis must consider psychiatric illness in both parents; data, however, often are available only from the mother's family. The stress of being an adoptee must also be considered as a diagnostic issue.

Family Genetic Methods

Currently these approaches benefit from better-structured interview methods and from careful choice of cases and control groups. Issues that are pertinent in family studies are heterogeneity and comorbidity. Estimates have been reported based on the severe presentation of a disorder or on a spectrum of disorder.

Genetic Considerations in the Childhood Onset of Mental Disorders

Genetic studies have been carried out to study the concordance of general behavioral deviance in twins. MZ-DZ differences in concordance indicate a genetic component with heredity greater than 50% (Graham and Stevenson 1985). However, for genetic counseling, findings in specific disorders are needed. The child and adolescent psychiatric conditions where genetic factors have been considered most likely are autism, schizophrenia, Tourette syndrome, and bipolar mood disorder. However, attention-deficit/hyperactivity disorder, anxiety disorders, conduct disorder, alcohol and drug abuse, anorexia nervosa, and learning disability are being actively investigated.

Infantile Autism

Autism is a rare disorder with a population prevalence of 4 in 10,000 or 0.04%; the rate is higher, 12–15 in 10,000, for more broadly defined autistic-like conditions (Wing 1993). The general population prevalence rate in siblings and for DZ twins for autistic disorder is 3% (Ritvo et al. 1989). The risk for a family having a second affected child is 8%–10% for male children and overall about 6%. In MZ twins the rate is approximately 50%, according to data pooled from several twin studies (Folstein and Rutter 1987). Since the base rate is so low for autism in the general population, Rutter (1991) suggested that it is one of the most strongly genetically influenced child psychiatric conditions. This concordance pattern points to the involvement of several genes that may act in combination. Because of their social disability, it is rare that an autistic individual marries, yet the disorder continues to be expressed. This may relate to there being a spectrum of autistic-like deficits and perhaps an as-yet unrecognized benefit to the heterozygote.

Schizophrenia

Schizophrenia affects approximately 1% of the population. It has been investigated using family studies, twin studies, and adoption studies. Qualitative modeling studies have not supported a specific mode of genetic transmission. Schizophrenia is a complex genetic disorder, and most support is for the multifactorial polygenetic model. However, a mixed genetic model with both a multifactorial component and a single major locus cannot be ruled out. Family studies support family transmission, but do not resolve environmental versus genetic mechanisms. Twin and adoption studies provide evidence for a genetic component and suggest that environmental components are much less important. There is little support for the single major locus genetic type of inheritance. Linkage studies are preliminary and inconsistent. Although localization on chromosome 5 has been suggested (McGillivray et al. 1990), it has not been verified in follow-up studies. Since schizophrenia is most likely a heterogeneous condition, the identification of potential subtypes is of importance. Clarifying risk factors that are distinct from genetic history is also essential. Table 22–1 provides the percentage of risk to relatives of schizophrenic patients.

Tourette Syndrome Spectrum

Recent investigations indicate that there is a pattern of disorders in family pedigrees with Tourette syndrome, which includes tics and obsessive-compulsive disorder (Pauls and Leckman 1986). Family study has identified tics and Tourette syndrome as occurring more often in males and obsessive-compulsive disorder as occurring more often in females. This Tourette/tic/obsessive-compulsive disorder phenotype is highly penetrant and is most likely inherited as an autosomal dominant condition with differential sexual penetrance. Con-

Table 22–1. Risk to relatives of schizophrenic patients

Relation	Risk (%)
First-degree relatives	
Parents	4.4
Brothers and sisters	8.5
Neither parent schizophrenic	8.2
One parent schizophrenic	13.8
Fraternal twins of opposite sex	5.6
Fraternal twins of same sex	12.0
Identical twins	57.7
Children	12.3
Both parents schizophrenic	36.6
Second-degree relatives	
Uncles and aunts	2.0
Nephews and nieces	2.2
Grandchildren	2.8
Half-brothers/sisters	3.2
First cousins (third-degree relatives)	2.9
General population	0.86

Note. These statistics include atypical cases. The risk may be lower using more strict criteria. However, even with criteria changes, the observed risk for first-degree relatives is 5–10 times the general population risk.
Source. Adapted from Tsuang and Vandermey 1980.

cordance in 30 MZ and 13 DZ twin pairs identified in a questionnaire study was 53% and 8%, respectively, but concordance for tic plus Tourette was 77% and 23% from questionnaires (Price et al. 1985). The rate approached 1.0 in MZ twins when cases were directly examined. When the full spectrum of presentation is considered, genetic analyses indicate that Tourette spectrum is inherited as a single gene (Pauls et al. 1986).

Mood Disorders

The risk for mood disorders for relatives of a depressed patient is greater than the risk for the general population. The risk increases with the proportion of genes that are shared with a parent or parents with a mood disorder. There is some evidence that increased genetic loading leads to earlier expression of depressive disorder in childhood (Weissman et al. 1987). Conversely, early onset is associated with increased risk in relatives, so it important to ask about the age at onset in family members when a parent indicates a family history of depression. The concordance rate among MZ twins is three times the rate in DZ twins. The MZ twin concordance rate is 0.7 for bipolar disorder and 0.5 for unipolar disorder.

The relatives of bipolar patients have a greater risk for both bipolar disorder and for unipolar disorder: a finding also noted in twin studies. Therefore, bipolar disorder has a greater familial component than unipolar disorder, but unipolar disorder may have a greater environmental component. Because women are at greater risk and transmission from fathers to sons is less frequent, an X chromosome focus has been suggested for bipolar disorder. This is being investigated but has not been confirmed by genetic studies, nor have other single genes been conclusively identified. No specific mode of genetic transmission has been consistently identified using mathematical modeling. Both multifactorial and mixed single-gene/multifactorial models have been suggested. However, since the condition is probably heterogeneous, analysis is unclear. Linkage studies are inconsistent, and although the X chromosome, chromosome 11, and chromosome 6 have been implicated, independent replication has not confirmed these findings. Biological markers such as transport of lithium into red cells and cholinergic supersensitivity have been suggested, but not confirmed. Pharmacogenetic study is consistent with similar drug responses in an identified patient when more than one relative is affected. Future investigations must deal with both genotypic and phenotypic heterogeneity. Genotypic heterogeneity suggests that more than one genotype can cause the disorder, and phenotypic heterogeneity indicates that a specific pathological genotype can be expressed in multiple behavioral phenotypes.

Attention-Deficit/Hyperactivity Disorder

Because of methodological problems, the initial studies suggesting genetic factors in the hyperkinetic syndrome have been supplemented by twin studies that compared MZ and DZ pairs. Concordance for hyperkinesis, when MZ and DZ pairs were pooled, was 50% in a questionnaire-based twin study carried out by Graham and Stevenson (1985) when one twin demonstrated pervasive hyperactivity at home and in school. However, the study of the genetics of attention-deficit/hyperactivity disorder has been complicated by the frequent co-occurrence of oppositional and antisocial behavior in these children. Children referred to psychiatric clinics often are referred for their behavioral difficulties rather than an attention-deficit/hyperactivity disorder alone. It has been suggested that there may be different family backgrounds for children with learning disabilities and hyperactivity in contrast to those with hyperactivity and aggressive behavior (August et al. 1981). No firm conclusions can be reached on heritability at this time. Systematic study is needed of children with pervasive hyperactivity and inattention beginning early in life, with careful attention given to oppositional and conduct symptoms and learning disabilities.

Anxiety Disorders

In adults, a familial loading for anxiety disorders has been reported (Noyes et al. 1987). Both generalized anxiety disorder and panic disorder with agoraphobia have been considered to have genetic components. Panic disorder with depression has been distinguished from depression alone. Whether these patterns are genetically based or the result of environmental or social transmission in the family is not clear. Twin studies have shown conflicting results; one recent study showed the importance of genetic factors in agoraphobia and panic disorder but not in generalized anxiety disorder (Torgersen 1983).

In children, an increased rate of separation anxiety in parents of children with school refusal (phobia) has been reported (Last et al. 1987). Mothers of children with overanxious disorder differ from those with separation anxiety disorder in their histories of past overanxious symptoms. The rate of separation anxiety has been reported to be increased in children whose mothers are agoraphobic (Berg 1976). Increased anxiety disorders have been reported in younger children of depressed mothers (Breslau et al. 1987). Family loading is then present for both children and adults, but additional research is needed to clarify the genetic and environmental interface.

Conduct Disorder

In adults, twin and adoptee studies suggest a genetic component in antisocial behavior and in criminality that is greatest for repeated minor crimes rather than for major crimes or violent antisocial behavior (Cloninger and Gottesman 1987). In twin studies, concordance rates are significant between MZ and DZ twins, with 26%–51% in MZ twins contrasted with 13%–22% for DZ twins (Rowe 1986). Adoption studies are also consistent in showing a genetic component, with associations between personality disorder and criminality in biological parents and similar conditions in their children who were placed in adoptive homes (Rowe 1986). This genetic risk may depend on exposure to risk environments (e.g., multiple placements, extended institutional care, and lower occupational status). In adolescence, there is an increased risk for delinquent behavior (Rowe 1986). Since rates are high in both MZ and DZ twins, the family environment is an important factor. Adoption studies suggest a weak genetic component (Rowe 1986). Although most children with antisocial behavior do not go on to develop adult antisocial disorders, those who do have the onset in childhood or adolescence. Therefore, in the group with persistent antisocial behavior, part of the risk may be due to a genetic component that is influenced by the environment where the child is reared. Furthermore, expression may be different in male and female children in that affected girls may have more somatic and mood complaints and boys more antisocial behavior. The underlying problems may be the child's social deficits, which lead to poor interpersonal relations and problems in social adaptation, which may lead to antisocial behavior in boys and somatic and mood symptoms in girls. Thus the phenotype to study is a broad one.

Alcohol and Drug Abuse

In adult studies, a significant genetic component has been suggested (Goedde and Agarwal 1987), but these findings are complicated in that there may be different types of alcoholism with different types of genetic influences. For example, there may be genetic factors in the amount of alcohol consumed once an individual begins to drink. Two paths have been suggested to substance abuse (Cadoret et al. 1986): an indirect route and a direct route. The indirect route may progress from alcohol problems in relatives to antisocial behavior to drug abuse. The direct route may progress from a family history of alcohol use to use and abuse. However, family environmental stresses such as divorce and psychiatric disorder (self-medication) must also be considered. Studies of children of alcoholic parents suggest an increased risk for both alcoholism and individual psychopathology (Cadoret et al. 1986). What might be inherited is an impulsive and sensation-seeking temperament that predisposes to antisocial behavior and alcohol use as well as a specific physiological response to alcohol. However, specific behavioral and physiological markers have not been conclusively established. Alcohol and drug abuse is an area of particular importance in regard to possible prevention; therefore, a careful family history is essential.

Anorexia Nervosa

Family studies are consistent with a genetic component in anorexia nervosa. Rates of 6% of combined anorexia nervosa and bulimia nervosa have been reported in first-degree relatives of anorexic patients in contrast to 1% in control subjects (Gershon et al. 1984; Holland et al. 1984). A twin study of 25 MZ pairs found concordance in 14, or 56%, compared with 5% (1 of 20) in DZ twins (Holland et al. 1984). A larger number of family members were found to have an eating disorder (anorexia nervosa, bulimia nervosa, subclinical anorexia nervosa), with a rate of 27% noted in family members compared with 6% of control families (Strober et al. 1985). Rates were higher in males than in females. Although a relationship with mood disorder has been suggested (Holland et al. 1984), it has not been demonstrated, suggesting that these are probably separate conditions. Further work is needed to determine whether the genetic factor is a predisposition to an eating disorder or to personality features that lead to vulnerability.

Mental Retardation Syndromes

Mental retardation refers to significantly subaverage intellectual functioning existing concurrently with deficits in adaptive behavior that are manifested during the developmental period. It is made up of a heterogeneous group of conditions that range from genetic and metabolic disorders to functional changes that follow trauma to the nervous system at birth or later in the developmental period. Mental retardation is not a disease or illness in itself; therefore, rather than mental retardation per se, we must consider whether there is a specific syndrome present (e.g., Down's syndrome or fragile X syndrome). In mental retardation, thinking is not characteristically disordered, and perception is not distorted unless there is a concurrent mental disorder. A mentally retarded person may have a diagnosis of a major psychiatric condition, although day-to-day problems ordinarily relate to difficulties in developmental functioning. However, a careful family history of mental illness is of particular importance when interviewing the families of mentally retarded persons. They have similar risks of developing major mental disorders as do the general population and may be doubly handicapped when both diagnoses are present.

The overall prevalence rate of mental retardation is estimated to be approximately 3% of the school-age population. In the adult population, the prevalence of mental retardation is about 1% since many of those who are mildly retarded may adapt in society following an appropriate education, and those who are more severely retarded with medical complications may not survive into adulthood. Of the mentally retarded population, 85% fall into the mildly retarded range, and the remaining 15% are more severely retarded.

There are four degrees of severity reflecting the amount of intellectual impairment: mild, moderate, severe, and profound. Although an intelligence test is not the sole basis for determining mental retardation, these tests are the accepted standard to measure the degrees of severity of mental retardation. Profound mental retardation is an IQ of 20 or less (adult mental age less than 3 years); severe is an IQ of 20–34 (adult mental age 3 to less than age 6 years); moderate is an IQ of 35–49 (adult mental age 6 to less than age 9 years); and mild is an IQ of 50–69 (adult mental age 9 to less than 12 years). Mental retardation is a permanent condition and is not curable, although the degree of habilitation that can be accomplished for the retarded person is considerable.

Genetic disorders were initially demonstrated in mentally retarded persons. In those who are mildly retarded, genetic influences are thought to be nonspecific and multifactorial. For those who are moderately, severely, or profoundly retarded (with an IQ of 49 or lower), approximately one-fourth have genetic etiologies. Of this group, chromosomal disorders make up the majority of cases (about 75%), followed by those having a single-gene disorder (approximately 20%). Table 22–2 lists the major mental retardation syndromes and their genetic bases.

Counseling

When conducting a counseling session, there is no simple answer to the question of what is a genetic disorder. Not all disorders that involve more than one family member are genetic, and not all genetic

Table 22–2. Mental retardation syndromes

Syndrome	Mode of inheritance
Down's syndrome	
95%	Trisomy 21
1.0%	Mosaic
4.0%	Robertsonian Translocation 21q/21q
Tay-Sachs disease	Autosomal recessive
Hurler's syndrome	Autosomal recessive
Hunter's syndrome	X-linked recessive
Phenylketonuria	Autosomal recessive
Rett's syndrome	Unknown
Lesch-Nyhan syndrome	X-linked recessive
Prader-Willi syndrome	Cytogenetic Deletion/genomic imprinting (maternal)
Fragile X syndrome	Trinucleotide repeat expansion (heritable unstable DNA sequences)

disorders involve more than one family member. In making the determination, the diagnosis is of particular importance and often can be made from careful clinical description prior to ordering tests. Genetic counseling must be individualized, taking into account the accuracy of the diagnosis, the type of genetic transmission, and known information about the natural history of the condition. However, each family is unique in how they will utilize the information provided to them. Working in close collaboration with a geneticist, a psychiatrist can assist the family in understanding the meaning and impact of the psychiatric disorder. The statistics for genetic risk for the same disorder may be interpreted differently from one family to the next, often depending on their life experience with affected family members.

The recognition of genetic disorders associated with conditions that follow Mendelian lines such as PKU is well known as are chromosomal disorders in children with mental retardation syndromes such as Down's syndrome and fragile X syndrome. Non-Mendelian modes of inheritance are now becoming apparent in some mental retardation syndromes. Recent work on genomic imprinting in Prader-Willi syndrome and Angelman's syndrome is of interest. (It is not yet known whether genomic imprinting occurs more often than previously suspected.) Specific detailed information can be given to families about the transmission of these well-studied conditions. This is best done by an experienced genetic counselor who appreciates the variable presentations of the particular conditions.

Genetic counseling is more problematic, however, for developmental neuropsychiatric disorders such as attention-deficit/hyperactivity disorder, autism, and psychiatric disorders such as depression, schizophrenia, and anorexia nervosa, where physical stigmata are generally not apparent, a specific biochemical marker is not available, and a genetic mechanism is not identified or agreed on. Each of these conditions may be a final common pathway; multiple subtypes that lead to the similar phenotypes may be present or the condition may be associated with another known medical disorder. In this sense there is an analogy to cerebral palsy and mental retardation, which are general terms for conditions that may have multiple etiologies. Because of this genetic heterogeneity, counseling in these conditions must be based on epidemiologic studies of prevalence of the condition. These are often found in family studies, which depend on the accuracy of the diagnosis and the methods used in analysis.

Consequently, depending on the criteria used, prevalence rates are ranges of prevalence, lower for the classic, most severe presentation and higher if the "spectrum disorder" is included in the estimate. At issue is what is inherited; is it a spectrum of social communication deficits as suggested in autism or a range of disorders in interpersonal functioning as seen in schizophrenia. One must be prepared to discuss prevalence of both the severe condition and the spectrum disorder while keeping in mind that subtypes may exist. Furthermore, there may be variable expression at different ages. More specifically, the multiple factors that go into multifactorial inheritance need to be reviewed with a family. The nature of the genetic contribution may be a vulnerability to stress, temperamental features that lead to choice of risk environments, or polygenetic risk of a disorder. For these conditions, the gene-environmental interaction is an important part of counseling.

Before the information is communicated to the person being counseled, an understanding of the person's emotional stage, the phase of acceptance of the disorder, and the person's intentions must be considered. In considering having another child, the burden of the illness can be presented, but the benefits of becoming a parent can be evaluated only by the individual being counseled. Counseling for siblings who have been found to be positive for a disorder on screening and will develop the disorder at a later age is particularly difficult and requires a careful assessment. It is essential to remember that counseling is an ongoing process and that the counselor should be available for support in follow-up sessions.

References

August GJ, Steward MA, Tsai L: The incidence of cognitive disabilities in the siblings of autistic children. Br J Psychiatry 138:416–422, 1981

Berg I: School phobia in the children of agoraphobic women. Br J Psychiatry 128:86–89, 1976

Breslau N, Davis GC, Prebucki K: Searching for evidence on the validity of generalized anxiety disorder: psychopathology in the children of anxious mothers. Psychiatric Research 20:285–297, 1987

Cadoret RJ, Troughton E, O'Gorman TW, et al: An adoption study of genetic and environmental factors in drug abuse. Arch Gen Psychiatry 43:1131–1136, 1986

Cloninger CR, Gottesman II: Genetic and environmental factors in antisocial behavior disorders, in Causes of Crime: New Biological Approaches. Edited by Mednick SA, Moffit TE, Sack SA. Cambridge, England, Cambridge University Press, 1987, pp 92–104

Folstein S, Rutter M: Autism: familial aggregation and genetic implications. J Autism Dev Disord 18:3–30, 1987

Gershon ES, Schreiber JL, Hamovit JR, et al: Clinical findings in patients with anorexia nervosa and affective illness in their relatives. Am J Psychiatry 141:1419–1422, 1984

Goedde HW, Agarwal DP (eds): Genetics and Alcoholism. New York, Alan R Liss, 1987

Graham P, Stevenson J: A twin study of genetic influences on behavioral deviance. Journal of the American Academy of Child Psychiatry 24:33–41, 1985

Holland AJ, Hall A, Murray R, et al: Anorexia nervosa: a study of 34 twin pairs and one set of triplets. Br J Psychiatry 145:414–419, 1984

Last CG, Phillips JE, Statfeld A: Childhood anxiety disorders in mothers and their children. Child Psychiatry Hum Dev 18:102–109, 1987

McGillivray BC, Bassett AS, Langlois S, et al: Familial 5q11.2–q13.3 segmental duplication cosegregating with multiple anomalies, including schizophrenia. Am J Med Genet 35:10–13, 1990

Noyes R, Clarkson C, Crowe RR, et al: A family study of generalized anxiety disorder. Am J Psychiatry 144:1019–1024, 1987

Pauls DL, Leckman JF: The inheritance of Gilles de la Tourette syndrome and associated behaviors: evidence for autosomal dominant transmission. N Engl J Med 315:993–996, 1986

Pauls DL, Towbin KE, Leckman JF, et al: Evidence supporting an etiological relationship with Gilles de la Tourette syndrome and obsessive compulsive disorder. Arch Gen Psychiatry 43:1180–1182, 1986

Price RA, Kidd KK, Cohen DJ, et al: A twin study of Tourette's syndrome. Arch Gen Psychiatry 42:815–820, 1985

Ritvo ER, Jorde LB, Mason-Brothers A, et al: The UCLA-University of Utah epidemiologic survey of autism: recurrence risk estimates and genetic counseling. Am J Psychiatry 146:1032–1036, 1989

Rowe DC: Genetic and environmental components of antisocial pairs: a study of 265 twin pairs. Criminology 24:513–532, 1986

Rutter M: Nature, nurture, and psychopathology: a new look at an old topic. Development and Psychopathology 3:125–137, 1991

Thompson MW, McInnes R, Willard HF: Genetics in Medicine. Philadelphia, PA, WB Saunders, 1991

Torgersen S: Genetic factors in anxiety disorders. Arch Gen Psychiatry 40:1085–1089, 1983

Tsuang MT, Faraone SV: The Genetics of Mood Disorders. Baltimore, MD, Johns Hopkins University Press, 1990

Tsuang MT, Vandermey R: Genes and the Mind. New York, Oxford University Press, 1980

Tsuang MT, Gilbertson MW, Faraone SV: The genetics of schizophrenia: current knowledge and future directions. Schizophr Res 4:157–171, 1990

Weissman MM, Gammon GD, John K, et al: Children of depressed parents: increased psychopathology and early onset of major depression. Arch Gen Psychiatry 44:847–853, 1987

Wing L: The definition and prevalence of autism: a review. European Child and Adolescent Psychiatry 2:61–74, 1993

Additional Readings

Beardslee WR, Bemporad J, Keller MB, et al: Children of parents with major affective disorder: a review. Am J Psychiatry 140:825–832, 1983

De Marchi N: The genetics of schizophrenia. Dev Med Child Neurol 33:452–458, 1991

Goodman R, Stevenson J: A twin study of hyperactivity, II: the aetiological role of genes, family relationships and perinatal adversity. J Child Psychol Psychiatry 30:691–709, 1989

Hodgson S: Genomic imprinting. Dev Med Child Neurol 33:552–556, 1991

Pauls D, Cohen DJ, Kidd KK, et al: Tourette syndrome and neuropsychiatric disorders: is there a genetic relationship? Am J Hum Genet 43:206–209, 1988

Rutter M: Children of sick parents: an environmental and psychiatric study (IOP Maudsley Monograph No 16). London, Oxford University Press, 1966

Rutter M, Bolton P, Harrington R, et al: Genetic factors in child psychiatric disorders, I: a review of research strategies. J Child Psychol Psychiatry 31:3–39, 1990

Rutter M, Macdonald H, LeCouteur AH, et al: Genetic factors in child psychiatric disorders, II: empirical findings. J Child Psychol Psychiatry 31:39–85, 1990

Strober M, Morrell W, Burroughs J, et al: A controlled family study of anorexia nervosa. J Psychiatry Res 19:239–246, 1985

23

Research Design, Measures, and Statistics

James R. Brasic, M.D., M.P.H.
J. Gerald Young, M.D.

Research Design: How to Ask the Question

Stages of Research

Despite the difficulty all clinicians experience when attempting to do research, it can be accomplished if the structure of research is understood and the clinician is sufficiently determined. Attempts to answer questions concerning the etiology and treatment of childhood neuropsychiatric disorders utilize both our understanding of the general process of acquiring knowledge (Polanyi 1962) and the stages of research in science (Merton 1973) and medicine (Fleck 1979). Clinical research generally begins with a conjecture based on personal clinical experience coupled with current theoretical knowledge, followed by a review of the published literature. Experiments must be designed to test the hypotheses generated, and new hypotheses formulated based on these results.

This work was supported by a grant from the Medical Fellows Program of the Office of Mental Retardation and Developmental Disabilities, State of New York.

The clinician often falters with an untested hypothesis, however, feeling unsure how to design and carry out a research protocol. Two factors contribute to this problem. First, research is a complex process, despite the fact that it is conceptually straightforward. The implementation of clinical investigation in child and adolescent psychiatry is burdened by many practical and technical pitfalls, as investigators strive to distinguish among the myriad contributing inherited and environmental influences or possible treatments. Second, the current state of clinical research is now sufficiently sophisticated that substantial resources may be required to mount certain types of protocols. If the research contemplated is to be carried out by a single clinician, the clinician must be able to construct a practical project that can be accomplished by an individual and still be a useful contribution to the field.

These problems for clinical investigators are reduced if the concepts and vocabulary of research are clearly understood. In addition, it is helpful if the stages of research are clearly differentiated as the clinician plans the project, even if there will be some temporal overlap in the implementation of these stages. In this chapter, we briefly review essential vocabulary, concepts, components, and stages of the research enterprise to orient clinicians attempting their own research or wishing to improve their understanding of terminology in scientific papers.

The development of a research protocol can be conceptualized according to two frames of reference: stages and components. The stages of research are conventionally considered in terms of the conceptual divisions of the research process. These include selecting a research hypothesis, developing the research protocol, using a pilot study to pretest and revise the protocol, conducting the research study, carrying out a statistical analysis of the findings, drawing conclusions, and preparing a manuscript for publication.

However, there is a pragmatic advantage to considering the written documents required for research as the six stages of research:

- Construction of a foundation for research: the development of trained staff and clinical research instruments
- Genesis of an hypothesis and its significance
- Preparation of a research protocol outline: 1–5 pages, utilized for

systematic planning, and later to serve as a checklist for completed activities

- Preparation of a research protocol: 5–50 pages, a comprehensive description of the research project and its organization
- Preparation of a protocol procedure manual: 50–200 pages, providing the detailed operational instructions that ensure that the protocol is carried out in a standard and accurate fashion despite its complexity
- Conduction of the research and preparation of a manuscript for publication describing the results

Utilization of these stages provides the quality control required for successful research. Regrettably, most investigators do not conduct their research according to these stages because of a variety of clinical, financial, and competitive pressures. However, awareness of this framework aids investigators in their efforts to improve the quality of the research product.

The components of clinical research include hypotheses and their significance, design strategies, subjects, independent and dependent variables, clinical and laboratory measures and the instruments used to obtain them, ethical guidelines, data management (acquisition, entry, verification, organization), and data reduction and analysis (Hulley and Cummings 1988).

Hypotheses

Research begins with an enjoyable phase: the genesis of an interesting hypothesis. The hypothesis should be both novel and relevant, but this is more difficult than it appears. First, interesting ideas are often repetitions of existing theories by the naive or are impractical. Second, at the opposite extreme, the investigator might design a feasible study that lacks sufficient relevance. This typically occurs when the investigator finds that specific methodological questions must be examined prior to answering conceptually broad principles; although often necessary, it also can lead to research that has limited relevance and interest. The research must be able to survive the question "Who cares?" The investigator must be able to present a rationale for the research that demonstrates that it is significant. Finally, the best research hypotheses tend to be precarious in the face of the requirement that they be feasible and practical. Determining how to design a research project within the invariably limited personnel and financial resources is an art, and most incipient research founders at this point (Hulley and Cummings 1988).

In practical terms, the hypothesis should be simple (not an unrealistically complex set of predictor and outcome variables) and specific (e.g., careful planning of sampling methods and operational definitions of measures). The formal procedure is for the investigator to formulate a *null hypothesis,* a statement that the proposed clinical factor (e.g., symptom, age, sex) or treatment has no effect. Typically the null hypothesis is a statement that the established theory is true (Bickel and Doksum 1977). The *alternative hypothesis* states that there *is* an effect or association; generally the alternative hypothesis is the new theory we seek to prove. A priori we do not know which of these two mutually exclusive hypotheses is true; if we did there would be no reason to conduct the experiment (Lehmann 1959). A *one-tailed alternative hypothesis* indicates the direction of the association between predictor and outcome variables, whereas a *two-tailed hypothesis* does not, proposing only that there is an association. The researcher then attempts to disprove the null hypothesis to conclude that the new treatment is effective; after the experiment the researcher examines the data and either accepts or rejects the null hypothesis. Of course, in clinical research there is rarely an absolutely definitive answer, so that results are always considered in terms of *probabilities*: the likelihood or probability that the finding is not simply due to chance. A probability of less than 1 in 20 (a value less than 5%) that the finding is due to chance is written as $P < .05$ and is commonly accepted as an acceptable risk in clinical research. This is the usual meaning of the statement that a finding is "statistically significant" or unlikely to be due to chance.

There is a standard method for examining the possibility of an error in experimental conclusions. Table 23–1 indicates the possible conclusions of a scientific experiment designed to test the null hypothesis. If the investigator accepts a true null hypothesis or rejects a false null hypothesis, the result is correct.

Two kinds of errors can result when testing null hypotheses.

Table 23–1. Hypothesis testing: conclusions and error types

		Truth of null hypothesis	
		Null hypothesis is true	Null hypothesis is false
Researcher's conclusion	Null hypothesis is true	No error	Type II error (false negative)
	Null hypothesis is false	Type I error (false positive)	No error

Rejecting a true null hypothesis is a *Type I error* (false positive), while accepting a false null hypothesis is a *Type II error* (false negative). A Type I error is generally considered to be more serious than a Type II error. Clinical studies are conventionally designed so that *alpha* (α), the probability of a Type I error, does not exceed 1 in 20 (symbolized as $\alpha \leq .05$), and *beta* (β), the probability of a Type II error, does not exceed 1 in 5 (symbolized as $\beta \leq .20$). Note that alpha is equivalent to the *level of statistical significance,* the probability (P) values mentioned above that are routinely reported in scientific papers (e.g., $P < .05$).

Design Strategies

Observational Studies

Design of observational studies. With a hypothesis in mind, the investigator must determine the structure for the research that best answers the investigator's questions. The research design that is usually optimal for answering research questions is the *experimental study,* in which the effects of an intervention are contrasted to results in subjects not receiving the intervention. However, experimental studies are more difficult to organize and carry out, so the investigator commonly collects other information initially, ensuring that the investigator is well prepared for the more demanding experimental study.

At the simplest level the researcher will only make observations about the subjects or events of the research without altering anything about them, conducting an *observational study.* This design is typical for epidemiological, diagnostic, assessment, and many biological types of clinical research. An initial step is often the collection of data about the events or subjects in an open-ended fashion without a carefully prepared design of the study. This type of *descriptive study* is used to obtain preliminary data in an exploratory manner, organizing subsequent research studies on the topic. A danger is that this often becomes the only study. The investigator then is tempted to try to repair design faults at the study's end. The same data might be used to conduct an *analytic study,* without a previous formal research design, by analyzing the associations among various measures in the data; the results are subject to the same risks as the descriptive study.

The investigator selects from among several subtypes of observational research:

- *Cross-sectional study*: The measures of the subjects or events are obtained at a single time. They will not be representative of the measures at other times.
- *Longitudinal study*: The measures are obtained on more than one occasion over a period of time. Longitudinal studies are conducted in two ways:

    - Prospective study: Following the initial measures of the subjects at a certain time, the subjects are followed for further measures in the future, as affected by intervening events. This is the optimal procedure.
    - Retrospective study: The measures of the subjects are obtained in the present and at selected times in the past from records of those past events. Although this is a less expensive, less time-consuming design, it has several limitations. For example, it is subject to bias; the desired measures might not be available in the records used; and the data might be difficult to interpret because they were not entered for the purposes of the current study.

These are the most common types of observational studies, but how the measures (or *variables,* as the characteristics of interest in subjects are usually called) are obtained determines the structure of further research designs for observational studies. For example, epidemiological research can use the observation of a population of individuals at a single time or over a period of time. Strategies commonly employed include cross-sectional, cohort, and case-control designs. A *cohort* is defined as a group of persons who possess a common trait and/or are followed together over time (e.g., all persons born in 1961). A *cohort study* is used particularly to establish *predictor variables* (subject characteristics that predict later outcome) and involves observing a cohort of subjects repeatedly over time. Predictor variables might be characteristics predicting onset of a disease (i.e., *risk factors*) or freedom from disease (i.e., *protective factors*), concepts used in *high-risk studies.* A *case-control study* involves identifying a group of cases, individuals with a certain characteristic (e.g., a disease), and control subjects who lack this characteristic, and examining selected variables in both groups. The case-control design is usually used when a researcher decides to start with the outcome, such as the presence or absence of a disease, and move back in time to compare the values of the predictor variables in the case and control subject samples.

Various other specific research designs for observational studies reflect modifications of these structures for specific research goals. Further information about the following examples can be found elsewhere (Hulley and Cummings 1988): prospective cohort studies, retrospective cohort design, nested case-control design, or double-cohort design.

Inferences and errors. Good research design requires that the investigator know the nature of the risks encountered in clinical research, so that they can be minimized. These dangers can be conceptualized by understanding the inferences involved in the study and knowing the types of errors that might undermine it. Two major types of inference are generally considered: *internal validity* (an estimate of the degree to which the study conclusions accurately describe the findings in the study sample) and *external validity* (an estimate of the degree to which the conclusions from the study sample are appropriate when generalized to the larger universe) (Kidder and Judd 1986).

The investigator attempts to minimize errors, which are described as random or systematic. *Random error* refers to erroneous results due to chance, those unknown sources of variation that plague any clinical investigation and can alter the results in either direction. The most straightforward procedure to reduce random error is to increase the sample size so that random error effects are minimized. *Systematic error* refers to erroneous results due to undetected bias; it consists of sources of variation altered in one direction. In this instance, increasing the sample size does not reduce the systematic error, so the investigator seeks to improve the study design to reduce the extent of the bias or provide information about the bias. Both types of error may contribute to specific types of errors at individual stages of research, such as *measurement error* (threatening internal validity) or *sampling error* (threatening external validity) (Hulley and Cummings 1988).

Assessment and diagnostic research. Accurate diagnoses constitute the foundation of many types of clinical research, such as those utilizing genetic or biological methods. Difficulties achieving accurate diagnoses in psychiatric research led to the generation of specific methods and terminology for this sector of observational studies. Methods for assessing diagnostic accuracy and precision are now standardized. This generally involves the evaluation of a procedure, such as the clinical interview (Young et al. 1987a, 1987b, 1990) or a new technology, such as single photon emission computed tomography (SPECT), as a diagnostic test (Young et al. 1991). Research on *diagnostic tests* uses the usual structure for observational studies: a predictor variable (the test result) and an outcome variable (the presence or absence of the disorder). However, diagnostic studies have two complicating features: first, there are special problems encountered in diagnostic research in psychiatry, because there is no "gold standard" (a definitive indicator of the presence of a disorder) to indicate the presence or absence of a disorder such as autism. Second, the investigator is not simply looking for associations between the predictor and outcome variables; instead, the investigator is determining which diagnostic test best discriminates the presence or absence of the disorder. Special statistics are used to express the possible results for a diagnostic test.

Sensitivity is defined as the percentage of subjects with the disease correctly identified; *specificity* is the percentage of subjects without the disease correctly identified. One important feature of diagnostic tests is that many use continuous variables, requiring a decision that an arbitrary value be selected (the *cutoff point*) beyond which all values indicate a positive test). There is a trade-off between sensitivity and specificity when selecting the cutoff point, so the relative importance of each determines how it is set (Young et al. 1987a).

Inferring cause in observational studies. Observational studies are usually not limited to descriptive data, and the examination of associations among variables brings inferences of possible cause-effect-relationships. Does an association indicate a true causal relationship? It might not. Competing possibilities include that this is a *spurious association* due to *chance* (random error) or *bias* (systematic error); other possibilities are that the association is real but the nature of the association is that of an *effect-cause relationship* (the causal influence acts in an *opposite* direction) or an *effect-effect relationship* (a *confounding effect* caused by a third, unidentified factor). Strategies used during the design or analysis phases can aid the likelihood that possible causal relationships are not misinterpreted. For example, confounding factors pose particular problems in clinical research. Strategies used to cope with this problem include 1) the *specification of inclusion criteria* for study subjects that exclude likely confounding factors; 2) *matching* (for each case, selecting a control matched to the same value of the confounding variable); 3) *stratification* (dividing subjects into strata or subgroups formed by the level of the possible confounding variable and then assessing possible cause-effect relationships in each stratum separately); or 4) one of various methods of *statistical adjustment* during the analysis phase. The techniques, strengths, and weaknesses of all these methods for enhancing causal inference in observational studies must be carefully considered (Hulley and Cummings 1988).

Experimental Studies and Intervention Research

When the investigator needs to enhance a study's capacity to infer a causal relationship, the investigator will commonly turn to an experimental design to control confounding variables. This is accomplished by actively manipulating the predictor variable by viewing it as an *intervention* and noting the effects on the outcome. This design is sometimes a more efficient means for answering a question, or the only design that can accomplish this. However, there are drawbacks to experimental designs. First, they are commonly more expensive and time-consuming. Second, some research questions are not suitable for this design. Third, generalizability may be restricted. Finally, the scope of the study hypothesis may be more limited. Therefore, it is conventional to withhold the use of an experimental design until the research hypotheses have been refined by obtaining basic descriptive data and likely causal relationships through observational studies.

In an *experimental design,* 1) a cohort of subjects is followed over time, while 2) associations among predictor and outcome variables are examined 3) in subjects grouped according to the presence or absence of an intervention (a predictor variable) to 4) demonstrate the likelihood of a cause-effect relationship by comparison of outcomes. In other words, to test the hypothesis that an intervention (such as psychotherapy, medication, or a behavior modification procedure) has an effect on patients, a researcher evaluates patients during periods of no treatment, symbolized by A, and periods of treatment, symbolized by B. Common research designs include AB, ABA, and ABAB. Two general forms of this design are to examine outcomes in groups that receive different interventions (*between-group designs,* the most popular design) or to compare outcomes in a single group before and after the intervention (*within-group designs*).

In fact, study of an intervention such as a pharmacological treatment often is initiated by an *open trial,* in which the drug is administered and the effects observed with no control subjects or rater blinding. This is done to examine possible benefits quickly and inexpensively and often is a response to emergent clinical needs for patients unresponsive to usual treatments. However, the information obtained is limited and very subject to random and systematic errors. Therefore, the classic intervention study design is preferred: a *randomized, double-blind, control trial.* In this design, study subjects are *randomly assigned* to groups receiving different treatments, preferably including a *placebo* (inactive agent) as the *control treatment.* Baseline and posttreatment measures are obtained by *blind raters,* where neither the patients nor investigators know which treatment is being administered, justifying the term *double-blind* (with the exception of the treating physicians not participating in the study ratings). The investigator then compares outcomes in the treatment groups when "unblinded" at the end of the study (Meinert 1986).

The stages of a randomized, double-blind control trial are 1) selection of a population sample for study; 2) measurement of baseline variables; 3) randomization of study subjects into two or more treatment groups; 4) administration of blinded interventions, preferably including a placebo; and 5) blind measurement of outcome variables and comparison of results among groups. A variety of problems must be considered, but chief among them are assuring *treatment compliance* by the patient and avoiding *subject attrition* (patient dropouts) during the study.

Other variations on this design include the run-in design, factorial design, matched-pair randomization, and group randomization (Hulley and Cummings 1988). The *time series* design follows a cohort of subjects, each of whom serves as his or her own control, during sequential treatment and control periods and compares outcomes before and after the treatment. *Carry-over effects* (residual intervention influences or practice effects) must be minimized, and *secular trends* (changes over time due to predictable influences, such as season of the year) must be considered when applying a time series design. A *crossover* design (the subjects are randomly assigned to one or the other treatment, and then each group is switched to the other treatment during the second intervention period) has many advantages, but the duration of the study is increased and carry-over effects can be a problem. The use of *repeated measures,* in multiple periods on and off treatment, aids the analysis of the outcome measures (Cochran 1983; Cochran and Cox 1957; Cook and Campbell 1979; Fleiss 1986).

Subjects

Inclusion and exclusion criteria. Research subjects are drawn from a *population* (the full set of people with the specific defining characteristics) in a *sample* (subset) of the population. The population can be conceptualized as consisting of the overall *target population* (the complete set) or the *accessible population* (the set actually available in geographical, temporal, and practical terms).

The salient characteristics that define the target and accessible populations are described as *inclusion criteria*—subjects must exhibit the inclusion criteria, which may be general characteristics such as age or treatment status, or characteristics drawn from a current classification system to be definite cases of the condition. The *exclusion criteria* describe features (e.g., demographic or diagnostic) of otherwise eligible subjects who are not to be included because they would undermine the quality or interpretation of the results in some manner. However, the findings then cannot be generalized to the population of excluded subjects. The need for operational definitions of criteria is discussed below.

Types of samples and sampling procedures. The investigator next defines the accessible population. The first of the usual two choices in medical research is a *clinic-based sample*. This is favored by ease of subject recruitment and fewer expenses, but is encumbered by significant *selection* or *ascertainment biases* (biasing factors determining who appears in the clinic and study, such as the typically more severe cases of Tourette syndrome seen in a specialty clinic). The second choice is the *population-based sample*, where subjects are selected in their homes, generating a representative sample. Obviously, the expense and inconvenience of a population-based sample restrict its use. Interviews might be conducted with each subject in person or by telephone, or a mail survey might be undertaken. Occasionally a preexisting data set may be available.

Two types of sampling designs are used: probability and nonprobability. A *probability sample* uses a scientific approach to estimate the degree to which the phenomena observed in the sample are representative of those in the population. It is obtained by a random process ensuring that each subject in the population has a specified chance of inclusion. Several types of probability sampling are available. *Simple random sampling* is achieved by identifying all subjects in the accessible population and then selecting a random sample; each subject has an equal chance to be selected. *Systematic sampling* uses a specified periodic selection procedure, such as every third child in a school. An advantage is that this sampling procedure is relatively easy to carry out. However, systematic biases may be introduced. *Stratified random sampling* is a procedure in which the population is separated into subgroups based on specific characteristics (e.g., age), then a random sample is obtained from each of the strata. Subsamples can be weighted to compensate for differences in the size of the strata while taking equal numbers from each stratum. *Cluster sampling* is a procedure in which a random sample of natural groupings, or clusters, of subjects in the population is obtained. For example, a random sample of schools in the state of New York is an efficient method of generating subjects for measuring some characteristic of students in the first year of high school when compared with a random sample of all of these students in the state. However, it is important to obtain a large number of clusters and to ensure that they are heterogeneous in relation to the target variables to minimize bias.

For all probability sampling techniques the essential challenge is *recruitment* of an adequately large sample that has sufficiently small bias due to technical errors or *nonresponse* (failure of potential subjects to participate).

A *nonprobability sample* may be more practical for the investigator, but statistical significance tests are based on the use of a probability sample, and investigators attempt to generate at least a facsimile. Several types of design are common. *Consecutive sampling,* probably the best and most practical, selects each subject meeting the inclusion and exclusion criteria over a specific number of patients or time interval. It is frequently the best option in clinical studies. *Convenience sampling* (haphazard sampling) simply selects easily available subjects in the accessible population without conscious planning. It is frequently used in clinical research because it is inexpensive and easily arranged, but there is a high likelihood of a biased sample. *Judgmental sampling* is similar to convenience sampling in advantages and disadvantages; the investigator selects the subjects that the he or she thinks are most appropriate for the study. A *volunteer sample* may be used when the evaluation process is uncomfortable in some respect.

Useful results may follow from nonprobability samples. However, since random selection is absent from nonprobability sampling, statistical inference theory cannot be applied. The results of nonprobability samples might not be representative, so they cannot be considered typical of the general population. The science of statistics is based on random selection, and it follows that statistical analyses are not appropriate for nonprobability samples (Cochran 1977).

Control and comparison (contrast) subject groups. A controlled experiment compares findings in a group of subjects with a group of individuals who are identical except that they lack the condition or intervention under study. In child and adolescent psychiatry studies, healthy control subjects are preferred. This is often not feasible in child psychiatric research because of ethical constraints related to the immaturity of the subjects (e.g., should otherwise healthy 7-year-olds be asked to agree to venipuncture for research purposes?). Instead, the investigator might consider one or more *comparison* or *contrast groups*, composed of subjects with a second condition or intervention for which the value of the variable of interest might not be expected to differ from healthy subjects.

The Single Subject Design

Child psychiatrists traditionally studied individual cases in depth, but theories spawned from this work drew increasing criticism. The controlled experiment is based on assumptions that are not valid for individuals (Fisher 1960), so the statistical techniques typically employed for group studies cannot be readily applied to single cases. Nevertheless, the design and analysis of single case studies has been reconsidered more favorably in recent years and is increasingly applied in clinical research (Barlow and Hersen 1984; Kazdin 1982; Kratochwill 1978). This approach is particularly useful in child and adolescent psychiatry for the study of a rare condition or a new and unusual treatment. Similarly, very complex cases not representative of a population or requiring extensive investment of the efforts of clinical personnel may be best studied through a single case design.

Ethics

It is essential that investigators acquaint themselves with the general principles of the ethical conduct of research (Levine 1981, 1991) and study the guidelines of their own institutional review boards for examining the ethical aspects of the proposed research. This is especially important in child psychiatric research because of the vulnerable status of potential subjects due to developmental immaturity, brain impairment, or mental illness. This requires that a parent or guardian give the essential consent for participation in research; the child may give additional assent to participation. In addition, it is often useful to have advocates who meet periodically with the investigators to review research proposals concerning a group of subjects, such as patients with mental retardation.

Research Measures: What and How to Measure

Clinical Measures

The clinical phenomena that are the subject of measurement must be 1) observable, permitting agreement among expert observers (i.e., they can be observed reliably when present); and 2) verifiable, indicating that they occur as hypothesized in the construct (i.e., they are valid). Clinical investigators aim for the optimal level of validity and reliability, and this requires knowledge about the development and use of clinical measures, which are gathered together in various assessment instruments.

Types of Variables

The effects of interventions clarify the meaning of, and mutual influences among, study variables. For example, the effects of two doses of antidepressant medication may be studied in relation to scores on depression rating scales, heart rate, and blood studies. In this instance, the variables play different roles in the research design. An *independent variable* (also known as a predictor variable or design variable) precedes the other variable and is the entity that is manipulated in the study. In this example, the dose of the medication is the independent variable. A *dependent variable* (outcome variable or response variable) changes according to the effects of manipulation of the independent variable. In this example, values on rating scales, heart rate, and blood tests are dependent variables. Independent and dependent variables are also essential concepts in an observational study, where the independent variable might be a risk factor, such as poverty, and the dependent variables outcomes such as poor academic performance, hyperactivity, and conduct disorders. A study typically has a single independent variable and multiple dependent variables (Kidder and Judd 1986).

Variables are usefully classified in another way, in relation to the procedure used to measure the variable. *Measurement scales* use differing types of measurements, producing the following types of variables. The simplest variables are *categorical variables,* such as gender or ethnicity, which are unsuitable for quantification but are instead placed into categories. If there are only two possible values (e.g., yes-no or true-false), then these are *dichotomous variables.* When more than two values are possible, further variable subtypes can be selected. *Nominal variables* are categories with no order; classic examples are the categories of blood types (type A, B, O) or ethnic group. *Ordinal variables* can be ordered grossly, but not in a quantitative manner; an example is a behavioral rating scale with categories such as never, rarely, sometimes, and so on. Both nominal and ordinal variables are straightforward to measure, but are not suitable for the more informative types of statistical analysis.

Continuous variables have values distributed across an infinite numerical scale, with intervals determined by the sensitivity of the measuring instrument and the requirements of the study (e.g., blood pressure or plasma norepinephrine values). *Discrete variables* are very similar, but the number of quantified intervals is finite (e.g., red blood cell count or number of offspring). Continuous variables are almost always preferred for measurements if they are appropriate, because they yield the most information in an efficient manner and allow meaningful statistical analyses (Hulley and Cummings 1988; Kidder and Judd 1986).

Assessment Instruments and Sources of Variance in Their Use

When thinking about a research hypothesis, a clinician might initially assume that, having decided on the variables of interest, they can readily be measured. Surprisingly, research protocols often fail because the measurement procedures are inadequate to the experimental demands (e.g., unreliable diagnoses invalidate a genetic linkage study); most often, they were poorly chosen because they were insufficiently considered at the outset. Psychiatric research lacks a gold standard, such as a tissue biopsy, so a range of measures are typically substituted to approximate the final measure of interest, such as diagnosis.

Measurements then become clinical assessment instruments, carefully prepared and standardized. Assessment instruments are meticulously constructed and continuously revised. Each instrument is devoted to a highly specific purpose, and together they constitute the backbone of much contemporary research in child and adolescent psychiatry. To characterize individuals as clearly as possible, researchers use different tools to measure a particular construct. The challenges of diagnostic research stand as the best example of the need for continuing efforts to improve clinical measures in psychiatry and exemplify available methods for solving problems concerning measures. Two major methods used in the development of diagnostic instruments are categorical and dimensional approaches to assessment, which conceptually correspond to the categorical and continuous variables employed.

Categorical methods of assessment. Diagnostic assessment instruments that place an individual in one of several classes within a diagnostic system exemplify the *categorical approach to diagnosis.* For example, the diagnostic categories for subtypes of mental retardation are defined by intelligence quotient (IQ) scores and adaptive level. Although assigning a diagnosis to a patient may seem like a straightforward and relatively simple procedure, clinical investigators recognize that it is fraught with dangers. The kinds of problems challenging the diagnostician are related to four types of bias, or variance, that must be considered when constructing an approach to a research diagnosis.

Lacking a gold standard for diagnosis (such as a definitive blood test), clinicians typically relied on their clinical judgment until recent years. This generally took the form of expert clinicians studying the scientific literature, building up years of clinical experience, and applying these perspectives to the diagnosis of individual patients. The deficiencies in this approach became apparent, however, because clinicians had different conceptions of a complex disorder (e.g., attention-deficit/hyperactivity disorder) and failed to achieve diagnostic agreement. Unintentionally, they actually used different rules (*diagnostic criteria,* as we now call them) for assigning the diagnosis. "*Criterion variance* is the disagreement associated with use of different definers or criteria for a diagnostic category" (Young et al. 1987a, p. 619, italics added). Current classification systems use explicitly stated inclusion and exclusion criteria for each diagnosis. This has markedly improved diagnostic agreement and has contributed to advances such as the recognition that single diagnoses must give way to the concept of *comorbidity*—patients often have more than one coexisting disorder.

Nevertheless, problems remain when the clinician attempts to apply the criteria in a clinical situation. For example, will two clinicians agree that a child has a restricted repertoire of interests and activities, or will one view the child as autistic and another as depressed? This problem has been partially solved by the use of operational definitions. "An *operational definition* provides a repeatable sequence of rules or steps to obtain a measurement, in this case a diagnosis" (Young et al. 1987a, p. 614, italics added). For example, DSM-III-R (American Psychiatric Association 1987) and DSM-IV (American Psychiatric Association 1994) are commonly employed instruments with operational definitions. Thus a classification system is constructed on the criteria and operational definitions used.

Another source of variability in diagnosis is the information on which the diagnosis is based. For example, different types of interviews (e.g., a psychodynamic interview examining habitual mechanisms of defense, as contrasted to a structured interview with predetermined questions covering a specific set of potential diagnoses) may result in different information obtained, generating different diagnoses despite using the same diagnostic criteria. To combat this problem, interview formats were constructed that increasingly defined how the information was obtained. Psychiatric diagnostic interviews may be structured, semistructured, or unstructured. In a *structured interview,* the wording of all questions is specified. They are read verbatim, and responses are coded in predetermined categories. In a *semistructured interview*, topics are listed; the interviewer must then formulate questions to elicit the information to be obtained in the interview (*probes*). In an *unstructured interview*, the interviewer may ask any questions judged to be pertinent, using language chosen by the interviewer and in any order. Of these three approaches, the structured approach is most likely to elicit the same information across interviews by different interviewers, therefore reducing information variance.

Two other types of variance affect diagnostic agreement. *Observation variance* is "the disagreement associated with circumstances in which observers perceive the same phenomena differently" (Young et al. 1987a, p. 619). For example, two child and adolescent psychiatrists may observe a videotape of a play interview. One takes copious notes; the other has eyes glued to the monitor. The psychiatrist taking notes may not observe a tear that is shed, a tic, or any other brief event. The descriptions of the play interview by the two observers may vary markedly. Observation variance reflects the professional training, level of professional experience, theoretical background, and personality characteristics of the interviewer, as well as the prevailing clinical practices of the interviewer's institution. Training in the use of specific structured diagnostic interviews helps reduce biases due to these aspects of interviewer response style. *Occasion variance* is "the disagreement associated with obtaining varying information from the same individual in different times and circumstances" (Young et al. 1987a, p. 619). Examples are the differences in reports of family and educators, as well as the differences in assessments by the same rater on the same patient at a 1-year interval. This *situational effect* was first thought to indicate fundamental problems with assessment instruments, but clinicians now expect that parents, teachers, and the child will all have different information to provide on rating scales. This reflects differing expectations in separate circumstances, as well as differing meanings and interpretations attached to the same behavior.

Dimensional methods of assessment. The second basis for clinical diagnosis is symptom grouping and enumeration, the *dimensional* or *multivariate approach to diagnosis*. A list of "all" symptoms of childhood psychiatric disorders is converted to a series of questions concerning their presence and severity. A patient is then determined to have whatever "disorders" correspond to high symptom frequencies (positive responses to specific groupings of related questions) as contrasted to expected frequencies according to age and sex in a multivariate analysis of the data. Clusters of these responses are given descriptive names (e.g., impulsivity, obsessions, anxiety) that correspond to concepts of symptoms or disorders. It must be recalled, however, that symptom designation is reliant on a more or less arbitrary selection of a cutoff point for inclusion or exclusion from a diagnostic category. As indicated previously, this cutoff point has an important effect on the assignment of a diagnosis to a patient and to the sensitivity and specificity of diagnostic procedures.

An example of the use of the dimensional approach at the more general conceptual level of diagnosis is the *multiaxial system of psychiatric diagnosis,* in which each person is simultaneously rated along several dimensions using both categorical and dimensional approaches, including primary and secondary psychiatric diagnoses, coexisting physical disorders and conditions, severity of psychosocial stressors, and global assessment of functioning (American Psychiatric Association 1987). Dimensional approaches are perhaps most often used in *specialized rating scales* constructed to monitor symptoms of a specific disorder, such as Tourette syndrome (Harcherik et al. 1984). These rating scales attempt to obtain highly reliable ratings of the common symptoms of the disorder, ultimately enhancing the validity of clinical assessment of the disorder and improving treatment outcome studies.

Research Statistics: Understanding the Results

For many years it was forgotten that the quality control procedures that hold for laboratory assay procedures also are necessary for clinical assessment procedures. *Quality control* can be monitored in clinical research using the same concepts and vocabulary as in the laboratory: accuracy (validity) and precision (reliability). "*Accuracy* is concerned with the relationship of a set of results to the true value" (Whitehead

1977, p. 9, italics added). Similarly, *validity* describes how well a test or instrument measures what it is supposed to measure (Young et al. 1990). "*Precision* measurements are concerned with the agreement between replicate analyses" (Whitehead 1977, p. 9, italics added). In the same way, *reliability* indicates the replicability, consistency, and stability of a clinical test or instrument when it is applied by multiple individuals in several circumstances and at different times; this yields an estimation of the "error variance" of the instrument (Young et al. 1990).

The following outline presents the major concepts defining the types of validity and reliability that are commonly used in clinical research, along with the measures used (modified from Young et al. 1987a, with permission).

Clinical Measures: The Examples of Reliability and Validity

Reliability of the interview. How accurately and consistently does the instrument measure what it measures? How well does the instrument reduce the chance variation (error variance) to a minimum?

- *Interrater reliability:* Do different raters obtain the same information from the same interview stimuli?
- *Test-retest reliability:* Does a repeat identical interview within a few days or weeks elicit the same information from the child or parent?
- *Internal consistency (split-half) reliability:* Do different sections of the interview give similar information? This is a measure of the extent to which the interview elements converge on a score assessed by means of correlations between those elements (halves of the interview or individual question responses).
- *Alternate-form (or parallel-form) reliability:* Does a nearly identical interview procedure give the same information?

Validity of the interview. Validity measures assess how well an instrument measures what it is intended to examine. In other words, validity describes whether the interview generates the type of information it is intended to obtain. No matter how precisely an interview measures a construct, if it is shown to be the wrong construct it is invalid.

- *Face validity:* Do most experts judge that the interview gives authentic diagnostic information, covering the criteria adequately?
- *Content validity:* Does the interview assess the intended range of diagnoses appropriately and accurately, as indicated by a match of questions or ratings to the specified criteria?
- *Construct validity:* Is the measure related in theoretically predicted ways to other measures, such as the course of the illness, impairment, risk factors, neurobiological measures, or familial aggregation?
    - Convergent validity: Does the measure agree (is it correlated) with scores obtained on other instruments thought to measure a similar construct?
    - Discriminant validity: Does the measure differentiate the constructs (diagnoses) of interest from other constructs (diagnoses)?
- *Criterion-referenced validity:* Does the interview give diagnostic information that agrees with the data contained in an independent, optimal method for diagnostic assignment? Although there is no final, accepted best method for assigning diagnoses available, the best estimate diagnosis, usually judged by expert clinicians from all available data, is most often used as criterion for assessing criterion-referenced validity.
- *Predictive validity:* Does the interview help us estimate future outcome, eventual differences, and optimal interventions?

Quantification of Reliability and Validity

Quantification of reliability

- *Percent agreement:* A simple method, but minimally informative, it indicates the proportion of instances in which the raters agree. It does not take chance into account, nor the specific frequency of a condition.
- *Specific agreement:* Cases in which examiners agree about the ab-

sence of the particular findings or diagnosis inflate levels of agreement. Those cases with no diagnosis are excluded when calculating specific agreement, so that it reflects agreement about the positive findings (e.g., agreement about diagnoses whenever one or more interviewers assigned a diagnosis).

- *Intraclass correlation coefficient:* This is a measure of within-class association often used to estimate reliability or consistency of assessment of scaled measures.
- *Kappa statistic:* A measure of interrater agreement in classification, it corrects for chance agreement and is the most widely applied measure in contemporary clinical diagnostic research (Cohen 1960).
- *Weighted kappa:* This measure allows for difference in the degree or level of disagreement. It provides partial credit when the disagreement is not complete.
- *The Y statistic:* Yule's Y is a measure of agreement independent of the base rate (prevalence) of the disorder.
- *Cronbach's coefficient alpha:* This measure is commonly used to indicate the degree of internal consistency of a scale. It is minimally used in diagnostic interviews because it requires at least two questions for each symptom, extending the length of the interview (Cronbach 1951; Novick and Lewis 1967).

Quantification of validity

- *Sensitivity:* The percentage of true cases correctly identified; false negatives detract from it.
- *Specificity:* The percentage of true noncases correctly identified; false positives reduce specificity.
- *Predictive power:* Sometimes termed predictive value or diagnostic confidence, it describes the percentage of total abnormal test results that are associated with (true positive for) the index illness.

Data Management

Even quite simple research requires meticulous data management. Consider including birthdays for 25 children in a longitudinal study to determine age at various time points. It would not be at all surprising to find at least one error among the 25 birth dates. Similarly, a carefully collected blood sample, one of five obtained that morning from a child with a rare disorder whom the clinician has studied for weeks, will often arrive in the laboratory with a label containing neither the date nor the time, causing the loss of an important and expensive set of data.

The typical procedures for *data management* include the construction of *precoded data collection forms* that specify the types of data and form of each variable to be entered. Management of data by pencil-and-paper methods is very difficult, so the investigator must select a *computer data-base program* for *data entry, editing,* and *organization.* Such programs are now much more accessible to clinical investigators because they have been developed for use on personal computers (microcomputers), and the ease of use of these programs has been markedly enhanced. An important step that is too often neglected is *data verification* following the original data entry. Anyone who does this for a moderately large set of data finds errors, emphasizing the danger of not validating the original data entered. Once the data have been entered in the database, there are usually a sufficient number of variables that it can be anticipated that a powerful program for data analysis will be required. To accomplish this, the data are "dumped" from the database into a *statistical package program,* which is a package of programs for statistical analyses that the investigator might use. Four programs currently in common use are BMDP (Dixon 1975), SAS (SAS Institute 1985), SPSS (Nie 1975), and SYSTAT (Wilkinson 1990). The clinician then selects the data analysis procedures that he or she chooses to employ.

Data Analysis

Data analysis is the process of organizing data and applying statistical procedures to understand the meaning of the data in relation to the research hypotheses. The first organizational step is often *data reduction,* through which the data are reduced into smaller manageable and coherent units. This is followed by two stages of data analysis: descriptive statistics and analytic statistics.

Descriptive statistics examine the distribution of variables one at a time. When the data fit the bell-shaped *normal distribution*, it is then possible to calculate basic statistics, such as the *mean* (or average value, the estimate of the central tendency) and the *standard deviation* and *standard error* (each indicating the variability or spread of the data). If the data include one or two extremely high or low values, they are described as *outliers* and cause an asymmetric distribution of data that requires a different statistic for the central tendency: the *median*, which is the middle value among all values in the distribution.

Analytic statistics examine two or more variables at a time. The associations among independent and dependent variables are examined by three steps:

- Inspecting and graphing the pattern of the association in the sample. Using *two dichotomous variables* as examples, the patterns of associations are visible by using *cross-tabulation* in a *two-by-two table* (utilizing the chi-square test). In contrast, *two continuous variables* can be graphed in a *scatterplot* to demonstrate the pattern of association between the variables.
- Calculating the magnitude of the association in the sample. The use of the *Pearson correlation coefficient* is the most common method for computing the magnitude of the association between two continuous variables.
- Estimating the probability that the association occurring in the sample would also occur in the population. *Tests of statistical significance* are mathematical procedures performed on quantitative data from experiments to determine if the results differ from chance occurrences. The *statistical significance* of an association is reported in terms of *probability values,* abbreviated as *P* values. As mentioned earlier, a result is arbitrarily considered statistically significant if the likelihood that it would occur by chance alone is less than 1 in 20; this probability value is abbreviated as $P < .05$. Correspondingly, results are sometimes reported in the form of *confidence intervals*: if a result falls outside a 95% confidence interval, then the likelihood of a chance occurrence is considered statistically significant.

When designing a study, it is important to consider the number of subjects needed to be able to prove or disprove the hypothesis. It was mentioned earlier in the chapter that alpha (α), the probability of committing a Type I error, is the same as the level of statistical significance. Beta (β) is the probability of committing a Type II error. The quantity $(1 - \beta)$ is known as the *power* of a study, the probability of rejecting a false null hypothesis (Bickel and Doksum 1977, p. 167). At the outset of a study, the investigator should determine the sample size necessary to attain specified power, alpha, and beta (Cohen 1988; Meinert 1986).

Many statistical tests are used in studies using multiple variables (requiring *multivariate analyses*) and group comparisons. The following describes the organization of statistical tests into parametric and nonparametric categories, with examples of each.

- *Parametric tests*: Mathematical procedures that use a *parameter*, an entity that describes a characteristic of the data, such as mean and variance. These tests assume that the populations of traits studied have a normal distribution.
    - *t* test: A procedure that assesses if the means of two groups are the same or different.
    - *F* test: A procedure that assesses if the variances of two groups are the same or different. This test is commonly encountered in regression analyses and the analysis of variance.

- *Nonparametric tests*: Mathematical procedures that do not use parameters. They frequently employ "ranks" of the items of data (*rank-ordered data*). The populations studied are not assumed to be normally distributed. These tests may be used for data that follow a normal distribution as well as for data that do not. They may also be used when the underlying distribution is not known.
    - Chi-square test: A procedure that contrasts the observed values and the expected values for two or more variables; that is, it determines if the observed data differ from data that would be expected by chance alone (Fleiss 1981).
    - Wilcoxon or Mann-Whitney test: A procedure that compares the ranks of items of two groups to determine if they are different (Lehmann 1975).

Clinical and Research Reality: Getting It Done

The most difficult challenge of research is finding the tenacity to follow through all the steps required to complete the research project and the meticulousness to do it well. Investigators are advised to seek clarity and simplicity of structure in their design. This is a demanding recommendation because a study that is expensive in time and resources is difficult to repeat as second- or third-phase follow-up studies; this tempts the researcher to attempt to answer many important questions simultaneously. Attention to detail is typically difficult for inexperienced investigators; experienced investigators who have seen research projects undermined by sloppiness have great respect for careful work. Finally, whether the goal is for a single clinician or a team to carry out research, the most important, and often ignored, requirement is to have the patience to build over time. Research projects contain many steps, and most interesting research questions actually require a series of studies to achieve an accurate answer. Build patiently and well, and your research will achieve clear and interesting results; will be replicated successfully by other investigators; and, most importantly, will contribute to the well-being of many patients.

References

American Psychiatric Association: Diagnostic and Statistical Manual of Mental Disorders, 3rd Edition, Revised. Washington, DC, American Psychiatric Association, 1987

American Psychiatric Association: Diagnostic and Statistical Manual of Mental Disorders, 4th Edition. Washington, DC, American Psychiatric Association, 1994

Barlow DH, Hersen M: Single Case Experimental Designs: Strategies for Studying Behavior Change, 2nd Edition. New York, Pergamon, 1984

Bickel PJ, Doksum KA: Mathematical Statistics: Basic Ideas and Selected Topics. Oakland, CA, Holden-Day, 1977

Cochran WG: Sampling Techniques, 3rd Edition. New York, Wiley, 1977

Cochran WG: Planning and Analysis of Observational Studies. New York, Wiley, 1983

Cochran WG, Cox GM: Experimental Designs, 2nd Edition. New York, Wiley, 1957

Cohen J: A coefficient of agreement for nominal scales. Educational Psychology Measurement 20:37–42, 1960

Cohen J: Statistical Power Analysis for the Behavioral Sciences, 2nd Edition. Hillsdale, NJ, Lawrence Erlbaum, 1988

Cook TD, Campbell DT: Quasi-Experimentation: Design and Analysis Issues for Field Settings. Boston, MA, Houghton Mifflin, 1979

Cronbach LJ: Coefficient alpha and the internal structure of tests. Psychometrika 16:297–334, 1951

Dixon WJ: BMDP: Biomedical Computer Programs. Berkeley, University of California Press, 1975

Fisher RA: The Design of Experiments, 7th Edition. New York, Hafner Publishing, 1960

Fleck L: Genesis and Development of a Scientific Fact. Edited by Trenn TJ, Merton RK. Translated by Bradley F, Trenn TJ. Chicago, IL, University of Chicago Press, 1979

Fleiss JL: Statistical Methods for Rates and Proportions, 2nd Edition. New York, Wiley, 1981

Fleiss JL: The Design and Analysis of Clinical Experiments. New York, Wiley, 1986

Harcherik DF, Leckman JF, Detlor J, et al: A new instrument for clinical studies of Tourette's syndrome. Journal of the American Academy of Child Psychiatry 23:153–160, 1984

Hulley SB, Cummings SR: Designing Clinical Research. Baltimore, MD, Williams & Wilkins, 1988

Kazdin AE: Single-Case Research Designs: Methods for Clinical and Applied Settings. New York, Oxford University Press, 1982

Kidder LH, Judd CM: Research Methods in Social Relations. New York, Holt, Rinehart & Winston, 1986

Kratochwill TR: Single Subject Research: Strategies for Evaluating Change. Orlando, FL, Academic Press, 1978

Lehmann EL: Testing Statistical Hypotheses. New York, Wiley, 1959

Lehmann EL: Nonparametrics: Statistical Methods Based on Ranks. Oakland, CA, Holden-Day, 1975

Levine RJ: Ethics and Regulations of Clinical Research. Baltimore, MD, Urban & Schwarzenberg, 1981

Levine RJ: Respect for children as research subjects, in Child and Adolescent Psychiatry: A Comprehensive Textbook. Edited by Lewis M. Baltimore, MD, William & Wilkins, 1991, pp 1229–1238

Meinert CL: Clinical Trials: Design, Conduct, and Analysis. New York, Oxford University Press, 1986

Merton RK: The Sociology of Science: Theoretical and Empirical Investigations. Chicago, IL, University of Chicago Press, 1973

Nie NH: SPSS: Statistical Package for the Social Sciences, 2nd Edition. New York, McGraw-Hill, 1975

Novick MR, Lewis C: Coefficient alpha and the reliability of composite measurements. Psychometrika 32:1–13, 1967

Polanyi M: Personal Knowledge: Towards a Post-Critical Philosophy. Chicago, IL, University of Chicago Press, 1962

SAS Institute: SAS User's Guide: Statistics, Version 5 Edition. Cary, NC, SAS Institute, 1985

Whitehead TP: Quality Control in Clinical Chemistry. New York, Wiley, 1977

Wilkinson L: SYSTAT: The System for Statistics. Evanston, IL, SYSTAT, 1990

Young JG, O'Brien JD, Gutterman EM, et al: Research on the clinical interview. J Am Acad Child Adolesc Psychiatry 26:613–620, 1987a

Young JG, O'Brien JD, Gutterman ED, et al: Structured diagnostic interviews for children and adolescents: introduction. J Am Acad Child Adolesc Psychiatry 26:611–612, 1987b

Young JG, Leven L, Ludman W, et al: Interviewing children and adolescents, in Psychiatric Disorders in Children and Adolescents. Edited by Garfinkel BD, Carlson GA, Weller EB. Philadelphia, PA, WB Saunders, 1990, pp 443–468

Young JG, Brasic JR, Kaplan D, et al: Advances in research techniques, in Child and Adolescent Psychiatry: A Comprehensive Text. Edited by Lewis M. Baltimore, MD, Williams & Wilkins, 1991, pp 1201–1228

Index

Page numbers printed in **boldface** *type refer to tables or figures.*